NATURAL TREATMENTS FOR LYME COINFECTIONS

"Stephen Harrod Buhner's new book *Natural Treatments for Lyme Coinfections: Anaplasma, Babesia, and Ehrlichia* is a brilliant follow up of his previous groundbreaking books *Healing Lyme* and *Healing Lyme Disease Coinfections: Complementary and Holistic Treatments for Bartonella and Mycoplasma*. This is a must read for medical practitioners and patients, providing a deep understanding of how these microorganisms have evolved and relate to their intricate ecosystems. Stephen insists that it is not possible to successfully treat these evolving microbes without a full grasp of this information. For example, knowing that *Babesia* requires red blood cells, endothelial cells, and spleen tissues to reproduce and understanding the biochemistry of how this happens allows him to provide a clear roadmap of how to approach treatment properly. This roadmap has not been available until now. Thank you, Stephen!"

NEIL NATHAN, M.D., BOARD CERTIFIED FAMILY PHYSICIAN AND
AUTHOR OF *HEALING IS POSSIBLE*

"Stephen Harrod Buhner is performing important work in disseminating this information to patients and their clinicians. Many with chronic Lyme suffer from undiagnosed coinfections and would benefit from the entourage effects and herbal synergies of medicinal plants. Relief is available in the natural world, a true alternative treatment, beyond the reach of the medical bureaucracy."

JULIE HOLLAND, M.D., AUTHOR OF
WEEKEND AT BELLEVUE

"In this newest volume of Stephen Buhner's exploration of Lyme and its coinfections, he again excels in presenting an enormous amount of detailed information in a thorough and accessible manner, offering what readers need most in such a tome: the knowledge to make their own informed decisions in addressing these issues."

JIM MCDONALD, HERBALIST

ALSO BY STEPHEN HARROD BUHNER

Ecological Medicine
Healing Lyme
Healing Lyme Disease Coinfections: Complementary and Holistic
*   Treatments for Bartonella and Mycoplasma*
Herbal Antibiotics
Herbal Antivirals
Herbs for Hepatitis C and the Liver
The Natural Testosterone Plan
Pine Pollen: Ancient Medicine for a New Millennium
The Transformational Power of Fasting
Vital Man

Nonfiction
Ensouling Language
The Lost Language of Plants
One Spirit Many Peoples
Sacred and Herbal Healing Beers
Sacred Plant Medicine
The Secret Teachings of Plants

Poetry
The Taste of Wild Water: Poems and Stories Found While Walking
*   in Woods*

NATURAL TREATMENTS
FOR **LYME**
COINFECTIONS

ANAPLASMA, BABESIA, AND EHRLICHIA

STEPHEN HARROD BUHNER

Healing Arts Press
Rochester, Vermont • Toronto, Canada

Healing Arts Press
One Park Street
Rochester, Vermont 05767
www.HealingArtsPress.com

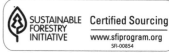

SUSTAINABLE FORESTRY INITIATIVE · Certified Sourcing · www.sfiprogram.org · SFI-00854

Text stock is SFI certified

Healing Arts Press is a division of Inner Traditions International

Note to the reader: *This book is intended as an informational guide. The remedies, approaches, and techniques described herein are meant to supplement, and not to be a substitute for, professional medical care or treatment. They should not be used to treat a serious ailment without prior consultation with a qualified health care professional.*

Library of Congress Cataloging-in-Publication Data
Buhner, Stephen Harrod.
  Natural treatments for lyme coinfections : anaplasma, babesia, and ehrlichia / Stephen Harrod Buhner.
     pages cm
  Includes bibliographical references and index.
  ISBN 978-1-62055-258-2 (paperback) — ISBN 978-1-62055-259-9 (e-book)
  1. Lyme disease—Alternative treatment. 2. Lyme disease—Complications—Alternative treatment. 3. Babesiosis—Alternative treatment. 4. Ehrlichiosis—Alternative treatment. 5. Anaplasmosis—Alternative treatment. I. Title.
  RC155.5.B86 2015
  616.9'246—dc23
                                                                            2014029051

Printed and bound in the United States by Lake Book Manufacturing, Inc. The text stock is SFI certified. The Sustainable Forestry Initiative® program promotes sustainable forest management.

10 9 8 7 6 5 4 3

Text design and layout by Priscilla Baker
This book was typeset in Garamond Premier Pro with Gill Sans, Legacy Sans, and Arial used as display typefaces

To send correspondence to the author of this book, mail a first-class letter to the author c/o Inner Traditions • Bear & Company, One Park Street, Rochester, VT 05767, and we will forward the communication, or contact the author directly at **www.gaianstudies.org**.

For Julie McIntyre,
whose caring for and dedication to her patients
is a continual inspiration to me.
And for everyone who has struggled with
any of these diseases—
there is hope,
don't give up.

Contents

I first wrote about Lyme disease in 2005 in my book *Healing Lyme*. In 2013 I followed up with *Healing Lyme Disease Coinfections*, which specifically deals with *Bartonella* and *Mycoplasma* infections. The book you have in your hands is another companion title, this one focusing on *Anaplasma, Babesia,* and *Ehrlichia* infections.

The issues and treatment considerations with Lyme apply to all coinfections. Therefore I have included in this book important summary information that you will also find in my other books on Lyme disease.

If you've already read some of this information before, you probably should still read it again. And again.

How to Use This Book and Who It Is For

In the spring of 2009, I was the 217th person ever to be diagnosed with anti-NMDA-receptor immune encephalitis. Just a year later that figure had doubled. Now the number is in the thousands. Yet Dr. Bailey, considered one of the best neurologists in the country, had never heard of it. When we live in a time when the rate of misdiagnoses has shown no improvement since the 1930s, the lesson here is that it's important to always get a second opinion. . . . While he may be an excellent doctor in many respects, Dr. Bailey is also, in some ways, a perfect example of what is wrong with medicine. I was just a number to him (and if he saw thirty-five patients a day, as he told me, that means I was one of a very large number). He is a by-product of a defective system that forces neurologists to spend five minutes with X number of patients a day to maintain their bottom line. It's a bad system. Dr. Bailey is not the exception to the rule. He is the rule.

SUSANNAH CAHALAN,
BRAIN ON FIRE: MY MONTH OF MADNESS

1

I did as much research as I could and I took ownership of this illness, because if you don't take care of your body, where are you going to live?

KAREN DUFFY,
MODEL PATIENT: MY LIFE AS AN INCURABLE WISE-ASS

Illness and death are not optional. Patients have a right to determine how they approach them.

MARCIA ANGELL, M.D.

Illness is the doctor to whom we pay most heed.

MARCEL PROUST

My first published exploration of Lyme disease and its coinfections occurred with the appearance of *Healing Lyme* (Raven Press) in 2005. In the years since that early work my increasing exposure to this group of emerging diseases, and the people who suffer from them, has significantly deepened my understanding of both Lyme and its coinfections. In consequence, mid-2013 saw the publication of an in-depth look at two crucial Lyme coinfections: mycoplasma and bartonella (Healing Arts Press). With the publication of this volume on babesia, ehrlichia, and anaplasma the five major coinfectious organisms of Lyme now have their own in-depth analysis and natural treatment protocols. (There are other, less common coinfections that may become more common in the future; Rocky Mountain spotted fever and various chlamydias are also [sometimes] spread by ticks.)

As with the earlier book on mycoplasma and bartonella, this book is meant to be used by specific groups of people, i.e., those who are suffering from a difficult-to-treat *Babesia* spp., *Ehrlichia* spp., or *Anaplasma* spp. infection, and/or clinicians who themselves treat those who are infected with any of these organisms.

IF YOU ARE INFECTED WITH *BABESIA*, *EHRLICHIA*, OR *ANAPLASMA*

This book is designed to help you understand the infectious organisms as well as some of the approaches that can be used to treat the diseases and the symptoms they cause.

Please understand that some of the book is fairly technical. That is for the clinicians (or for you if you want to delve that deeply into it). You can skip the really technical bits if you want. They are not necessary in order for you to treat either of these conditions effectively. However, I do think, if you are up for it, you will find the overview chapters on these infections useful. I have found that once someone understands what the bacteria do in the body, it tends to lessen the fear that these diseases engender. Understanding what the organisms do during infection also makes it easier to understand the treatment regimens I recommend, i.e., just why they help to turn the conditions around. Still, that being said, the deeper technical look at the cytokine cascade and the minutiae of what the organisms do in the body are not really necessary if you just want a cursory overview of the diseases and how to treat them.

This book also explores just how widespread these kinds of infections are. And, as usual, the real figures are very different than those indicated by Centers for Disease Control (CDC)—generally by a factor of anywhere from 100 to 1,000. During research for the previous coinfection book (*Bartonella* and *Mycoplasma* spp.) I found that scores of research articles, easily located in peer-reviewed journals, continually reported mycoplasma and bartonella infections to be *very* common throughout the world. In fact it turns out that between one-tenth and one-third of the United States population (as an example) is asymptomatically infected with at least one of those organisms. *Babesia, Ehrlichia,* and *Anaplasma* infections are apparently less widespread but research still finds them to be far more common than the CDC reports. Technological medical treatment for these latter three conditions is often difficult and, as with Lyme, bartonella, and mycoplasma, many physicians don't understand how to treat or diagnose them very well. Thus, as an aid to physicians and their patients, in addition to natural protocols, this book also examines which antibiotics (and tests) research has found useful (and which ones are not).

Again, this book contains an extensive look at the natural protocols that are effective for each of the diseases. Please note: *These protocols are designed to be used along with antibiotics if you wish to do so.* I don't think you necessarily have to give up either pharmaceuticals *or* natural medicines to find health. However, if you have tried antibiotics and they have failed to help you, the protocols in this book can be used by themselves to treat all three infections.

Also, a note: *The herbs and supplements in this book are **not** the only ones in the world that will help.* Please use the protocols outlined herein *only* as a starting place, a guideline. Add anything that you feel will help you and delete anything that you feel is not useful. Microorganisms, when they enter a human body, find a very unique ecosystem in that particular person. Thus the disease is always slightly different every time it occurs. That means that a pharmaceutical or herb that works for one person may not work or work as well for another. *There is no one-size-fits-all treatment for these particular organisms.*

Again . . . there is no one-size-fits-all treatment for Lyme or *any* of its coinfections.

Anyone who says there is, is either trying to sell you something or doesn't really understand this group of infectious organisms. *There is no one way to health such that in all times and in all places and with all people it will always work.* Life, and disease, and the journey to wellness are much more complex and sophisticated than that. So, trust your own feeling sense and pay attention to what your body is telling you. *You* are the best judge of whether something is working for you or not, whether you need to add something else or not, whether you are getting better . . . or not.

Now, a comment on dosages: I will often suggest a *range* of dosages for the herbs and supplements that can help these conditions. If you have a very healthy immune system, you will probably need smaller doses; if your immune system is severely depleted, you may need to use larger doses. If you are *very* sensitive to outside substances, as some people with Lyme and these coinfections are, then you might need to use very tiny doses, that is, from one to five drops of tincture at a time. (This is true for about 1 percent of the people with these infections.) I have seen six-foot-five, 280-pound men be unable to take more than five drops of a tincture and a tiny, 95-pound woman need a tablespoon at a time. *Dosages need to be adjusted for each person's individual ecology.*

**Again . . . dosages need to be adjusted for
each person's individual ecology.**

And . . . *please be conscious of how you respond to the medicines you are taking. If something disagrees with you, if you feel something is not right in how you are responding to a medicine,* **stop taking it.** Remember: you will always know yourself better than any outside physician. And, just a tiny rant here . . .

||||||||||||||||||||||||||||||||||||||||||||||||||||||

Tiny Rant
People Get Sick, Not Stupid

I have been told by a number of clinicians, both herbal and medical, that the majority of people with Lyme and/or its coinfections are too uneducated to understand this series of books, that they are not intelligent enough to determine which herbs to use and which herbs not to use (and, in fact, that many herbs should be discussed or dispensed *only* by properly trained and credentialed herbalists—and yes, they mean that most community herbalists and all those who are ill should not), that people with this group of diseases cannot in fact be trusted to be in charge of their own health and journey to wellness, and that I am remiss, even foolish (i.e., stupid, silly, idiotic, witless, brainless, vacuous, mindless, unintelligent, thoughtless, half-baked, harebrained, imprudent, incautious, injudicious, unwise), in supporting members of the Lyme community in their self-empowerment. My feelings about that kind of thinking (and the people who promulgate it—you know who you are and yes, I still know where you live) can be captured in a number of common one-syllable words normally not used in polite company. (Please insert your own favorites here.)

Thus, while it *can* help to have a sophisticated clinician to aid in the journey to welless, it is not always necessary. Further, the truth is, for many people, finding such a person is sometimes impossible, hence taking charge of their own journey to wellness is the *only* option. That is most likely why the Lyme community is as potently informed as they are (much to the dismay of many physicians and paternalistic medical herbalists and naturopaths).

I do not agree with those clinicians who think you are too stupid to orchestrate your own journey to wellness, that you are too unintelligent or uneducated to understand these books, that you should not be allowed to engage in your own healing without some licensed person overseeing your regimen. In fact, I disagree with that kind of condescending attitude quite strongly. If you do feel you need a health professional to help you, then by all means find one. If you do not feel that you need someone, or that your past efforts with professionals have been unsatisfactory, then again, trust yourself to find what works for you and what does not. In fact, even if you do work with a health professional, I highly recommend that you trust yourself to determine what you are willing to take as medicine and what you are not, to determine for yourself if something is working or if it is not, to engage in self-determination on your journey to wellness. Or as Paul Krugman once put it . . .

> When everyone—tout le monde, as Tom Wolfe used to put it, meaning a relative handful of people, but everyone who supposedly matters—is saying something it takes a real effort to step outside and say, wait a minute, how do we know that? It's especially hard if you spend your time hanging out with other Very Serious People. . . . This is what you need to know: important people have no special monopoly on wisdom; and in times like these, when the usual rules . . . don't apply, they are often deeply foolish, because the power of conventional wisdom prevents them from talking sense about a deeply unconventional situation. (Krugman, 2010)

IF YOU ARE A CLINICIAN

I have gone into these organisms in depth so that you can begin to understand just how complex their actions in the body are. It is my hope that Western herbal medicine can begin to emerge as a highly sophisticated form of healing, one *understood* to be highly sophisticated, and one that can deal with the kinds of complexities that are now commonly found in emerging infections. To that end I have introduced the idea of thinking about the synergies that exist between coinfections as well as the concept of examining the kind of cytokine cascades bacteria create during infection. Cytokines are messenger molecules that act as intercellular mediators during the body's immune responses. Each stealth pathogen, during infection, releases certain cytokines to facilitate its infection of the body and, further, to stimulate the breakdown of specific tissues to gain nutrients. Each pathogen decreases the activity of certain parts of the human immune system (interfering with an effective immune response) and activates others (stimulating inflammation and cellular breakdown). So while some parts of the immune system become less functional, others become overactive. The overactivity comes from an organism-initiated cascade (think "domino effect") of inflammatory cytokines. Each stealth pathogen creates a different kind of cascade; that is, they stimulate certain kinds of inflammation in the body through using the body's immune response for their own ends. This is why infection with these organisms often mimics an autoimmune disease dynamic. This is important to understand when designing any kind of elegant, interventive treatment strategy. If you *know* what is happening in the body you don't have to guess what to do—you *know* what to do.

And while I don't go into it in any depth in this book, the idea of the complex synergies that exist between herbal medicines is crucial, as is the understanding of herbal synergists. These concepts are developed in more depth in the revised and expanded second edition of my book *Herbal Antibiotics* (Storey Publishing, 2012). If you wish to look deeper into plant synergists and herbal synergies, I think you will find that book useful. As well, time and space limitations made the inclusion of *in-depth* monographs on many of these herbs impossible to include in this volume. I have developed in-depth monographs on many of these herbs elsewhere . . . the only ones included in this book are those not included in other books I have written. If you would like to see them they can be found in *Healing Lyme, Herbal Antibiotics* (second edition), *Herbal Antivirals,* and *Healing Lyme Disease Coinfections: Complementary and Holistic Treatments for Bartonella and Mycoplasma.* (For specifics, see chapter 9.)

Please note that along with *Babesia, Anaplasma, Ehrlichia, Bartonella,* and *Mycoplasma* there are a number of other coinfections that are sometimes encountered, generally with less frequency (at least for now). One, tick-borne encephalitis or TBE, is dealt with in some depth in *Herbal Antivirals.* Others such as Rocky Mountain spotted fever will be covered in the revised edition of *Healing Lyme,* due out, hopefully, not too long after this book.

HOW I ARRIVED AT THE HERBAL PROTOCOLS IN THIS BOOK

The protocols in this book were developed by exploring the dynamics of the diseases themselves, their impacts in people, the experience of clinicians treating them, protocols that those with the diseases have successfully used, many hundreds of journal papers, a look at the plants' history of usage around the world for treating these and similar conditions, and my own experience with plant medicines over a nearly 30-year period. But please note . . .

The plants herein are just guidelines. The protocols themselves are just guidelines. The dosages are just guidelines. Again: there is *no* one-size-fits-all way to treat these diseases. The intent of this book is to give those who wish one an understanding of the diseases so that they can be treated more effectively and with greater sophistication. This is just a beginning, a starting place so we no longer have to grope along in the dark.

Feel free to alter, add, delete, innovate, think outside the box, argue, insist, and never settle for less than being healthy in the way that you understand it.

And remember: *all* plants are useful as medicinals.

Again, *all* plants are useful as medicinals.

The secret, as always, is in the dose, the timing, and the combination that is used. Just because a plant is not mentioned in this book does not mean it is not useful.

One of the things I have learned from the ill people I have worked with since 1986 (especially those in the Lyme community) is that when a lot of people with a lot of motivation begin looking around themselves, searching for answers, they come up with some truly amazing things. If you lock people in a room with only four ways out, someone will find a fifth way out. *Always.*

Trust yourself, and remember, only *you* know what health is for you.

1

Emerging Diseases and Coinfections

The New Epidemics

Hosts that are coinfected by multiple parasite species seem to be the rule rather than the exception in natural systems.
A. L. GRAHAM, I. M. CATTADORI,
J. O. LLOYD-SMITH, ET AL.,
"TRANSMISSION CONSEQUENCES OF COINFECTION:
CYTOKINES WRIT LARGE?"

Patients with immunocompromised systems are at greater risk for a more prolonged and severe course of illness, especially with multiple infectious etiologies, illustrated here with Lyme disease and babesia. In these patients, reasoning to the single most likely cause of illness may not be the best approach to diagnosis and empiric treatment. Familiarity with tick-borne diseases is important and may become more so as the habitats of humans and ticks increasingly intersect.

Y. ABRAMS,
"COMPLICATIONS OF COINFECTION WITH BABESIA
AND LYME DISEASE AFTER SPLENECTOMY"

Coinfections could, thus, increase vulnerability to the emergence of new parasites by facilitating species jumps, if the coinfected portion of a population provides favourable conditions for an emerging parasite to adapt to a new host species.

A. GRAHAM, I. M. CATTADORI,
J. O. LLOYD-SMITH, ET AL.,
"TRANSMISSION CONSEQUENCES OF COINFECTION:
CYTOKINES WRIT LARGE?"

I first became interested in bacterial diseases in the early 1990s after reading about the emergence of resistant bacteria in hospitals. Having studied mathematics, I well understood what an exponential growth curve meant. I could see as well as anyone that we had only a short period of time in which to begin to address the problem.

As I studied more deeply, I began to be aware not only of resistant bacteria, the majority of which flow from hospital settings (and large, commercial farms) into the general community, but also of diseases emerging in the human population due to overpopulation and the environmental disruption that causes. Lyme was among the earliest of the emerging diseases that caught my attention and, as time went on, the coinfections that accompany Lyme (initially thought to be extremely uncommon) did so as well.

It became clear, the more I learned, that many of these emerging diseases were difficult to treat with conventional technological medicine, that the diagnostic tests were often unreliable, and that many of the organisms did not respond well to antibiotics. As well, and most regret-tably, it slowly became obvious that many physicians had little knowl-edge of, or much interest in, these diseases.

I have been deeply immersed in the study of emerging and resistant bacteria for over two decades now. It is clear that while technological medicine still has a role to play, sometimes an important one, evolution-ary changes are occurring that make many of our assumptions about such diseases and their treatment obsolete.

I was born in 1952 into an extended family that included many physicians, among them a surgeon general of the United States. For my family, "modern" medicine was *the* way to approach disease—the *only* way. Penicillin had become widely available in 1946, just after World War II, and new antibiotics were being discovered (seemingly) every day. Vaccines, too, were making history. The year I was born there were 58,000 new cases of polio, more than 3,000 of those infected with the disease died, and many of the others were permanently disabled—some terribly so. The next year, Jonas Salk announced the successful testing of his vaccine against polio. Then, in 1962, Albert Sabin introduced his oral vaccine, something that made mass vaccina-tion easily possible. I still remember that long walk to the lunch room in elementary school, the long wait in line, and the sugar cube in the tiny, white paper cup.

The excitement of those days is very hard to explain to newer gen-erations, but for people then, it seemed as if infectious diseases were going to be permanently eradicated. In fact, many researchers and phy-sicians in the late 1950s and early 1960s, including my great-uncle Lee Burney, then surgeon general of the United States, and my grandfather David Cox, president of the Kentucky Medical Association, went so far as to loudly proclaim that the end of all infectious disease was upon us. A 1963 statement by the Australian physician Sir F. Macfarlane Burnet, a Nobel laureate, is typical. By the end of the twentieth century, he said, humanity would see the "virtual elimination of infectious disease as a significant factor in societal life" (Levy 1992, 3). And in 1970, one of my great-uncle's successors, Surgeon General William Stewart, testified to Congress that "it was time to close the book on infectious diseases" (Levy 1992, 3). With satisfaction, physician David Moreau observed in a 1976 article in *Vogue* magazine that "the chemotherapeutic revolution has reduced nearly all non-viral disease to the significance of a bad cold" (Griggs 1991, 261).

They were wrong, of course, the victims of their own hubris and a deep lack of understanding of the natural world, most especially of bacteria. By the time Moreau's comments appeared resistant bacterial diseases were already on the rise. A short 30 years later, with infectious diseases from resistant bacterial strains become rampant, the world came to face the specter of epidemic disease outbreaks more dangerous than any known in history. As bacterial resistance researcher and physician David Livermore recently put it, "It is naive to think we can win" (Bosley 2010).

There are two factors that have stimulated the emergence of potent bacterial disease organisms. The first is the tremendous overuse of antibiotics over the past 70 years. The second is the severe ecological disruption that increasing human population is causing.

In an extremely short period of geologic time the earth has been saturated with hundreds of millions of tons of nonbiodegradable, often biologically unique pharmaceuticals designed to kill bacteria. Many antibiotics (whose name literally means "against life") do not discriminate in their activity but kill broad groups of diverse bacteria whenever they are used. The worldwide environmental dumping, over the past 65 years, of huge quantities of synthetic antibiotics has initiated the most pervasive impacts on the earth's bacterial underpinnings since oxygen-generating bacteria supplanted methanogens 2.5 billion years ago. It has, according to medical researcher and physician Stuart Levy, "stimulated evolutionary changes that are unparalleled in recorded biologic history" (Levy 1992, 75). Bacteria *had* to evolve resistance. If not, due to their crucial role in the ecological functioning of this planet (and our own bodies), all life, including the human species, would already have been killed off by those very same antibiotics.

Ecological disruption has also played an extensive role. For example, the damage to wild landscapes, intrusions into forest ecosystems, the cutting of those same forests to make way for suburbs, and the damage to plant diversity and its crucial homeodynamic functions by suburban and agricultural intrusions have all had a place in stimulating the emergence of new disease groups. A study from the State University of New York is representative:

> This study examined 11 years of surveillance data in New York State to measure the relationship between forest fragmentation and the incidence of human babesiosis. Adjusted Poisson models showed that increasing edges of contact between forested land and developed land, as measured by their shared parameters, was associated with a higher incidence of babesiosis cases, even after controlling for the total developed land area and forest density, and temperature and precipitation. Each 10-km increase in perimeter contact between forested land and developed land per county was associated with a 1.5% increase in babesiosis risk. Higher temperature was also strongly associated with increasing babesiosis risk, wherein each degree Celsius increase was associated with an 18% increase in babesiosis risk. (Walsh, 2013)

Human movement into previously unoccupied forest lands significantly increases the risk of infections, from both the ecological pressure put on the infectious organisms and the increasing numbers of people in that habitat. For example, studies of forest ticks in southern Poland have found that 77 percent carry *Anaplasma*, 60 percent *Babesia*, and only 3 percent *Borrelia*. Coinfection with *Anaplasma* and *Babesia* was found in 50 percent of the ticks. The more that such locations are inhabited by people, the more likely it is that they will get bitten and develop disease. Too, the unique grouping of the infectious organisms in that ecological zone determines the kinds of coinfection complex people will develop. Thus in that part of Poland there is a much higher chance of becoming infected with *Babesia* and *Anaplasma* than Lyme. This is something that physicians should understand: they live in a particular ecological habitat and the grouping of disease organisms in that habitat's ticks is always going to be unique—as is the immune health of that region's people.

Also crucial to the emergence of these coinfections is the reduction of wild predator populations (not only of mountain lions, for example, but of the bird species that eat insects and mice). This creates subsequent increases in the deer, mice, and insect populations that carry those bacterial pathogens, which in itself increases the movement of disease into human populations.

And finally, the reduction of large, wild mammal populations in undisturbed forest habitats plays its own important role. As fewer and fewer wild animal populations are available as hosts for the bacterial diseases that once were (mostly) limited to those populations, the bacteria have had no choice: they have had to jump species in order to find hosts in which to live. Because human beings now live in the habitat formerly occupied by those animals, many of the bacteria have moved into us. We are *not* inadvertent hosts. We are becoming primary reservoirs for many of these emerging diseases.

Unfortunately, bacterial resistance and ecological disruption can't help but intersect—with, of course, terrible ramifications. Many of the primary coinfections of Lyme are closely related to some of the most potent resistant bacterial organisms known. They are all members of the Proteobacteria phylum, a large and closely related group of bacteria.

One branch of the Proteobacteria includes *Bartonella* spp., and another includes *Ehrlichia* spp., *Anaplasma* spp., Rocky Mountain spotted fever, and the other rickettsia—all of which are coinfections of Lyme. A different but closely related branch includes *Klebsiella* spp., *E. coli*, cholera organisms, *Pseudomonas* spp., *Salmonella* spp. (including *Salmonella enterica*, the cause of typhoid fever), and *Shigella* spp.—all now resistant to many antibiotics. It also includes *Yersinia*, the organism responsible for the plague, a bacteria transmitted by fleas much as *Bartonella* is. Still another branch includes the bacteria responsible for gonorrhea infections (also resistant), and another includes both *Helicobacter* and *Campylobacter* organisms.

There is strong evidence that both resistance and virulence factors are being shared among all members of this phylum. In other words, the various bacteria are teaching each other how to resist antibiotics and how to more easily infect people, thus making them sicker. They do this, usually, through sharing segments of DNA that have within them resistance and virulence information. *Bartonella* organisms, as an example, are often coinfective with many of the bacteria in this phylum and, in many instances, these kinds of multiple infections show a remarkable synergy during the disease process. In other words, the bacteria work together to reduce the effectiveness of the immune response and thus enable long-term infection.

In practical terms what all this means is that a great many more diseases are emerging out of the ecological matrix of the planet and infecting human beings. As well, many of them possess, or soon acquire, resistance to the majority of antibiotics that people use to treat bacterial diseases. And what they do together in the body is a great deal more complex than what any one of them does alone. The unique nature of the Lyme group of emerging infections, for example, is causing many researchers to refer to them not only as stealth pathogens but as second-generation pathogens. That is, they are very different than the bacteria (first-generation pathogens) for which antibiotics were created in the latter half of the twentieth century.

One of the most important understandings now facing us is accepting the limits of pharmaceuticals in the treatment of many of these emerging diseases. While antibiotics do still have a role, sometimes a very important one, they can no longer be relied on to provide the *sole* response to these kinds of infections as they spread through the human population. We have to approach treatment with a more sophisticated eye.

There are two important aspects to this. The first is realizing that single-treatment approaches, most of which were developed out of an inaccurate nineteenth- and early-twentieth-century bacterial paradigm and were based on identifying the bacterial pathogen involved and killing it (i.e., monotherapy), are going to have to be abandoned as the primary method of treating these kinds of diseases. (Something that newer generations of physicians, especially in countries other than the United States, are beginning to understand.) The second is coming to understand just *what* the bacteria do in the body and then designing a treatment protocol that is *specific* in counteracting what the organisms do. In essence this means designing treatment protocols that address bacterial cytokine cascades, the particular health or non-health of the person's immune system, and the specific symptom picture that is reducing the quality of the person's life. Combined with antibacterials, of whatever sort, this creates the most sophisticated basic approach to the treatment of bacterial diseases. (If you add to that approach sophisticated human-to-human interactions oriented around deep caring and personal presence, something most physicians do not understand, you have the core of the most elegant and potent paradigm of healing disease that can occur.)

Some additional sophistications can occur for those who wish to go even deeper. Among them are the synergy that occurs among the healing agents that are used *and* the synergy that exists between the different bacteria. The use of healing agents (pharmaceuticals *or* herbs) always involves synergy between the agents used—though this is rarely addressed in a positive light. It's usually the side effects of a drug combination or drug/herb combination that are highlighted. However, herbs are synergistic with each other and can be synergistic with pharmaceuticals. For example, Chinese skullcap (*Scutellaria baicalensis*) root and licorice (*Glycyrrhiza* spp.) are synergists; they enhance the action of other herbs with which they are combined. They can, as well, enhance the action of pharmaceuticals. For example, Japanese knotweed (*Polygonum cuspidatum*) root, when used along with formerly ineffective antibiotics, can enhance the drugs' actions enough to make them effective.

As well, the microbial pathogens are often synergistic with each other. That is, when an infection involves two or more Lyme-group organisms, the impacts on the body are often more severe. And this increase in severity is not additive, it is synergistic. This means that a simple linear approach will not give you an understanding of what the pathogens are doing in the body. As Telfer et al. (2010) comment:

> Most hosts, including humans, are simultaneously or sequentially infected with several parasites. . . . Indeed, effects are typically of greater magnitude, and explain more variation in infection risk, than the effects associated with host and environmental factors more commonly considered in disease studies. We highlight the danger of mistaken inference when considering parasite species in isolation rather than parasite communities. . . . Single parasite studies may yield incorrect or incomplete conclusions. Nonetheless, most epidemiological studies, in animals and humans, still focus on single species.

COINFECTION DYNAMICS

To generate sophisticated, reliable inverventions with these second-generation bacteria, there are a number of important dynamics to understand. The primary ones are understandings of the specific cytokine cascades that occur, the immune health (and preexisting conditions) in the host, the synergy between the various microorganisms, and their synergy with the vector of transmission.

Cytokines

The past several decades have seen a shift in the way many researchers (but regrettably few physicians) are approaching disease, nowhere more so than with the stealth pathogens that, due to their nature, often cause a wide range of symptoms. Researchers Ian Clark et al., for example, have done some marvelous work on the dynamics of cytokines specific to various disease conditions, especially malaria and its close relative babesiosis. They note:

It is our view that focusing on malaria [and babesiosis and Lyme] in isolation will never provide the insights required to understand the pathogenesis of this disease. How can the illnesses caused by a spirochete and a virus be so clinically identical: typhoid readily diagnosed as malaria and malaria in returning travelers so commonly dismissed as influenza? . . . Understanding why these clinical confusions occur entails appreciating the sequence of events that led up to the cytokine revolution that has transformed the field over the last 15 years. (Clark et al., 2004)

Again, cytokines are small cell-signaling molecules released by cells that are damaged, cells of the immune system, and glial cells of the nervous system that are important in intercellular communications in the body. As it turns out, many disease organisms have learned to use cytokines for their own purposes.

In practical terms: When bacterium touches a cell, the cell gives off a signal, a cytokine, that tells the immune system what is happening and what that cell needs. This calls on the immune system to respond (initially, the innate immune system), which then sends specific immune cells to that location to deal with the problem. Stealth pathogens utilize this process to enable their successful infection of the body. Instead of waiting for the host's cells to release a cytokine, the microorganism does it as soon as it enters the body.

As the microorganism enters the body an initial, and very powerful, cytokine (for example, tumor necrosis factor, a.k.a. TNF) is released into the body. That initial cytokine stimulates the production of others, and those generate still others—all of which have potent impacts on the body. Thus a *cascade* of cytokines occurs. This cascade (and any subsequent immune response) is carefully modulated by the pathogen to produce the exact effects it needs to facilitate its spread in the body and its sequestration inside our body's cells (thus hiding it from the immune system), to break apart particular cells in order to get nutrients, and to shut down the parts of our immune response that can effectively deal with the infection. It is this cascade of carefully modulated cytokines that, in fact, creates most of the symptoms that people experience when they become ill.

The cytokine cascade dynamics and its impacts alter depending on the animal host and its immune health. Clark et al. found that parasite load—that is, the numbers of organisms in the body—counterintuitively, did not correlate to severity of illness, something that plays havoc with older bacterial theories of disease. They comment:

> Since *P. falciparum* and *Babesia microti,* another hemoprotozoan protozoan, infect both humans and another host (the owl monkey, *Aotus* sp., and the mouse, respectively), it was possible to establish that the relationship [between severity of illness and parasite density] depended on a characteristic of the host, not the parasite species. This provided, for the first time, a plausible explanation for the long-standing puzzle that, although very low parasite densities cause onset of illness in first infections of human malaria and babesiosis and bovine babesiosis, mice withstand high parasite densities of several species of either causative genus before onset of illness. In other words, previously unexposed humans become ill after exposure to very few hemoprotozoan parasites whereas mice do not become ill until exposed to many organisms. Similarly inexplicable had been the observation that incredibly high malaria parasite densities (sometimes reaching a peak of 35,000 parasites per 10,000 red blood cells) do not cause illness in reptiles. (Clark et al., 2004)

And in fact, very low densities of babesial (and ehrlichial and anaplasmal) organisms in people can (and do) cause serious disease. (This is also why diagnosis is sometimes so difficult; there are so few organisms they just can't be found.) In some people high densities occur but they remain asymptomatic; in others low densities exist along with multiorgan failure, coma, and death. The belief that a high density of infectious organisms is correlated with severity of disease turns out to be inaccurate. The thought that very few organisms could cause death did not, in older models of disease (and still for many physicians), compute. Instead of parasite density, something else is involved in the development and seriousness of the disease and its symptoms. And that something is cytokines. Clark et al. (2004) note:

> The long-postulated malaria toxin did not cause illness directly, as had been assumed since the late 19th century, but did so through inducing the host to release a shower of LPS-inducible cytokines that, at lower concentrations, are an essential part of the host immune response.

They continue . . .

> Serum TNF level in East African and West African children at time of admission correlated with the severity of disease and mortality, even though serum TNF levels varied greatly. . . . Patients with complicated malaria (combined organ dysfunction, hypotension, thrombocytopenia, and the highest parasite densities) and the longest durations between onset of clinical symptoms and diagnosis had significantly higher TNF levels than those in whom malaria ran a more benign course.

Cytokine researchers have found that even tiny alterations in existing cytokine profiles will cause significant shifts in disease symptoms. Clark et al. (2004) comment, "In one IL-2 [interleukin-2] study, 15 of 44 patients developed behavioral changes sufficiently severe to warrant acute intervention and 22 had severe cognitive defects."

Although the news has not yet reached most medical doctors, many researchers are insisting that the most important thing is not the microbial source of infection but rather the cytokine cascade that is generated. This is especially true during coinfections with multiple stealth pathogens. One of the better articles on this is "Transmission consequences of coinfection: Cytokines writ large?" by Andrea Graham et al. (2007). The authors comment, "When the taxonomic identities of parasites are replaced with their cytokine signatures, for example, it becomes possible to predict the within-host consequences of coinfection for microparasite replication" as well as symptom picture, treatment approaches, and treatment outcomes.

(This, by the way, is the approach I use when exploring how best to treat the complex of Lyme-group coinfections. After more than a decade of experience, it turns out that interrupting the cytokine cascade these organisms initiate does in fact reduce or even eliminate both symptoms and infection.)

Immune Health and Preexisting Conditions

Lyme-group parasites, like many stealth pathogens, utilize the immune responses of whatever mammal they infect as part of their infection strategy. As Graham et al. (2007) note: "The influence of cytokines on effector responses is so powerful that many parasites manipulate host-cytokine pathways for their own benefit," as is indeed the case with *Babesia, Ehrlichia*, and *Anaplasma*. Most crucially, they continue, "the magnitude and type of cytokine response influence host susceptibility and infectiousness. Susceptibility to a given parasite will be affected by cytokine responses that are ongoing at the time of exposure, including responses to pre-existing infections." In other words, the parasites utilize inflammatory processes that are already occurring in the body (e.g., if you have preexisting arthritis) to facilitate successful infection.

But equally important is the overall *immune health* of the infected person. Telfer et al. (2008) comment:

> There is mounting evidence from experimental studies that the outcome of interactions during co-infections (for either the host or the parasite) is context dependent, potentially varying with different host or parasite genotypes or environmental conditions. Perhaps most critically, outcome can depend on the timing and sequence of

infections. . . . Susceptibility is a property of an individual host at a given time. . . . The ability of a parasite to establish an infection successfully will depend on the initial immune response of the exposed host. On entry into the host, a parasite will experience an "immunoenvironment" potentially determined by both previous and current infections, as well as intrinsic factors such as sex, age, nutritional status and genotype. The immediate immuno-effectors in a naive host will be dominated by cells and molecules that comprise the innate immune response, and thus the efficiency of this arm of host immunity at reducing and clearing an infection will be influential in determining susceptibility.

Resto-Ruiz et al. (2003) emphasize this as well, as do so many other researchers. They note that people with "intact" immune function who become infected with *B. henselae* usually do not experience severe symptoms. However, they continue, "the reduced ability of the host's immune response to control bacterial infection apparently results in a bacteremia of longer duration." In other words, the immune status of someone with coinfections *must be* addressed as part of any treatment protocol. Due to the synergistic nature of coinfections an inescapable truth exists: the weaker or more compromised the immune system, the more likely someone is to become infected and the more likely they are to have a debilitating course of illness.

Improving the immune status of those with chronic coinfections allows the immune system, refined over very long evolutionary time, to do what it does best, which is to use very elegant mechanisms to control and clear infection. Eventually, the healthy immune system begins to identify the outer membrane proteins of the bacteria and create antibodies to them. Due to the sophistication of the bacteria's subversion of the host immune system during coinfections, this can take anywhere from four to eight months. In those whose immune systems are very compromised it may take longer; how long is directly proportional to the health of the immune system. Once the immune system creates the proper antigens, the bacteria are then eliminated fairly rapidly from the body. Reinfection is difficult as the antibodies remain in the body for some time.

Immune system health is a crucial element in the treatment of coinfections and it is one that technological medicine is generally unable to address. It is most definitely *not* a subject in which most physicians are trained.

Parasite Synergy

Symptoms, length of illness, and its severity are all generally worse if infection occurs by more than one organism. The research of Graham et al. (2007) confirmed that, as the researchers put it, "coinfection increases the reproductive number for the incoming parasite species and facilitates its transmission through the host population." In other words, while the immune system is often compromised by the cytokine dynamics initiated by one type of bacteria, multiple, simultaneously initiated cascades are more potent in their impacts; infection is much more easily accomplished. This is, as Graham et al. comment, more common than otherwise: "Hosts that are coinfected by multiple parasite species seem to be the rule rather than the exception in natural systems and some of the most devastating human diseases are associated with coinfections that challenge immune response efficacy."

Another very fine paper on this, by S. Telfer et al. (2008), echoes Graham et al., with its authors noting, "In natural populations 'concomitant' or 'mixed' infections by more than one parasite species or genotype are common. Consequently, interactions between different parasite genotypes or species frequently occur. These interactions may be synergistic or antagonistic with potential fitness implications for both the host (morbidity and/or mortality) and parasite (transmission potential)." In other words, if you want to successfully treat someone who is infected with a vector-borne infection you need to realize up front that it is usually the case that coinfection has occurred and you have to look at the interactive picture, not merely single infectious agents. We can no longer assume that bacterial organisms exist in a vacuum. They can't be studied in isolation.

Telfer and his associates, in another paper, explored the interactions and infection risks between cowpox virus, *Babesia microti*, *Bartonella* spp., and *Anaplasma phagocytophilum*. They note:

> We found that this community of parasites represents not four independent infections but an interconnected web of interactions: Effects of other infections on infection risk were strong and wide-spread, and connectance within the parasite community was exceptionally high, with evidence detected for all possible pair-wide interactions. (Telfer et al. 2010)

They found, as they note, that "the sizes of the effects of other parasites on infection risk were also similar to, and frequently greater than, other factors." Specifically here, seasonal effects. That is, infection with Lyme-group coinfections is generally higher in certain months, e.g., three times higher for anaplasmal infections and 15 times higher for babesial. However, this is matched by the synergistic effects of multiple coinfections on host susceptibility. As they comment, "The most likely explanation for these effects is that interactions between these microparasites with individual hosts have a large impact on host susceptibility."

The synergistic effects also contribute to symptom picture. If *Bartonella* is a coinfection with Lyme, for example, what you then get is assault on and resultant degradation of the collagen systems of the body by the Lyme spirochetes while a simultaneous assault on red blood cells occurs with a concomitant subversion and abnormalization of endothelial cells and their functions. So, the infected person is battling not only Lyme arthritis or neurological Lyme (both caused by collagen degradation) but a red blood cell infection (with potential anemia and lowered oxygen availability in the blood) and abnormal endothelial cell growth in the blood vessels themselves.

But the *Bartonella* bacteria also use what the Lyme bacteria are doing for their own purposes. This, as Telfer et al. (2010) noted, also affects host susceptibility. Once Lyme spirochetes damage collagen tissues, for instance in the joints of the knee, the body sends CD34+ cells to that site to help repair the damage. This is a normal part of the healing process when collagen is damaged. But *Bartonella* typically invade CD34+ cells, so some of those CD34+ cells will be infected and the *Bartonella* will take advantage of the local inflammation to establish a colony of their own in that location. The existing inflammation actually facilitates their growth. Once established, the *Bartonella* bacteria will begin their own cytokine cascade, which will itself contribute to even more collagen degradation at that location.

The more coinfections, the more stress on the immune system. As Telfer et al. (2008) comment, "Attempts by the immune system to simultaneously counter the multiple parasite species involved in a co-infection can lead to immunopathological disease and pathology that are more than the simple additive pathogenic effects of the different parasite species." This is a crucial point. *The impact of multiple coinfectious organisms is **not** additive.* They are synergistic. They create effects that are more than the sum of the parts.

For example, infections with both *Babesia* and *Bartonella* are synergistically impactful on red blood cells and can reduce red blood cell counts up to 25 percent, leading to anemia, fatigue, breathlessness, and general weakness. In the immune-competent, neither parasite will normally create this severe an impact by themselves. (One positive note: Because both parasites are competing for red blood cells, longer studies have found that the *Babesia*, over time, tends to clear the *Bartonella* infection by outcompeting the latter organisms. Also: If someone is already infected by *Bartonella*, they are less likely to be infected with *Babesia*, and vice versa. Nevertheless, during infection with both, in the initial stages, the impact on red blood cells is immense.)

Babesia species sequester themselves in the capillary networks of the spleen and liver. *Bartonella* species sequester themselves in the endothelial cells of the capillary networks of the spleen and liver. Both then seed the bloodstream from those locations at regular intervals. The impacts of infection with both parasites on the spleen and liver are much greater than either alone and this has to be taken into account in any treatment approach. In other words, you have to design spleen- and liver-supportive interventions that are tightly focused on normalizing functioning in those organs. This protects them from cytokine damage *and* begins to reduce habitat for the parasites, thus reducing bacterial/protozoal load and presence in the body.

Studies of coinfection with *Anaplasma* and *Borrelia* species have found that the deleterious impacts on immune function from such a double infection enhance the pathogenicity of the Lyme spirochetes and long-term infection. Researchers note, "These effects may have a significant impact on the persistence of *B. burgdorferi* and the immunologic selective pressure it is subjected to" (Moro et al. 2002). Coinfection with Lyme spirochetes and anaplasmal bacteria produces synergistic effects on cytokine expression. Interleukin-12 (IL-12), interferon-gamma (IFN-γ), and tumor necrosis factor alpha (TNF-α) are more inhibited during early infection than with either bacteria alone; IL-6 levels are higher. Coinfection with these two organisms also produces more significant impacts in the brain and on brain function. There is a synergistically increased production and release of matrix metalloproteinases (MMPs) in the brain, specifically MMP-1, -3, -7, -8, and -9. IL-10 levels (which reduce effective innate immune responses and which are induced by the bacteria during initial infection) are significantly higher, and IL-8 and MIP-1α (macrophage inflammatory protein 1-alpha) levels increase. Along with the MMPs, this leads to increased vascular permeability in the brain and central nervous system. This produces more inflammation deeper in the brain, with increased brain dysfunction and more serious neurocognitive defects. There is an increased bacterial burden throughout the body; the symptom picture is generally worse.

Coinfection with *Borrelia* spirochetes and *Babesia microti* shows similar impacts and results in both increased severity of Lyme arthritis and longer duration.

Telfer et al. (2010) also found that infection with *Anaplasma* (for example) made subsequent infection by *Babesia* much easier—in fact, twice as likely. Reversing the order of infection found the same rate of increase—each organism paves the road for the other. Telfer et al. also found that animals infected with one *Bartonella* species who were also infected by other *Bartonella* species were much more likely to have long-term infections—that is, a chronic illness.

An *Ehrlichia* infection, when combined with *Bartonella* (or *Babesia* or a hemoplasma), is often much more severe in its impacts than would be expected by looking at either alone. In this situation, both white and red blood cells are infected. Specifically, *Ehrlichia* infect neutrophils, the most abundant form of white blood cell in the body and an essential element of the innate immune system. Thus the immune system is fighting not only bacteria in the red blood cells and vascular tissues but bacteria inside its own immune cells. To make it worse, the bacteria cross-talk and engage in mutual support of each other, actually enhancing each other's impacts on the host and their resistance to antibiotics.

During coinfection with both *Mycoplasma* and *Bartonella*, there are going to be severe effects on the endothelial cells, the red blood cells, and the brain and central nervous system that are out of proportion to infection by either organism alone. Thus the cytokine impacts on those areas of the body are going to be stronger, synergistic, and more debilitating; treatment regimens must be designed to reverse much stronger effects than would occur by either alone. This often calls for larger doses, longer treatment duration, and more sophisticated intervention for symptom management. As only one example, such a double infection *may* simultaneously cause a form of regular epileptic seizures *and* periodic bouts of homicidal rage. Herbs that reduce the cytokine cascades involved *and* are specific for these types of seizures *and* are particularly calming to the nervous system, thus reducing extreme rage events, need to be used and the doses need to be largish, continual, and very focused. (Chinese skullcap is a specific example, and it tends to be synergistic with several others such as motherwort and pasqueflower that are also specific for these kinds of conditions, although in slightly different ways.)

Vector of Transmission

The vector of transmission—that is, the tick, flea, mosquito, and so on in which the bacteria live before they are injected through a bite into a human being—plays a crucial part in the disease as well.

Bacteria have learned to take advantage of the biologically active components in their vector's saliva in order to facilitate avoidance of the immune system. For example, tick saliva itself contains highly active compounds that reduce nerve signaling, thus allowing the tick to remain embedded for long periods. The saliva also reduces swelling at the bite location and inactivates immune responses, again allowing the tick to feed for longer periods. Similar though unique dynamics occur for every insect vector in this group. The Lyme group of bacteria take advantage of this in order to more successfully infect a new host. There is in fact a synergy between the vector's inactivation of the immune system and the bacterial inactivation of immune responses. This makes penetration of the host and long-term infection much easier. Studies have consistently shown that infection through a vector of transmission produces longer and more serious infections than direct infection, that is, through hypodermic injection (by researchers). This kind of synergy is not limited, it appears, to saliva.

Although little research has occurred on louse and flea feces, two main routes of infection for *Bartonella*, researchers comment that a similar dynamic might be playing out here as well: "It is also quite likely that under natural conditions components of the flea feces other than *B. henselae* may enhance the development of *Bartonella*-induced lymphadenopathy and thus enable the onset of disease at a lower dose of infection in humans" (Kunz et al., 2008) Given the very long evolutionary relationship between ticks and Lyme or fleas and *Bartonella*, it is not surprising that the bacteria have learned to utilize both to assist their infection of new hosts.

PRACTITIONER ORIENTATION AND
APPROACH TO TREATMENT

In my experience, the technological medical community tends to downplay both the impact and occurrence of coinfections in the people they see while the natural medicine community tends to exaggerate them. Oddly, despite their training, most physicians don't really understand bacterial organisms very well, nor how to treat them. They tend to look in textbooks (or drug company brochures) for a pharmaceutical that is active for the bacteria in question and apply it, a fairly superficial approach that is increasingly failing in practice. If they have not definitively *identified* the bacterial cause of the condition they will generally prescribe a broad-spectrum antibiotic that will, as often as it helps, do more harm than good (the literature is full of such blunders). They are also very poor at developing a broad, synergistic, and human view of the people they treat, the disease conditions that occur, and the pharmaceutical interventions they commonly use. Most of them stopped *reasoning* a long time ago and simply act as if the worldview they were trained in, in school, really is an accurate map of the world around them—despite current events and research clearly showing it is not.

The natural medicine community, on the other hand, often tends to be somewhat hysterical about resistant or emerging infections, commonly fails at rigor of analysis, and too often lacks the focus, and courage, needed to confront deadly or life-debilitating infections. Both communities (often) make too much money off people's suffering—though, in fairness, most (not all) of the alternative community tends to make much less; I just don't see that many herbalists with their own private airplanes. (Nevertheless, overall, the natural medicine community is much safer—and less expensive, irrespective of their level of training—and they very rarely kill their patients. *Properly* prescribed pharmaceuticals are the fourth leading cause of death in the United States.)

When approaching the treatment of coinfections, the approach should be depth based with rigor of analysis. The bacterial infections need to be identified (muscle testing is not reliable enough, and no, ELISA is not either—neither should be relied upon as diagnostically definitive).

Once a diagnosis is achieved, a treatment protocol should be initiated. This seems obvious but in the actual world, not the theoretical one in people's heads or in books, most people are not diagnosed competently, or accurately. Many physicians and herbalists (including most naturopaths) simply look at the symptoms and *guess* at the underlying condition. In acute conditions where something must be done immediately this is a legitimate approach but *at the same time,* in the background, there needs to be a concerted effort to correctly diagnose. Physicians, counterintuitively, are often not very good at this—as a number of the case studies in this volume make clear. For many of them the problem lies in their internalized paradigms about disease, the structure of their practice, and, frankly, tremendous hubris. Those of us concerned with Lyme and its coinfections have heard scores of stories about physicians insisting that Lyme could not be the cause of a person's symptoms simply because Lyme isn't endemic in that location (so the physician refused to test for it), or that the person had already used antibiotics so the disease was cured and all the symptoms must now be in that person's head, or that the physician just did not have time for the kind of neediness that the Lyme-infected often present. Most physicians are not in the healing business but the pharmaceutical-dispensing business—these are not the same things.

Still, it is clear that in some cases antibiotics are very effective and with diseases as debilitating as Lyme and its coinfections they should be considered. However, if that kind of superficial approach fails, then an in-depth understanding of the cytokine cascades and the likely interactions between the coninfections should be developed and a treatment protocol initiated that addresses all that in depth. The most important thing in treating coinfections is to reduce the inflammatory processes the bacteria initiate, basically by counteracting the cytokine cascade they initiate. That stops pretty much all the symptoms right there, especially if treatment protocols are also begun that are designed to protect the areas of the body that are affected. And again, the immune system must be strengthened. As Telfer et al. (2010) observe, "An immune response that effectively cleared the infection from endothelial cells would therefore ultimately control an infection [by *Bartonella*]." Importantly, this observation applies as well to *any* intervention that will protect endothelial tissue from the bacteria, not just immune response. So if you use Japanese knotweed (*Polygonum cuspidatum*) or epigallocatechin gallate (EGCG) as an interventive, abnormal endothelial cell inflammation would cease. The bacteria *can't* survive if they are not able to initiate their particular form of inflammation in the body; it is how they make habitat and scavenge food. If you simultaneously enhance immune function, the body is then able to deal with the infection on its own. The addition of protocols to reduce acute symptoms and help restore quality of life are also very helpful. Not only does this help support the body's health at that particular location but the quality of life of the infected person is enhanced. The importance of this on outcomes cannot be stressed enough.

And finally, the *human* response of the healer toward the patient is essential. People who are ill *need* deep, caring contact with another human being. It is an essential aspect of healing. Physicians (and herbalists, including naturopaths) who don't take the time for this are, in my opinion, engaging in malpractice of the most egregious sort and, in effect, betraying their duty to their patients. I have continually seen, and numerous studies have found, that this one thing, in and of itself, contributes significantly to the successful resolution of illness. Genuine caring *is* medicine and it is time, more than time, that we, as a culture, recognize that. We absolutely *have to abandon* the paradigm that insists we not touch our patients, that we not love them, that we not spend time with them, that we not act as guides for them on their journey through illness. We must abandon the training, and the teacher, that tells us that we should *not* care, that somehow, as healers, we must keep our emotional distance from those who come to us.

Antibacterials *can* help but comprehensive treatment protocols must be more complex than that simple, monotherapeutic approach. Relying on a "kill the invaders" approach is becoming increasingly ineffective. Soon, if the world's major epidemiologists and researchers are to be believed, it won't work at all.

The bacteria are *evolving*. We should, too.

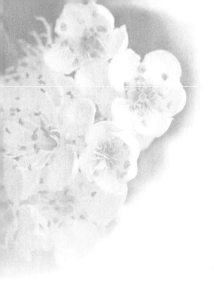

2

Babesia

An Overview

The number of reported cases in humans is rising steadily worldwide. Hitherto unknown zoonotic Babesia spp. are now being reported from geographic areas where babesiosis was not previously known to occur.

A. HILDEBRANDT, J. S. GRAY, AND K. P. HUNFELD,
"HUMAN BABESIOSIS IN EUROPE:
WHAT CLINICIANS NEED TO KNOW"

Genetic diversity was very high and infections with multiple genotypes were frequently found for both [Babesia] parasites in outbreak samples.

E. GUILLEMI, P. RUYBAL, V. LIA, ET AL.,
"MULTI-LOCUS TYPING SCHEME FOR *BABESIA BOVIS*
AND *BABESIA BIGEMINA* REVEALS HIGH LEVELS
OF GENETIC VARIABILITY IN STRAINS
FROM NORTHERN ARGENTINA"

Babesia microti, which has long been considered a single species [but is not], demonstrates a high degree of genetic diversity.

A. ZAMOTO-NIIJURA, M. TSUJI, W. QIANG, ET AL.,
"DETECTION OF TWO ZOONOTIC *BABESIA MICROTI*
LINEAGES, THE HOBETSU AND U.S. LINEAGES,
IN TWO SYMPATRIC TICK SPECIES, *IXODES OVATUS*
AND *IXODES PERSULCATUS*, RESPECTIVELY, IN JAPAN"

Babesia organisms are protozoa, not bacteria, as everyone surely knows. Still, if you try to find a really usable definition of what protozoa are, and why the differences between bacteria and protozoa matter, you are going to be unhappy. Inevitably you will find yourself reading such linguistic tours de force as this one (from Wikipedia, which has apparently been taken over by inarticulate reductionists). Protozoa, they note, are "organisms formerly classified in the Kingdom Protozoa." Unsurprisingly unhelpful so far; still, as the authors (insistently) continue:

> The species traditionally collectively ["traditionally collectively"?] termed "protozoa" are not closely related to each other, and have only superficial similarities (eukaryotic, unicellular, motile, though with exceptions). The terms "protozoa" (and protist) are usually discouraged in the modern biosciences. However, this terminology is still encountered in medicine. This is partially because of the conservative character of medical classification, and partially due to the necessity of making identifications of organisms based upon appearances and not upon DNA. (Wikipedia, under "protozoan infection," Jan. 12, 2013)

In other words, he looks like a duck, therefore he is a duck. Nevertheless, if you remain undaunted, and decide to travel deeper into Wikipedia-think by clicking on "Protist," you get the following descriptive:

> Protists are a large and diverse group of eukaryotic microorganisms, which belong to the kingdom Protista. There have been attempts to remove the kingdom from the taxonomy but it is still very much in use. The use of Protoctista is also preferred by various organizations and institutions. Molecular information has also been used to redefine this group in modern taxonomy as diverse and often distantly related phyla. The group of protists is now considered to mean diverse phyla that are not closely related through evolution and have different life cycles, tropic levels, modes of locomotion and cellular structures. Besides their relatively simple levels of organization, the protists do not have much in common. They are unicellular or they are multicellular.

"They are unicellular or they are multicellular"? Alrighty then.

This hasn't been a lot of help so far, though it does give you an experience of the current state of taxonomy (and science in general) when it comes to the natural world. Taxonomists, in other words . . .

people who are taxing, that is, burdensome, onerous, difficult, laborious, exhausting, grueling, oppressive, rigid, toilsome, wearing, stressful

really are a pain.

And no, it's not just a Wikipedia problem. This same kind of definitional fog about protozoa, and unfortunately most living organisms, can be found wherever taxonomists reside. So, let's try again . . .

Babesia organisms are protozoa, like malarial parasites, rather than bacteria (not that I am sure it really matters for our purposes). And according to current taxonometric classifications, bacteria are prokaryotes while protozoa are eukaryotes. (Hmmm, not very enlightening so far but let's soldier on.)

Protozoa, it turns out, possess a nucleus while bacteria do not. The term *prokaryote* (which bacteria are) means "pre-nucleus" or rather more exactly "before the nut," while *eukaryote* (which protozoa are) means "easily formed nut," if that helps any.

> *Taxonomists then would be eukaryotes, that is, easily formed nuts, as in "insane, unbalanced, a state of mind that prevents normal perception, behavior, or social interaction; seriously mentally ill."*

Bacteria have, instead of a nucleus, a *nucleoid* where they keep their DNA. ("These are not the nucleiods you are looking for. Move along, move along.") A nucleoid, it turns out, *is* a kind of nucleus but it doesn't have a membrane around it—thus nucleoid. It's a sort-of nucleus, a baby nucleus, a semi-nucleus, a pretend nucleus. Again, this is not very useful. Hmmmm, maybe then this will work:

Protozoa are bigger, some ten to one hundred times larger than bacteria, so much so that they sometimes feed on bacteria. This is why protozoa were originally considered to be the simplest form of animal (*protozoa* actually means "first animal") while bacteria are, well, just bacteria. Hmmmm. Still, if we look deeper, and despite all the definitional posturing by VSP (very serious people), it turns out that the particular protozoa we are concerned with here, that is, *Babesia,* are more similar to bacteria than these definitions would have us believe. Researchers note:

Due to its origin, this [babesial] organelle has bacterial characteristics, and the metabolic pathways it contains have been shown to be vital for parasite survival. Therefore it can be targeted by bacterial antibiotics which, as has been demonstrated in *Plasmodium* and *Toxoplasma*, result in a delayed-death response. Hence, particularly antibiotics that target the bacterial-like protein biosynthesis within the plastid like azithromycin, clindamycin, and tetracycline, are commonly used to treat human babesiosis. (Schnittger et al. 2012)

Ultimately, if you stay with it long enough, you will find out that protozoa, like bacteria, are simply microorganisms that sometimes infect people, and I don't know why they just can't say that to begin with.

There are some 30,000 different types of protozoa that have been identified so far in a variety of genera (genuses?). Each protozoal genus has from one to hundreds of different species within it. In the genus *Babesia* some 110 different species have been found so far. Like many of the Lyme group of infections, members of the *Babesia* complex, irrespective of what animal they infect, are parasites. They don't live in the wild but always inside another organism. Like their relatives, the malarial organisms, they colonize (infect) red blood cells (which is why they are sometimes referred to as hemoprotozoans—as if we didn't need another term and yes, they are sometimes called piroplasmids, too). It is from those cells that they gather the nutrients they need to survive. Babesial organisms infect pretty much everything with red blood cells: mammals, birds, and almost certainly reptiles and amphibians—although no one has spent any time looking for the ones that do. In fact, every mammal species tested has been found to harbor babesial infections, often specific to themselves. That is, lions and tigers and bears (don't say it) all tend to be infected, usually subclinically, with one babesial organism unique to themselves. Each different than the others. (But as current research is finding, this is not as cut-and-dried as was once thought.)

Babesial parasites have been around for hundreds of millions of years. In fact, genome studies have found that the ancestors of babesial organisms existed inside the early ancestors of ticks. Both evolved together into their current forms; they have had a very long coevolutionary mutualism. As new species of animals emerged from the ecological background of the planet, and as each was fed upon by ticks (or their ancestors), the *Babesia* protozoa altered their genome to make infection of those new animals possible. Some sources still insist that the various members of the genus *only* infect specific animals (and specific vectors) and that humans are incidental hosts. However, as leading babesial researchers Schnittger et al. (2012) comment:

Although a single tick species is typically the principal vector of a certain *Babesia* or *Theileria* species, this transmission capacity is usually extended to the whole genus. Moreover, often two or even more tick genera can transmit any one piroplasmid species. It has also been reported that a given tick species transmits two or more different piroplasmid species (e.g. *Hyalomma a. anatolicum* can transmit *Babesia* sp. Xinjinang, *T. annulata*, and *T. lestoquardi*). One vertebrate host may be infected by several different piroplasmid species, and likewise "vertebrate host specificity" is not a reliable taxonomic criterion. Some *Babesia* spp. have a broad host range.

And, as they go on to say:

During the last decade, it has become clear that *B. microti* infects a large variety of different hosts worldwide (many different small rodent species; carnivores, such as raccoon, skunk, canine, fox, river otter; macaque; and humans) and does not constitute a single species as previously assumed, but a variety of different species currently referred to as the *B. microti*-species complex.

Gaffer et al. (2003) as well note that "*B. bovis* merozoites invade and develop in multiple species in contrast to the host specificity observed in nature." And as Schnittger et al. (2012) conclude, with their usual gift for understatement, "These findings suggest that our picture of the species that harbor babesia parasites is far from complete." In fact, it appears that babesial protozoa can infect a much broader range of animals than is currently supposed, essentially anything with red blood cells.

Analysis of piroplasmid genomes has found that there has been frequent switching of their vertebrate hosts over millennia. That is, they can alter their genome under environmental pressure to allow them to infect any life form that possesses red blood cells. They jump species. These organisms have in fact been around for so long that in one form or another they have infected everything they could infect. Long ago they infected dinosaurs, and as mammals emerged, they began to infect them, too. This, of course, includes the primates, of which humans are a member.

Those that specialize in humans tend to be a bit smaller in size than those that infect other mammals (but not always). There are currently twelve species of babesia that are known to infect people. Still, the research on babesial organisms is, as with most of the Lyme group, only a few decades old, so the knowledge base is actually very thin. As researchers look more deeply at the genus, more species that infect people are being discovered. And, to make matters more complex, while there are twelve species that are currently known to infect people, there are scores of different genotypes of those species. In other words, to hide from the human immune system, during infection each species produces offspring that possess slightly different exterior protein structures, i.e., genotypes. So, what you get during infection is, as is the case with most of the Lyme group, an infectious swarm of similar but not identical organisms. This is why successful treatment can sometimes be difficult and why, even after antibiotic treatment, the organisms may remain and disease symptoms recur.

HUMAN INFECTION

Transmission of babesial parasites is primarily by tick bite (with various different ticks carrying different or multiple species of the organisms). Still, infection through transfusions of infected blood are becoming an increasing problem (blood donors are rarely tested for the parasites) and placental transfer from an infected mother to an unborn child has also been documented.

The main endemic areas for infection are the northeast (New Jersey upward), northern California up through Washington State, the geographical area around Wisconsin, and the southeast, with Georgia as the epicenter. For the most part, the usual Lyme-endemic areas.

The majority of clinicians believe that there are only four *Babesia* species that infect people: *Babesia microti, B. duncani, B. divergens,* and *B. venatorum.* But as is common with the Lyme group (and much medical knowledge), that information bears little relation to reality. There are at least twelve currently known: *Babesia microti, Babesia duncani* (formerly called *Babesia* WA1), *Babesia* CA1, CA3, and CA4, *Babesia* MO1 (also called *Babesia divergens*-like), *Babesia divergens, Babesia venatorum* (formerly *Babesia* EU1), *Babesia bigemina, Babesia vinsonii* subspecies *arupensis,* and *Babesia* KO1 and TW1. (There are also others that have been found, noted by the terms WA2, CA5, CA6. They might be unique species or simply a subtype of, for example, *Babesia duncani;* the research is still too new to say for sure.)

Each of the species identified by letters such as CA1 and so on are currently named for where they were first identified. In other words, California (CA1, etc.), Missouri (MO1), Europe (EU1), Korea (KO1), and Taiwan (TW1). These species have been found to infect people throughout the world but have not yet been given their own species name. Again, and importantly, each of these species generates multiple genotypes during human infection.

And, irritatingly for determinists, *Babesia microti* is not just one species. It turns out that it is a group of similar but not identical species. The various *B. microti* species, like many of the human-infecting *Babesia* complex, at present only possess casual identifiers. The four primary *B. microti* lineages or subtypes (U.S. type, Munich type, Kobe type, and Hobetsu type), which tend to infect people in different regions of the planet, have discrete genome differences. They are, in fact, each unique. Each creates slightly different symptoms and responds slightly differently to pharmaceuticals. They, too, generate multiple genotypes. And it turns out that this is not uncommon. *Babesia canis,* which normally infects canines, is not in fact a single species either but rather three distinct ones.

Unfortunately, to continue making things difficult, some people (taxonomists with OCD, a well-known subgroup of the genus) are beginning to call babesial organisms piroplasms and the infections they cause piroplasmosis. *Piro* means "pear-shaped" and *plasm* essentially means "substance of a living cell." In essence, a pear-shaped cell. (Scientists like to use big words; when translated most of them are just this mentally simplistic.) While some researchers like to call *Babesia* "pear-shaped" they are in fact only sometimes pear-shaped, and at other times they are oval, and sometimes round. So, again and with monotonous regularity, not a very useful descriptive.

There are three types of piroplasms (it seems): organisms in the genera *Babesia*, *Theileria*, and *Cytauxzoon*. But there is a lot of infighting going on among researchers. Some taxonomists, inevitably, are now insisting that *Babesia microti* is not a *Babesia* but belongs among the *Theileria*, hence you may see *Babesia microti* also referred to as *Theileria microti*. (This is why no one likes taxonomists.) Other researchers disagree, and with reams of genetic data trailing behind them, they snicker, point to their data, and make geek jokes.

> *Two theoretical physicists are lost at the top of a*
> *mountain.*

Still other taxonomists are (of course) insisting that some of the *Theileria* are really *Babesia*.

> *Physicist one pulls out a map and peruses it for a while,*
> *then says, "Hey, I know where we are!"*

The arguments are heated and unrelenting. (Fisticuffs at eleven.) *Cytauxzoon*, however, has so far been left alone (there is only one, so not much to fight over).

> *Physicist two says, "Okay then, where are we?"*
> *Physicist one points and says, "You see that*
> *mountain over there?"*
> *"Yes."*
> *"Well, that's where we are!"*

Uh, oh, I feel another rant coming on.

|||||||||||||||||||||||||||||||||||||||||||||||||||||

Tiny Rant
Monological Antipathies

The problem is that most scientists don't know much about the real, living world. They don't spend much time in it and, to make things worse, their paradigm is inaccurate; it's much too simplistic. These organisms do not fit into, as Buckminster Fuller once put it, monological descriptions of Universe. In other words, there is no one-picture answer to either the Earth or organisms this complex. The Lyme group of microorganisms are called stealth pathogens for a reason. They are highly sensitive nonlinear life forms with tremendous genetic flexibility, a flexibility that has been honed over billions of years. They perform unique and highly sophisticated functions within the ecological network of the planet. As Lynn Margulis once put it, "They have lots better things to do than sit around figuring out how to make us sick." (Even if a few of them do so from time to time.) Hence, when reductive researchers approach organisms with this kind of complexity, they are often at a loss. There is in fact no one word that can be used to describe an organism that is sometimes pear-shaped, sometimes oval, sometimes round; sometimes has one genetic structure, sometimes another; sometimes infects this mammal, sometimes that one; and sometimes responds to this antibiotic, while sometimes not.

The Lyme group, along with other resistant bacteria, are forcing a truer picture of the world into our awareness, whether we wish it or not. Younger researchers (those not so firmly embedded within a reductive framework) are beginning to let go of their presuppositions and look at what is right in front of them. They are finding that the simplistic descriptives that fill medical texts are very much inaccurate compared to what they are seeing. For example . . .

> On one hand, piroplasms can be distinguished into two groups by their diameter: theileria and small babesia, and large babesia parasites. However, species identification can be hampered due to developmental changes in the form and size of parasitic stages in the erythrocyte [red blood cell], and due to the observation that some piroplasmid species may differ in form and size when infecting different vertebrate hosts. (Schnittger et al. 2012)

In other words, the organisms can alter their physical form depending on the habitat within which they find themselves; they are genetically responsive to any alterations in their environment. To put it another way, any environmental pressure can stimulate alterations in their genome. And among environmental pressures are such things as vaccinations against *Babesia* (in cattle), antibiotics (and their prevalence in water supplies and soil), and ecological disruption (such as cutting of forests and people inhabiting formerly undeveloped habitat). The various babesial species also engage in highly prolific genetic exchanges between themselves (and other bacteria), which enhances the emergence of unique genotypes. Thus . . .

In one study, 31 cattle were examined over a six-month period. Of the 31 animals, 20 showed babesial genotype alterations. Within those 20 cattle, 28 different genotypes were found. New genotype innovation was continual. The researchers note:

> Genetic exchange is frequent in *Babesia* as well as in *Theileria* parasites, and it may have the following significance with respect to disease control. First, drug resistance, if it occurs, will most likely spread rapidly in the entire population. Second, inter-genetic recombination between and intra-genetic recombination within

polymorphic surface antigen-coding genes should highly promote the diversity of the parasite surface and its surface antigens.
This may result in continuous creation of immune escape variants
in a given parasite population, advocate vaccine breakthroughs,
and complicate vaccine development. (Schnittger et al. 2012)

In fact, both resistant forms and vaccine breakthroughs
have already occurred and are becoming problematic. And it is
well recognized among most medical researchers that immune
escape variants (that is, the immune system can't "see" them)
are common in a substantial number of people who are infected
with the organisms. Babesial organisms, it turns out, are so
adaptable that the same species may take on forms that make
them unrecognizable from one host to the next. This, inevitably, screws up successful diagnosis . . . and simplistic mental
approaches to the organisms.

Despite desires to the contrary, a simple, and useful, descriptive of the organisms is very hard to create. *Babesia* do have a core
identity but the organisms' physical expression is highly variable.
Their gene structure (genotype) is in constant flux, giving rise to
multiple phenotypes (physical and behavioral forms). This means
that they can truly be unrecognizable from one host to the next,
even if you do manage to see them under a microscope.

There seem to be only three constants: they are parasitic
microorganisms, they are primarily transmitted by ticks, they
infect red blood cells, inside of which they (primarily) reproduce.

SYMPTOMS OF INFECTION

As with many microorganism infections, most people are and remain
asymptomatic; that is, they have the parasites in their blood but show
no symptoms. This is most commonly because their immune function

is healthy. The human and the babesial organisms become relatively stress-free joint tenants in the body. (It is this group of people who often donate infected blood. People receiving the blood, if their immune function is low, are at risk of a symptomatic infection.) However, if immune function in the asymptomatic falls for any reason the organism can, and often does, begin to cause problems.

For others, once infected, they merely experience a bout of the "flu." (The "flu" we think we have is often not the flu but can be nearly any infection at all; it is just what many infections feel like at onset.) After a week or two the "flu" is gone and the person feels fine once more. This group of people sometimes then become asymptomatic carriers themselves. (Other times, the organism actually is eradicated from the body.) And again, if immune function falls later on in their lives, the disease can bloom once more. Generally, symptoms arise one to four weeks after a tick bite, though up to nine weeks has been reported. Here is the symptom breakdown among those who show symptoms.

Symptom	Outpatients	Inpatients
Fever	68 %	89 %
Fatigue	78 %	79 %
Chills	39 %	68 %
Sweats	41 %	56 %
Headache	75 %	32 %
Myalgia	37 %	32 %
Anorexia	24 %	24 %
Cough	17 %	23 %
Arthralgia	31 %	17 %
Nausea	22 %	9 %

The symptoms for those who successfully process the disease on their own mostly consist of the general aches and pains, low-grade fever, fatigue, and chills that accompany "the flu." For those who need hospitalization, the symptom picture is generally more severe, especially the fever, fatigue, chills, and sweats. Malaise, abdominal pain, and diarrhea, though not included in the chart, may also occur among both groups.

As with malaria, a relapsing form of the infection is common. The disease appears to be a simple flu, and the person recovers, then relapses months later, recovers, relapses, and so on ad nauseum. This is moderately common among those with Lyme-group infections, especially with *Babesia*.

To be more specific: all babesial infections commonly present with malaise and fatigue followed by intermittent fever accompanied by (one or more of the following) chills, sweats, general pallor, mild hepatosplenomegaly (liver and/or spleen enlargement and/or pain), headache, lightheadedness, arthralgia, myalgia, anorexia, cough, vomiting, nausea, GI tract problems, depression, and/or emotional lability. In some the illness may last weeks to months; prolonged recovery can last more than a year.

In those in whom the disease becomes more severe, fever may increase to 105°F, shaking chills are common, and hepatosplenomegaly (liver and spleen inflammation and damage) increases. Other symptoms include noncardiogenic pulmonary edema, hypotension, hemolysis (ruptured blood cells), jaundice, hemoglobinuria (hemoglobin in the urine), dark urine, proteinuria (excess protein in the urine), mild neutropenia (low numbers of neutrophils in the blood), leukopenia (low numbers of leukocytes in the blood), atypical lymphocytosis (an increase in lymphocytes in the blood), thrombocytopenia (abnormally low levels of platelets in the blood), retinal infarcts (a blockage of the central retinal artery leading to sudden vision loss), anemia, ecchymoses (a kind of bruising that spontaneously occurs on the skin from ruptured blood vessels), petechia (small red or purple spots on the body caused by hemorrhage in small blood capillaries), and hyperesthesia (abnormal sensitivity to sensory inputs). Hepatic transaminases may become elevated. The lymph nodes rarely become enlarged.

Neurological problems can occur in some people, in part from decreased red blood cell presence in the brain and subsequent damage to various areas of the organ caused by intravascular coagulation and endothelial cell damage. The brain capillaries can become packed with parasitized erythrocytes, interfering with proper blood flow to differing regions of the brain, with resultant problems in mental functioning. Stroke can occur if coagulation is severe.

During very severe infections, further complications may arise: severe acute respiratory distress syndrome, disseminated intravascular coagulation, acute kidney injury, organ failure (renal, heart, liver), splenic rupture, septic shock, coma, and death.

Those most at risk for severe disease are those without a spleen, the elderly (over 50), and the immunocompromised. As an example of the importance of the spleen during a *Babesia* infection: parasitemia (organism numbers) in those *with* a spleen runs around 5 percent, but in those *without* spleens it's 85 percent. As *Babesia* specialist Peter Krause, MD, observes, the spleen "helps to clear organisms in the blood that shouldn't be there. It produces antibodies that attack the protozoans, which are then gobbled up by macrophages, and it acts like a sieve, screening out *Babesia*-infected red blood cells, which are too big to get through and back into circulation" (Brody 2012). For some people, during severe infection, the spleen is so strongly affected that it may rupture.

Because the spleen performs an essential function during the body's response to babesial infection and because of the heavy impact on its functioning, it must be supported during treatment. (Removal of the spleen is often performed after splenic rupture. Because that patient population tends to live in *Babesia*-endemic areas, future infections are very dangerous. The spleen should not be removed unless it absolutely must be. And yes, splenic rupture can be, and has been, successfully treated without spleen removal.)

General mortality among those who are hospitalized due to babesial infection is about 5 percent, among those who are immunocompromised about 10 percent, and among those who have no spleen 21 percent.

Infection rates are increasing in endemic areas (as studies over the decades from 1990 to 2010 have shown) and are spreading outward from those centers. Over a 10-year period researchers found that infections on Block Island (off the coast of Rhode Island) were increasing substantially, from minimal levels when the study began to nearly the same levels as Lyme infection by the study's end. Sixty percent of the children tested, at one time or another, were found to be symptomatic, as were 81 percent of the adults. The rest of those tested were infected but asymptomatic. The children experienced the same range of symptoms as adults; they just recovered faster and better due to their better immune health.

DIAGNOSIS

As with Lyme disease, many physicians refuse to entertain the thought that a *Babesia* infection is present if someone has not traveled to what is considered an endemic area within the past four to nine weeks. The organism, however, is rapidly spreading into what are considered non-endemic areas. And because *Babesia* are regularly transmitted through blood transfusions the disease commonly appears in atypical and non-endemic areas.

The poor medical understanding of *Babesia*, the numerous species and multiple genotypes that can be found during infection, and the variety of different shapes the organisms take on make clear diagnosis difficult. To make matters worse, diagnostic tests are often unreliable, poorly administered or read, and not sensitive to the wide range of species and genotypes now known to exist.

Simplistically, during a tick bite, some tick saliva and babesial parasites are injected into the bloodstream of the new host. The organisms use the compounds in the tick saliva to facilitate their entry and bypass immune responses. Once in the bloodstream they immediately infect red blood cells, then begin to divide inside those cells. They usually form two or four new babesial organisms inside those cells, depending on the babesial species. When mature, these burst out of the red blood cells, killing them, and infect new cells (which is why anemia, shortness of breath, and fatigue are so common in the condition). A few of the microorganisms do not divide but remain inside red blood cells in order to be picked up by ticks during feeding and thus spread to new hosts.

Blood Smear Analysis

The primary approach to diagnosing a babesial infection has been to microscopically examine the red blood cells (blood smear analysis) and literally look at the structure of the reproducing babesial cells. (During blood smear analysis, daughter cells, free in the blood, are also examined.) Many *Babesia* (the smaller ones) form what is called a Maltese cross, similar to a plus sign. Once seen inside the blood cells, the diagnosis is certain. Larger forms, when replicating inside cells, form two daughter cells that resemble two pears hanging together (hence the name *piroplasmosis*). Still, as Schnittger et al. (2012) comment, relying on that is problematic; the organisms don't always form these shapes and some *Babesia* form other patterns during reproduction. Specifically, they note that "corresponding to their size classification, all small *Babesia* as well as all *Theileria* parasites divide into four merozoite daughter cells (a maltese cross formation), while large *Babesia* bud into two merozoite daughter cells. However . . . exceptions do occur."

Diagnostic problems also arise using this procedure because the organisms are often present in the blood in extremely low levels; as few as 1 percent of the red blood cells may be infected. (And even so, symptoms can be severe.) Case studies are common in which people are admitted to a hospital with signs of infection but no parasites are noted in blood smears. These studies regularly contain comments such as "There were no blood parasites or schistocytes noted on blood smears performed at that time. Over the next two months, the patient remained on the increased dose of steroids, but had worsening of his anemia and rising values of serum lactate dehydrogenase, suggesting a hemolytic process" (Lubin et al. 2011). It was another month, after symptoms refused to resolve, before protozoa were found in blood smears of that particular patient. (In this instance, the babesial parasites were transmitted via stem cell transplantation.)

Added complications of blood smear diagnosis include: 1) *Babesia* and malarial parasites may at times be indistinguishable from each other; and 2) blood smear readings generally cannot differentiate between different species or genotypes.

Polymerase Chain Reaction (PCR)

Rapid real-time PCR is perhaps the best of all the tests for babesial organisms, especially when combined with blood smear analysis. A "tick panel" is often the best approach as it can test for *Babesia, Ehrlichia, Anaplasma,* and *Borrelia* at the same time. PCR tests are increasing in their sensitivity to the various babesial species though there is not yet one that can test for all those that may infect people.

Indirect Fluorescence Assay (IFA)

IFA is considered to be the third best test to use; however, it possesses a number of problems that make it suspect. The primary problem is that it tests for antibodies in the blood and antibodies do not always appear during the early stages of infection. False negative and false positive results are common. Positive diagnosis from various laboratories has been found to range from 69 to 100 percent in accuracy, from 88 to 96 percent in sensitivity, and from 90 to 100 percent in specificity (for the species tested). Of the IFA tests used, IgM is the most reliable as a diagnostic.

Indirect Enzyme-Linked Immunosorbent Assay (ELISA)

Relatively useless, nevertheless still sometimes used.

The best diagnostic approach is considered to be symptom picture combined with blood smear analysis and PCR. Researchers Chan et al. (2013) comment:

Accurate diagnosis of various tick-borne diseases is problematic, due to similar clinical manifestations. Currently available serological tests are neither cost-effective, nor sensitive or specific for diagnosis of infections by these three pathogens [*Borrelia, Anaplasma, Babesia*] transmitted by ticks, especially at early stage of infection. . . . *A. phagocytophilum* and *B. microti* infect white and red blood cells, respectively, but are not easily detectable in blood. This offers additional risk since they can also be transmitted through blood transfusions and potentially vertically from mother to infant. The presence of *Babesia* species is usually visualized by microscopic examination after Giemsa staining; however, it is frequently overlooked, because of the infection of less than 1% of erythrocytes or due to hemolysis during the sample transport. . . . PCR has been found to be more sensitive for its detection.

PHARMACEUTICAL TREATMENT

Pharmaceutical treatment does work for many people. However, both genotypic variation and increasing resistance are causing more failures among the pharmaceutically inclined. One of the main causes of resistance is the use of antibabesial drugs in farm animals. Babesial infections are a common, and serious, problem in cattle throughout the world. In consequence many ranchers include antibabesial drugs in animal feed to try to prevent infection. As researchers note, "The indiscriminate use of anti-*Babesia* prophylactic agents, including the administration of the drug at sub-lethal blood levels to animals, can produce the development of drug resistant parasites" (Mosqueda et al. 2012). And in fact, it has. Thus, physicians are seeing more treatment failures in general practice.

The standard treatment for people is atovaquone, 750 mg orally twice daily, *plus* azithromycin. Dosage for the latter is 500 to 1,000 mg on the first day, and 250 to 1,000 mg on subsequent days. Both drugs usually are given for 7 to 10 days. Resistance to this combination has been reported in the literature.

Some people utilize an older treatment approach, especially if the first approach fails. This is the use of clindamycin (600 mg orally three times daily, or by IV four times daily) *plus* quinine (650 mg orally three times daily). The combination is, again, usually given for 7 to 10 days. This combination is generally used for the more severely ill, but is, however, frequently associated with unpleasant side effects: tinnitus, vertigo, and GI tract upset. The combination often fails when used in those without a spleen, those with HIV, or those on corticosteroid therapy. Resistance to this combination has also been reported in the literature.

In those who are immunocompromised, no one treatment approach has been found to be effective and pharmaceutical treatment for a minimum of six weeks with an additional two weeks of treatment after the last positive blood smear has been found to be essential.

The literature contains reports of people "successfully" treated with pharmaceuticals whose blood showed no organisms who nevertheless were still infected and experienced relapsing episodes of infection. As Krause et al. (1998) comment, "Although treatment with clindamycin and quinine reduces the duration of parasitemia, infection may still persist and recrudesce and side effects are common."

Numerous studies are indicating that a longer treatment duration than 7 to 10 days is necessary, in general six to eight weeks. As an example: Atovaquone administered for 7 days to dogs infected with *B. gibsoni* initially cleared the parasites. However they reappeared in blood smears 33 days later. The recurring parasites were more strongly resistant to the drug during the second antibacterial treatment. This same outcome has been reported in dogs when using an atovaquone/ azithromycin combination. As well, a rather large percentage of people treated for 7 to 10 days with either of these drug combinations have been found to experience a reemergence of the disease. As researchers comment:

In a prospective study, DNA evidence of parasitemia persisted after 7 days of treatment in approximately 40% of subjects who received azithromycin plus atovaquone and in approximately 50% of subjects who were treated with clindamycin plus quinine. (Florescu et al. 2008)

In the case of the man infected through stem cell transplantation, once he was correctly diagnosed, he was treated with azithromycin and atovaquone. His symptoms improved but did not resolve; blood smear showed the continued presence of parasites, though reduced in number. After two months on the protocol symptoms worsened, with increasing hemolysis and persistent parasitemia. He was switched to clindamycin and quinine for the usual 7- to 10-day treatment. Infection cleared and he was discharged from the hospital. He was readmitted one month later, again with worsening symptoms. This time he was given *both* pharmaceutical protocols. After 7 days, with significant symptom resolution, he was discharged but left on the combined protocol for another six weeks. Clindamycin/quinine was discontinued due to side effects; he remained on azithromycin/atovaquone for an additional six weeks. It was only then that PCR failed to detect babesial infection. The necessity for such lengthy treatment times, again, is common in approximately half of the infected. Failure to treat for longer than 7 to 10 days risks disease recurrence, often with worsening symptoms, including death. For example, Florescu et al. (2008) report the death of a woman, aged 75, who was hospitalized with symptoms of fever, fatigue, and night sweats and was treated with the usual 7- to 10-day regimen.

Upon initial examination her spleen was enlarged, and lower leg edema and anemia were present. Ceftazidime, filgrastim, and epoietin alfa were administered prophylactically before diagnosis. Blood smears for malaria and babesiosis were negative. Due to persistent anemia and fever, after 25 days of hospitalization additional blood smears were taken. Babesial protozoa were found. Initial treatment was with azithromycin and atovaquone and then altered to clindamycin, quinine, and doxycycline. After 7 days symptoms resolved and blood smear was negative, and after 3 more days of treatment she was discharged. Ten days later she was readmitted with similar but more severe symptoms. Blood smears showed babesial infection. Treatment was resumed but the organisms did not respond to any drug course utilized. Severe lung edema, sepsis, and multiorgan failure followed over the next six weeks until death occurred.

The opinion of researchers who reviewed that case is that a longer duration of therapy would have prevented a recrudescence of the disease. However, due to CDC guidelines only a 7- to 10-day course of therapy was pursued. As the researchers note, "In this case relapse was most likely associated with delayed clearance of parasitemia, which has been observed in a substantial portion of treated patients" (Florescu et al. 2008).

Given that some 40 to 50 percent of those treated with the standard pharmaceutical regimens show relapses, a more responsible treatment regimen would entail at minimum 30 days of drug therapy.

OTHER USEFUL DRUGS

Heparin is emerging as a possible adjunct to the common pharmaceutical treatments for *Babesia* infection. For severe babesiosis it should be considered, especially during infection with cerebral impacts. It has a number of relevant actions for treating the disease. It inhibits blood coagulation, suppresses replication of the parasites, and significantly decreases the penetration of red blood cells by the organisms. Heparin has been successfully used in the treatment of cerebral malaria infections and found to be effective in vitro and in vivo for *Babesia*. Also of note:

- Epoxomicin and its analog carfilzomib have been found effective in reducing babesial parasitemia.
- Other apicoplast-targeting antibacterials, similar to clindamycin, have also been found effective for babesial organisms: ciprofloxacin, thiostrepton, and rifampin.

- Antifungals such as nystatin, clotrimazole, and ketoconazole have been found effective against various *Babesia* species.
- Mefloquine is also effective.
- So is fusidic acid, an oldie but goodie.

In those in whom infection is severe, a complete transfusion of the blood has been used, sometimes successfully.

3

Babesia

A Deeper Look

The modulation of host immune and inflammatory responses by various bioactive molecules present in the tick saliva facilitates pathogen acquisition and transmission.

O. Hajdusek, R. Sima, N. Ayollon, et al.,
"Interaction of the Tick Immune
System with Transmitted Pathogens"

Parasites invade host red blood cells where they multiply asexually, rupture the host cell and invade new ones. Invasion is one of the critical steps of the life cycle that is vulnerable to the immunological response of the host.

F. R. Gaffar, F. F. Franssen, and E. de Vries,
"*Babesia bovis* Merozoites Invade Human,
Ovine, Equine, Porcine and Caprine
Erythrocytes by Sialic Acid-Dependent
Mechanism Followed by Developmental
Arrest after a Single Round of Cell Fission"

The spleen is a critical effector organ functioning, in haemoparasitic diseases like babesiosis, to destroy the pathogen and clear the host of infected erythrocytes. It has an important role in both innate responses and adaptive immune responses.

W. L. Goff, R. G. Bastos, W. C. Brown, et al.,
"The Bovine Spleen"

The pursuit of the LPS-inducible soluble factors (later called cytokines) appeared to be the best way to understand disease pathogenesis in malaria and babesiosis.

I. A. Clark, L. M. Alleva, A. C. Mills, et al.,
"Pathogenesis of Malaria and
Clinically Similar Conditions"

Babesia are tremendously sophisticated when it comes to infecting their hosts. To understand what they do in the body, and how to interrupt it, it's first helpful to look at the role the ticks play in transmission. Ticks are not simply carriers; they fulfill a much more active role, one refined over long evolutionary time. They, in fact, facilitate babesial invasion of the body.

TICK FACTORS DURING INFECTION

Many of the Lyme group of stealth pathogens can be transmitted by a number of vectors, from mosquitoes to fleas to ticks, and, in some instances, a great many others. Babesial organisms are, at least so far as is currently known, much more limited. They are restricted to tick transmission in the wild. (Though their close relatives, the malarial parasites, are spread by mosquitoes, very little research has occurred on mosquito or other forms of babesial transmission.) Ticks are generally divided into two families, hard ticks and soft ticks, each with somewhat different life cycles, host preferences, and (as the family names imply) exoskeletons. While it is generally true that *Babesia* are primarily transmitted by hard ticks, it turns out that soft tick transmission has been demonstrated in laboratory experiments. (Soft ticks primarily spread viruses.) Hard ticks usually attach for much longer than soft ticks, from two days to two weeks; soft ticks may attach and feed for only a few minutes to an hour and, in rare instances, for up to two days. As with the other coinfections, which are spread by vectors from ticks to mosquitoes to biting flies to lice, mutualistic organisms such as babesial parasites alter their infection dynamics depending on which vector or tick species is spreading them.

As Hajdusek et al. (2013) comment:

> The length of feeding, that strikingly differs between the hard and soft ticks (days vs. minutes, respectively), definitely shape the course of pathogen transmission. Pathogens transmitted by the hard ticks (*Ixodidae*) usually undergo several days of development until they infect the host. On the contrary, pathogens transmitted by the soft ticks (*Argasidae*) are ready for transmission immediately after the feeding starts.

Babesia, when they are first ingested by a tick that is feeding on an infected host, immediately travel to the tick midgut. There the parasites undergo sexual development and multiply. Their offspring then spread to different tissues, primarily the ovaries and salivary glands. This readies the microorganisms for transmission to newer generations of ticks (transovarial transmission) and, when the tick takes a blood meal, to a new vertebrate host. Hard ticks go through three different stages of development and the babesial organisms survive each transformation (something called transstadial transmission). Because the babesial protozoa are capable of transovarial transmission, they are present in the eggs the ticks lay and in the offspring as they hatch.

Due to their long mutualism, the ticks themselves (apparently) never become ill with the disease. They have a number of compounds in their bodies that limit the impact of the parasites upon them, such as longicin, longipain, and cystatin-2. All inhibit the proliferation of the protozoa and reduce their impacts on tick physiology.

ACTIVE COMPOUNDS IN TICK SALIVA

Babesia, because they have coevolved with ticks over such long timelines, have learned to use many of the compounds in tick saliva to foster their infection of a vertebrate host. More than 3,500 different compounds have been identified in the world's tick species so far, all of them with unique functions. As Francischetti et al. (2010) comment:

> The adaptation to blood feeding involved evolution of a complex cocktail of salivary compounds that help the [tick] parasite to overcome their host's defenses against blood loss and development of inflammatory reactions at the feeding site that may disrupt blood flow or trigger host-defensive behavior by the sensation of pain or itching. Accordingly, saliva of blood-sucking arthropods contain anti-clotting, anti-platelet, vasodilatory, anti-inflammatory and immunomodulatory components, usually in redundant amounts.

"Usually in redundant amounts." As with plants, the levels of produced compounds are more than the tick itself needs. In this instance, the redundant amounts facilitate the transmission of bacterial and protozoal parasites into new vertebrate hosts. (In return for this, the ticks receive benefits, too. Among them: the protozoa create compounds, similar to antifreeze, that help protect the ticks from freezing during cold weather.)

Ticks have to overcome a number of very difficult responses to their bite, their lengthy attachment to a host, and their many days of feeding. The natural sensitivity of the skin to bites, the processes of blood coagulation and wound healing, and the immune responses that occur during injuries have to be deactivated.

As soon as a capillary is cut, the tick immediately encounters the suite of physiological responses that occur during any vascular injury: platelet aggregation, vasoconstriction, and coagulation. When the endothelial cells that line a blood vessel are damaged, cells and cell fragments are freed to flow into the blood. This exposes collagen, von Willebrand factor, and platelet tissue factor (thromboplastin) from the subendothelium to the bloodstream. Platelets, present in the blood, come into contact with them and immediately begin a coagulation cascade. The platelets cluster at the damage site and release chemical communication factors signaling that damage has occurred (and what kind) so that the body can begin to repair itself. Compounds such as adenosine diphosphate or ADP (which stimulates coagulation), activated leukocytes (which release platelet-activating factor), and thromboxane A2 (from the activated platelets) all flow into the system. These trigger the activation of phospholipase C, which stimulates the expression of chemicals that activate a compound called fibrinogen. Fibrinogen acts to form a bridge between the activated platelets, creating what is called a platelet plug. This stops the bleeding, closes the wound, and begins repair of the damaged tissues. The process is very fast; within four seconds of injury, platelet plugs have already begun to form. This helps stop the bleeding and acts as an initial matrix for the wound healing that begins some four days after injury.

Ticks use their salival compounds to stop the coagulation cascade. This keeps the blood liquid and flowing, enabling them to get the blood meal they need to survive. Tick saliva, in fact, contains anticlotting compounds that shut down every step of the coagulation cascade. The compounds deactivate ADP, inhibit platelet aggregation, prevent their binding to fibrinogen, and even prevent the formation of fibrinogen itself. Over 200 anticlotting agents have been found in various tick species' saliva during the past few decades.

At the same time coagulation is inhibited, other tick compounds (such as prostaglandin E2—PGE2—and PGF2α) increase vasodilation and vascular permeability. This gets more blood into the area of the tick bite, so more food is available. Then there is wound healing . . .

Wound healing is composed of a number of processes, among the most important of which are inflammation, proliferation, and remodeling. Inflammation occurs when specific chemical messenger molecules (cytokines) are released into the bloodstream; these flow to the injury site (proliferation) and begin the process of wound repair. The swelling and redness (a.k.a. inflammation) that nearly always occurs at a wound site are an integral part of this process. The cytokines trigger chemical signals controlling the migration, proliferation, and differentiation of cells at the wound site. In other words, a lot of wound repair chemicals all congregate around the wound and begin to fix the damage (remodeling). Because blood capillaries have been damaged with this type of wound, angiogenesis, the stimulation of new blood vessels, also occurs. Tick compounds deactivate the cytokine cascade that produces inflammation and also inhibit angiogenesis. The ticks also actively shut down skin sensitivity.

During a skin injury, nerve impulses are sent to the brain, letting the organism know an injury has occurred. In extreme instances we experience this as pain; with less intense damage we feel an itch. This calls our attention to the site of the wound and we either scratch or focus on the wound, working to decrease the pain. Mast cells, which are recruited to this kind of injury site by the immune system, release histamine, which produces pruritus (itching), which stimulates scratching. Tick salivary compounds called lipocalins sequester (bind) histamine, inhibiting itching and stopping the scratching response. Pain responses are shut down through multiple channels. Adenosine triphosphate (ATP), an early mediator of pain impulses, is inhibited by a number of enzymes in the tick saliva. Serotonin, commonly released by platelets, can also act as a pain-signaling chemical. This is inhibited by the lipocalins that also bind histamine. TNF-α, an immune response to the injury of cells, activates the release of interleukin-1 (IL-1) and IL-6. These compounds cause increased sensitivity to pain and are a part of the cascade of cytokine-mediated pain stimulation. Compounds in tick saliva actively depress TNF-α production. Tick saliva also shuts down many other immune responses.

Leukocytes (e.g., mast cells, eosinophils, dendritic cells, macrophages), present in the epidermis and dermis, are activated once a wound occurs. They are part of the automatic or innate immune response to skin injury of any sort. The cells release pre-formed chemicals immediately when an injury occurs and also produce chemotactic compounds that recruit inflammatory cells to the site. Tick salival compounds inhibit various types of eosinophils, dendritic cells, and macrophages as well as many basophils, T cells, and B cells.

To be more specific, tick saliva inhibits immunoglobulin G (IgG), IL-1, IL-2, IL-8, IL-10, IL-12, TNF-α, IFN-γ, MCP-1 (monocyte chemoattractant protein 1, a.k.a. CC chemokine ligand 2 or CCL2), MIP-1α (CCL3), RANTES (CCL5), and various eotaxins (CCL11, 24, and 26). The maturation of dendritic cells is strongly inhibited (by PGE2 and PGF2α), and CD40 white blood cell and CD4+ T cell production is significantly decreased (CD8+ is sometimes significantly increased). Tick saliva tends, in general, to polarize the immune response to Th2 rather than Th1. (This is important in that it is a predominantly Th1 response that clears babesial infection.)

A Very Brief Look at Th1 and Th2
Immune Responses

One of the primary strategies of the Lyme group of microbes is their ability to shift human immune responses from Th1 to Th2. T helper cells (abbreviated Th) are a kind of T cell (so-called because they mature in the thymus and tonsils—you didn't get your tonsils out did you?). T cells are white blood cells that become active during certain kinds of infections; there are a number of different kinds, among them T helper cells. Th cells, well, they help other white blood cells do their job, hence "helper." (They are also known as CD4+ T cells—because they have a CD4 glycoprotein on their cellular surfaces—

just to make things more complicated.) Once stimulated, they rapidly reproduce and begin generating a range of cytokines to help deal with infections. There are, of course, a number of different subtypes: Th1, Th2, Th3, Th9, Th17, and so on. Each subgroup has evolved to deal with different kinds of infections. Th1 cells are specific for intra-cellular infections; that is, infections from microbes that like to hide inside other cells. Specifically, this includes most of the Lyme group of coinfectious agents. It is not surprising then that these pathogens learned long ago to shift the body's immune response away from Th1 and into Th2. (Th2 immune responses are designed, primarily, to deal with intestinal parasites such as nematodes; they also act to limit overactive Th1 responses.) This shift facilitates infection by the Lyme group of intracellular pathogens, strongly inhibiting an effective immune response. A polarized Th2 immune profile is present in a number of autoimmune diseases such as lupus and systemic sclero-sis. This is why so many long-term infections from the Lyme group appear to be an autoimmune disorder. (To be clear here, it is not an "auto" immune disorder. In this instance it is microbially initiated and can be reversed.) Unsurprisingly, each Th group possesses a different cytokine profile. Th1 cells, for instance, generate interferon-gamma, interleukin-12, and TNF-α; Th2 produces IL-4, IL-5, IL-10, and IL-13. This is why inducing IFN-γ and inhibiting IL-10, as examples, can reverse many of the problems with these coinfections.

As researchers comment, studies conducted during the years 2007 to 2013 found that tick

saliva has a much broader complexity than anticipated, having hun-dreds of different proteins, many of which are novel, in the sense that they produce no similarities to other proteins in large databases. . . . Another surprise is that the most abundant tick proteins are members of multi-gene families. For some of these protein families, it is known that they are differentially expressed as feeding progresses, thus, at the last day of feeding the tick is producing a different family member in saliva than that produced on the first day and may thus be evading the host immune response. . . . We cannot anticipate at all the function of the majority of the tick salivary proteins. Indeed for any tick species with a known transcriptome, less than 5% of the proteins have been expressed and their function verified. (Francischetti et al. 2010)

In other words, the ticks carefully modulate their release of salival proteins over the feeding period, playing the immune system like a virtuoso would a concert violin. They adjust their salival compounds to keep the immune system and the body's wound healing inactive for as long as they wish to feed, despite the body's response over time. And they have access to a lot of compounds. In the soft ticks, over 200 salival proteins have been found so far, and well over 500 in hard ticks. A further complexity is that there is also a different grouping of proteins present in tick saliva at each stage of tick development.

There is, as one group of researchers put it, a lengthy and sophisticated "molecular dialogue" between the tick and vertebrate host, a dialogue of which the babesial parasites take great advantage. They, in essence, use the impacts of the tick salival compounds to facilitate their stealth entry into the body.

BABESIAL LIFE CYCLE AND PENETRATION OF THE HOST

As soon as you begin looking more deeply at the life cycle of babesial organisms, you (unfortunately) once more enter the world of taxonometric minutiae and unnecessarily obscurant terminology. Hence the emergence of sporozoites, gametocytes, merozoites, and even of ookinetes. And, as usual, if you try to find a useful definition of any of those terms you begin a journey that takes you to overly intimate experiences of unnecessary linguistic obfuscation. Thus, this definition of sporo-zoite: "the motile infective stage of certain protozoa that results from sporogony."

Sporogony, I am pretty sure, is either agony caused by spores or a town in Latvia; my sources are unclear.

Turning to etymology in search of clarity, let us seek the roots of the word *sporozoite*. *Sporozoite* emerges, it turns out, from a combination of the ancient Greek terms *sporos* (for seed) and *zoon* (for animal), thus animal seed. (I am thinking they are going for "baby protozoa" in their meaning here but let's soldier on and find out for sure . . . if we can.)

To see if we can find something more useful, let's look at *sporogony*. . . . Hmmm, let's see, that is "the asexual process of spore formation in parasitic sporozoans." Which takes us, inevitably, to *sporozoans*. Hmmm (types frantically). Ahhh, *sporozoan*. "Any of numerous parasitic proto-zoans of the class Sporozoa, most of which produce sexually and asexu-ally by means of spores." (Tears hair.) Aaaargh. ("Never give up, never surrender.") How about Sporozoa . . .

The older taxon Sporozoa was created by Joseph Schrevel in 1971 and grouped the Apicomplexa together with the Microsporidia and Myxosporida. This grouping is no longer regarded as biologically valid and its use is discouraged.

Geesus. (Takes deep breath, begins muttering, "Taxonomists suck," over and over.) Okaaaaay. Let's try *spore*.

In biology, a spore is a unit of asexual reproduction that may be adapted for dispersal and for survival, often for extended periods of time, in unfavorable conditions. By contrast gametes are units of sexual reproduction. [So, now we are units? Have these guys ever actually had sex?] Spores form part of the life cycles of many plants, algae, fungi, and protozoa. [Finally!] In bacteria, spores are not part of a sexual cycle but are resistant structures used for survival under unfavorable conditions. [Hence the encysted, unsexy forms of Lyme bacteria.]

And finally, let's check the etymology of *spore*. Hmmm, "developed in the mid-19th century." Okay, uh huh, let's see . . . "from the ancient Greek," okay . . . "to sow, specifically to sow seeds." Ah. A picture is beginning to emerge. A sporozoite then is a kind of encysted or seedlike or spore form of the babesial parasites, better able to withstand environmental pressures than unencysted forms.

> *This kind of seedlike formation, by the way, to those who work deeply in Earth systems functioning, is what is called a metapattern, that is a pattern that Earth uses over and over again because it is so successful. Viruses, bacteria, protozoa, seeds, nuts (in the shell), eggs . . . all are utilizing that underlying metapattern as part of their reproductive or survival process. The round shape is one of the strongest known; it protects the embryo or encysted organism from deleterious environmental forces.*

Sporozoites are, apparently, one of four (or more according to some, irritating, sources) stages of development that the babesial parasites go through while living in their hosts and vectors.

Hmmm (takes life in hands and types once more into Google search), *Babesia* "replicate via ways of multiple fission (also known as schizogony) [the agony of schizophrenics?]. These ways include gametogony, sporogony, and merogony, although the latter is sometimes referred to as schizogony, despite its general meaning."

> *General meaning? There is no general meaning to that word. (As opposed to, say,* automobile *or* towelette.*)

The obfuscation of taxonomists is deleterious to successful habitation of this planet. Nevertheless . . . let's take a stab at the process of babesial development and see if it makes any sense now.

The babesial forms that are stored in the tick ovaries and salival glands are sporozoites (a.k.a., oversimplistically, encysted forms, spores, seeds). They remain relatively somnolent, that is, in a kind of comatose or inactive state, like a plant seed. This shape makes them better able to survive extended periods of cold storage, sequestered in unique locations, until needed to spread the disease. In essence, they are a form of stored genome, intended for later use.

During a tick bite, as host blood flows into the tick, the tick body uploads a large number of chemicals into its saliva in order for it to maintain attachment to the host. That chemical alteration of saliva *and* the influx of a warm-temperature blood into a cold-blooded arthropod (tick) stimulates the sporozoites to become active. That is, they begin to wake up from their long sleep.

Even though in a dormant form, the sporozoites, much like plant seeds, actively analyze their environment, in this case the red blood cells being ingested by the tick, determining the type of animal (soil or ecosystem) they will be entering. The sporozoite genome then alters itself so that the particular phenotype (bodily form and accompanying behavior) that can live in that host will be generated. The sporozoites in the saliva awaken from their comatose state readying themselves to infect the blood cells of the new host. Then, during the blood meal, along with tick saliva, they flow into the blood capillaries of the new vertebrate host. It takes a sporozoite about 30 seconds to find a host red blood cell. Within 45 seconds 70 percent of the sporozoites will be encapsulated inside host cells. By 10 minutes all are enclosed; infection happens very quickly.

A sporozoite, as soon as it attaches to the outside of a red blood cell (RBC), releases compounds that cause the cell walls to become more porous. This allows easier penetration into the interior of the cell. Once inside the RBC, the sporozoite unencysts, altering its form, becoming what is called a merozoite—the next developmental stage of the protozoa. (Very little is known about this process, so let's jump ahead . . .) After transformation, the merozoite uses the red blood cell's constituents as nutrients in order to reproduce. The merozoite engages in what is called asexual reproduction (also known as taxonomist sex), forming new nuclei inside itself (two or four depending on the kind of babesium it is). The merozoite cell then divides (fission) into two or four new cells (as the case may be), each containing one of those nuclei.

The term merozoite, *ridiculously, comes from the*
ancient Greek meros *for "thigh" and* zoon *for "animal."*
Thigh animal? Animal thigh? (Ah, teenager protozoa.)

During this process, the parent merozoite generates multiple genetic variants in its daughter cells in order to facilitate protozoal survival in the host. Specifically, the exterior cell walls of the new merozoites contain slightly different compounds than that of the parent. This helps protect the new cells from discovery by the immune system.

Sometimes this genetic alteration is referred to as
antigenic variation. Foreign substances in the blood
are also known as antigens, against which the immune
system makes antibodies.

Even a tiny variation of the chemical structure of the cell wall will allow the organism to remain invisible to the previously activated immune response.

Once they are fully formed, the merozoites burst open the red blood cell, enter the bloodstream, and seek out new RBCs. Merozoites are capable of more motility than sporozoites; they actively move through the blood and along the vascular walls (using gliding motility) to find RBCs (and occasionally endothelial cells as well). Once they find a red blood cell, they use powerful chemoattractant compounds to attach to its exterior. Specifically, the merozoites bind themselves to sialic acid glycoproteins in the red blood cell membrane, primarily glycoproteins A and B. Pretreatment of red blood cells with neuraminidase, an enzyme that dissolves (or catalyzes) sialic acids from the cell membranes, inhibits babesial penetration of the red blood cell by 80 to 97 percent. As well, mice without glycoprotein A in their blood cell membranes are resistant to infection by babesial protozoa. In other words, when a red blood cell has no sialic acid glycoproteins in its membrane, the protozoa can't bind to the cell.

The merozoites have highly specialized tiny organs (organelles) located at the apical or forward end of their cellular membrane. Some of them contain and exude a unique babesial protein, apical membrane antigen 1 (AMA1), that is similar to but unique from the protein used by malarial parasites. The babesial AMA1 concentrates on the surface of the apical end of the merozoite and binds to trypsin- and chymotrypsin-sensitive receptors on the red blood cell. This is why both trypsin and chymotrypsin-A, two pancreatic enzymes, act to inhibit babesial binding to blood cells, by up to 40 percent (in vitro). One of the ways the immune system creates immunity to babesial infection is to make an AMA1 antibody.

Ultimately, then, the merozoites utilize *two* binding processes for attaching to red blood cells, one involving sialic acid glycoproteins, the other chymotrypsin/trypsin-sensitive cells, both of which are located at the red blood cell membrane surface. The sialic acid adhesins seem to be the most crucial since the removal of those glycoproteins from the blood cell membrane reduces infection of cells by at minimum 80 percent, while the removal of the chymotrypsin/trypsin-sensitive cells reduces infection by only 20 to 40 percent.

To facilitate its entry into a RBC, the babesial merozoite actively works to shut down the RBC immune response. Normally, when a parasite attaches to a red blood cell, the RBC releases nitric oxide (NO) as one of its major defense responses. NO, a gas, surrounds the cell when it is released, forming, in essence, a toxic gas cloud. This burst of gas only lasts a few seconds but that is all it usually needs to last.

NO is toxic to many bacteria and intracellular RBC parasites, including *Babesia, Plasmodia,* and *Leishmania.* To counteract this, the protozoa have developed a defense: they release a compound very similar to the arginase that naturally occurs in our bodies. Arginase is an enzyme that downregulates the production of NO by the RBCs; it inactivates the L-arginine that is used to generate the NO. (Babesial parasites are very susceptible to NO. This is why supplementation with L-arginine helps inhibit babesial infection.)

Once it has stopped the NO defense, the protozoan attaches to and then analyzes the RBC, determining if it is suitable for penetration. If it is not, then the babesial organism moves away from the RBC, breaking the bond.

> *There is, in fact, a wide diversity among red blood cells and their exterior cell walls. Babesial protozoa cannot easily infect every type. Some red blood cells are too old, becoming senescent, while some are simply not suitable.*

The chemotactic compounds that create a bond between a red blood cell and the protozoal organism are so strong that, under magnification, it is possible to see the red blood cell wall distort, pulling outward with the babesial organism before the bond suddenly lets go. (It looks similar to a soap bubble when you try to pull your finger away from it.)

Once it finds an RBC it likes, the protozoan uses unique enzymes to make the RBC cell wall more porous. (These enzymes have not been identified, which is unfortunate, as an inhibitor of whatever enzyme the organism uses would help prevent entry into the cells.) Once the cell wall becomes porous, the merozoite uses a kind of screwing motion to move into the cell's interior. As it does so, it creates what is called a parasitophorous vacuole (PV), using special organelles near the front tip of the merozoite. In other words, as the merozoite enters the red blood cell, a membrane forms around it. The membrane is formed from fats (lipids) released from inside special organs (a.k.a. organelles) at the tip of the merozoite as well as some lipids gathered from the red blood cell membrane during entry. A special enzyme, sphingomyelin synthase, is then released by the merozoite into the expanding PV. This generates sphingomyelin, a major component of many cell walls, which strengthens and expands the PV.

Once the merozoite is inside the red blood cell, other alterations in both the RBC and the merozoite occur, all of them poorly understood.

Not all that much is understood about how the babesial
organisms act in the body or in nature. As with most
of the Lyme group of organisms, research is only a
few decades old.

The PV is then broken down, normally within 10 minutes, which releases the envacuoled merozoite into the interior of the red blood cell. The merozoite creates its new nuclei, does its fission thing, and produces two to four new babesial cells.

Importantly, cell division in eukaryotes (which *Babesia* are) is strictly regulated by what are called cyclin-dependent kinases (CDKs); replication cannot occur without them. CDK inhibitors (and there are many of plant origin) bind to CDKs and stop them from being used by the parasites. They can effectively block RBC invasion and the intraerythrocytic development of babesial parasites, thus counteracting infection. (Some useful ones are licorice, artemisinin, *Scutellaria barbata*, ginger, *Peganum harmala*, *Eurycoma longifolia*, *Magnolia officinalis,* and *Dunaliella salina*.)

If the numbers of merozoites are very high, many more blood cells will be invaded and destroyed, thus producing anemia. If the *Babesia* are infecting blood capillaries close to the surface of the skin, they may cause petechia, that is, small red or purple spots caused by minor hemorrhages in the blood capillaries.

During an active infection there will always be some merozoites free in the blood, seeking new cells, and some inside red blood cells in various stages of reproduction. (The analysis of these free and red blood cell–enclosed merozoites in blood smears by microscopic examination is how a babesial infection is usually diagnosed.) Although it is the impacts in the blood and on blood cells that gets most of the attention, babesial organisms do much more than simply infect red blood cells. They can also infect many of the body's organs, including the spleen and the endothelial cells that line blood vessels.

Superficially, the spleen is composed of two parts, simplistically termed red pulp and white pulp. The red pulp acts as a blood filter, removing damaged and worn-out red blood cells as well as foreign material (e.g., bacteria) from the blood. It also stores iron, platelets, and healthy red blood cells for later insertion into the bloodstream. (This is the part of the spleen usually infected by babesial parasites.) The white pulp is a primary immune organ and contains about one-fourth of the body's lymphocytes. This part of the spleen initiates responses to blood-borne antigens (i.e., bacteria, protozoa, viruses, pollen, chemicals, bacterial toxins, and so on, or certain parts of their cell walls). It produces antibodies to any of those substances that are detected in the blood. (This is the part of the spleen whose actions are inhibited by tick saliva and babesial anti-immune compounds.)

The spleen is the major immune organ that acts to limit the degree of babesial infection and ultimately clear it from the body. As researchers comment, successful immune response to babesial infection is "spleen-dependent and age-related" ("age-related" refers to the age-dependent strength of the immune system). To reiterate: the spleen must be supported during any babesial infection, and, yes, there are herbs that are very good for this. (*Salvia miltiorrhiza* and red root—*Ceanothus* spp.—are two of them.)

Because of their continual contact with the spleen, liver, and blood vessels (as the blood circulates through them), babesial protozoa have learned to infect them in very specific ways. To accomplish this, some of the merozoites undergo further development, forming what is called a gamont (or pre-gametocyte, as if we didn't need more useless words in our heads). The altered merozoite elongates and forms, on one end, a spikelike arrowhead organelle (a tiny organ, and no, not the kind you are imagining either). The organelle is designed for contact with endothelial cells in the spleen's blood vessels (as well as sometimes in the liver and general vascular system), and, once it makes contact, it releases an enzyme which causes the endothelial cells to become more porous. (And, no, researchers don't know what enzyme is used here either.) The gamont then enters the endothelial cell, where it develops into a third babesial form, a gametocyte. Gametocytes may be either male and female and once they form, as all such gendered organisms do, they immediately begin to have sex. Their offspring, like the offspring of the RBC-infecting merozoites, will be genetic variants.

This is part of the reason the protozoa are so successful:
they utilize multiple mechanisms to continually create
new genotypes.

The offspring of the gametocytes are called, unfortunately for us, ookinetes (there is a joke in here somewhere but it escapes me at the moment), which simply means a motile egg, that is, an egg that can move around. This is the fourth primary developmental form of the protozoa. (Sometimes, just to irritate the rest of us, they are also called kinetes.) These ookinetes can, when they find suitable host tissues (in the tick these are the ovaries and the salivary glands), also alter their form, becoming once again semi-comatose seeds, a.k.a. sporozoites. In essence, they once again form protozoal seeds or (to misuse the term again) encysted forms. And they are very small; an infected cell can contain thousands of them.

Once the protozoa infect endothelial cells, they begin to emit compounds that call free merozoites to that location. The merozoites cluster along the infected endothelial surface and use their chemotactic compounds to, in essence, glue large numbers of red blood cells to the merozoite membranes. The clustering of RBCs to the endothelium performs multiple functions. The RBCs that cover the site of the infection hide it from the immune system, are part of an expanding colony of the organisms, and act as food storage for the parasites. (If the formation grows too large, the blood vessel may be blocked. This is what creates the spontaneous ruptures of the smaller blood vessels that produces the petechia—red or purple spots on the skin—or ecchymoses—the bruising—that can appear on the skin during babesiosis. If it is too severe, in the larger organs it can cause rupture, or in the brain stroke.)

Thus, in the spleen's vascular tissues (and sometimes in many other organs, most commonly the liver and the body's blood vessels) the parasite sequesters multiple forms of itself. In consequence, in every infected host, in various parts of the body, there will be merozoites, (gamonts, a.k.a. pregametocytes), gametocytes, ookinetes, and sporozoites. This is why, even after "successful" antibiotic therapy (that is, upon blood smear analysis the blood is found to be clear of parasites), the disease can recur. Within anywhere from two weeks to a month, from their sequestered locations the protozoa release new sporozoites that infect new red blood cells. These form new merozoites once more and the entire cycle begins again.

Pharmaceutical treatment after "successful" drug treatment is, however, often more difficult. The protozoa have, by this time, often had exposure to the pharmaceuticals used to treat them and, as studies show, have developed increased resistance to them, usually through the creation of genetic variants. Again, the protozoa, under environmental challenge, engage in pleomorphism; that is, they alter their genetic structure and their subsequent bodily shape. This can occur from the use of pharmaceuticals or even normal human immune responses. As Chauvin et al. (2009) comment, "Immune responses led to the appearance of intracellular 'crisis' forms." The various "crisis" forms found so far are pyriform, globular, budding, ring-like, and amoeboid.

After parasite reemergence from sequestered sites, the new infection may remain asymptomatic (as it does in many cases) or it can become symptomatic or it can become a relapsing form of the disease. During relapsing forms, the merozoites invade the blood cells, but the body's immune system is effective enough that after a few days to several weeks it eliminates the merozoites. There is a pause, usually around a month, and then the sequestered protozoa make more sporozoites and the cycle continues.

The infection of the spleen and liver endothelial cells is why there will sometimes be inflammation in those organs. Examination of spleen and liver tissues of those with severe infections has found immune complex–mediated tissue lesions throughout the organs. (In the liver hyperplasia of Kupffer cells and cytoplasmic vacuolation can occur.) Vacuolation, lesions, and inflammation in the spleen can be so severe that the organ may spontaneously rupture, or burst open.

BABESIAL CYTOKINE AND IMMUNE MODULATION

Because compounds in tick saliva actively depress the immune response, sporozoites can enter the bloodstream relatively unimpeded. Again, 70 percent of them have entered red blood cells within 45 seconds and are already converting to merozoite forms. Once these merozoites reproduce, burst out of the red blood cells, and move into the bloodstream (often within 30 minutes of infection), they too begin actively modulating the immune response of the host organism.

The merozoites release factors into the blood that immediately stimulate B cells in the spleen to begin producing large amounts of interleukin-10 (IL-10). (Transforming growth factor beta—TGF-β—is also upregulated.) IL-10 strongly downregulates the specific immune responses that would, under normal circumstances, clear the body of a babesial infection. Specifically, IL-10 (and TGF-β) downregulates the spleen's production of IL-12, IL-18, interferon-gamma (IFN-γ), and nitric oxide (NO).

An essential aspect of the innate immune response at the moment of infection is the presence in the body's phagocytes (monocytes, macrophages, and neutrophils) of inducible nitric oxide synthase (iNOS). As soon as an infection begins, the body's cells release IFN-γ, which stimulates iNOS release from the immune cells. The iNOS interacts with the body's L-arginine to generate nitric oxide—again, one of the most potent antimicrobial substances the body produces. The babesial organisms' reduction of IFN-γ keeps NO levels low, thus protecting the parasites from the immune response and allowing their spread in the body.

The IL-10 that is upregulated during infection also stimulates the body's release of arginase. Arginase, again, is an enzyme that catalyzes L-arginine, breaking it apart into other molecules so that it can't be used by the body. In essence, a babesial infection causes a form of arginine depletion to occur. (Supplementation with L-arginine counteracts this depletion state.)

There are, in fact, multiple mechanisms the parasites utilize to reduce NO levels in the host. TGF-β, for instance, which is upregulated during infection, also acts as a powerful suppressant of NO production. Merozoite destruction of RBCs also plays an integral role. When the merozoites burst out of the RBCs, this immediately releases a number of important compounds (generated from the destroyed RBCs) into the bloodstream, specifically arginase, hemoglobin (Hb), and asymmetric dimethylarginine (ADMA). Again, the arginase reduces L-arginine levels. The Hb helps because it reacts with the nitric oxide produced by the body's endothelial cells, converting NO to biologically inactive nitrite (NO_2), while the ADMA, through its own unique mechanisms, interferes with L-arginine in the production of NO.

The reduction of NO is one of the major actions of the parasites in the body. Stimulation of NO is a primary mechanism for clearing a babesial infection; there are many plants and supplements that can help facilitate this process. (One is L-arginine, of course, while another is *Salvia miltiorrhiza*, which upregulates endothelial nitric oxide synthase, stimulating endothelial cells to produce NO.)

As the parasites attach to endothelial cells, they release more arginase, which inhibits endothelial NO production. Endothelial cells are major producers of nitric oxide. They use it to, among other things, relax the blood vessels, increasing vasodilation. Nitric oxide also inhibits platelet aggregation and adhesion of cells to the endothelium, keeping the blood vessels free of any obstructions.

> *Nitric oxide inhibits the adhesion of parasitized RBCs to the vascular endothelium. This clustering of RBCs to the endothelial cells has been found crucial for maximizing TNF production and illness during babesiosis. Stopping it by enhancing NO production and protecting endothelial cellular integrity goes a long way toward reducing disease symptoms and severity.*

The reduction of NO allows the parasites to enter the endothelial cells and, by allowing aggregation, enables merozoites to adhere to the endothelial cells, forming the colony clumping that is common during babesiosis. The infection deeply affects endothelial cell function, including that of the endothelial cell's mitochondria. As researchers comment, "These findings provide conclusive and unbiased evidence that mitochondriopathy represents an early manifestation of endothelial dysfunction, shifting cell metabolism toward 'metabolic hypoxia'" (Addabbo et al. 2009). This "metabolic hypoxia" is part of what causes the fatigue so common during babesial infection. (Endothelial and mitochondrial support and protection can help alleviate this. There are a number of plants that are specific for these, e.g., *Polygonum cuspidatum* for endothelial cell protection and *Leonurus cardiaca* for mitochondrial protection.)

The mechanism that the babesial parasites use to decrease L-arginine and thus the body's nitric oxide levels—and the impact this has on health—is nearly identical with that of malarial parasites. Dowling et al. (2010) comment that during these kinds of parasitic infections, studies

> reveal nearly complete depletion of L-arginine levels. . . . Low levels of L-arginine correlate with decreased immunity and nitric oxide

(NO) 1 production. . . . Increased arginase activity characterizes the alternative immune response, which downregulates inflammation and tissue damage while upregulating angiogenesis and tissue repair mechanisms. Such conditions favor parasite growth through suppressed T cell and inflammatory responses to pathogens and increased concentrations of L-ornithine-derived polyamines, which facilitate cellular proliferation.

The shift of the body away from NO production to that of L-ornithine has strongly deleterious effects on bodily health; it also supports parasite reproduction. L-ornithine stimulates the production of polyamines (and collagen), and the polyamines, it turns out, are essential for the intracellular replication of the parasites. TGF-β, by the way, is an integral player in the induction of L-ornithine-derived polyamines. (Herbs that inhibit TGF-β and counteract this are *Artemisia* spp., *Astragalus* spp., *Schisandra chinensis, Salvia miltiorrhiza, Scutellaria baicalensis, Scutellaria barbata, Ginkgo biloba, Magnolia officinalis,* and *Paeonia lactiflora.*)

The parasite-stimulated shift from a Th1 immune response to Th2 contributes to the formation of fibrosis and granulomas in the organs affected by the parasites. Arginase is most strongly released during babesial infection in the liver, kidneys, prostate, and small intestine. Overproduction, due to parasite infection, in the liver and kidneys—and the eventual formation of fibrosis due to the increases in L-ornithine (creating collagen and polyamines)—is part of what causes the damage to those organs. As granulomas form, large numbers of arginase-expressing macrophages accumulate in and around them, exacerbating the problem. Intravascular coagulation also occurs at the site of endothelial infection and the merozoite colonies on their surface. This can lead to coagulative necrosis; unchecked, the damage to organs can be severe.

Numerous studies have shown that successful resolution of babesial infections is dependent on the spleen's IFN-γ and the body's NO production. Nitric oxide is primarily generated by L-arginine and IFN-γ; IFN-γ depends on both IL-12 and IL-18 to be upregulated. However, once IFN-γ and NO are inhibited, the babesia can spread relatively easily throughout the host system. As researchers Jeong et al. (2012) note, "Bregs, Tregs, and IL-10 production induced by *B. microti* infection are required to facilitate the growth and survival of the parasite." And as researchers Chauvin et al. reveal, the upregulation of IL-10, and subsequent repression of more effective splenic responses, is a primary strategy of all members of the *Babesia* genus:

> During acute infection with *B. bovis,* the innate immune response seems to be essential and requires the production of interleukin-12 (IL12) and interleukin-18 (IL18). These stimulate natural killer (NK) cells to produce high levels of gamma interferon (IFNγ), which induce the production of nitric oxide (NO) by the macrophages. During chronic infection, lysis of the infected red blood cells (iRBC) is also mainly mediated by the NO produced by splenic macrophages activated by IFNγ and Tumor Necrosis Factor alpha (TNFα). This mechanism is then regulated by type 1 cytokines and is inhibited by interleukin-4 (IL4) and interleukin-10 (IL10). . . . The evolution of acute infection depends on the timing and location of production of the inflammatory and type 1 cytokines and on the quantities produced. A comparison of the immune response of calves and adult cattle against *B. bovis* showed that the innate response is only protective if the IFNγ and the IL12 are produced early on, before IL10 production. When IL10, IL12, and IFN-γ are produced at the same time, the type 1 response and the production of NO in the spleen are delayed or decreased, which allows disease expression. (Chauvin et al. 2009)

Other studies (with a variety of hosts) have found that IL-1β, TNF-α, and CD4+ and CD13+ cells are also important in the induction of IFN-γ and NO. The more mature and numerous the splenic dendritic cells, the better the resolution of infection. (Dendritic cells, again, are specifically inhibited by the organisms.) As well, during most successful resolutions, there is a CD8+ cellular proliferation in the spleen. Researchers have found that neutralization of IL-12, irrespective of the host species, "resulted," as Shoda et al. (2001) comment, "in increased parasitemia and mortality." Increasing IL-12, IFN-γ, and NO production in the body are essential in treating babesial infections. Again, there are many natural compounds and plants that will do this. (Some examples include *Withania somnifera*, which will regulate IL-10 levels and increase IL-12, and *Eleutherococcus senticosus* and *Astragalus* spp., which will upregulate IL-12.)

As a reminder, compounds in tick saliva inhibit IL-1β, IL-8, IL-12, TNF-α, and IFN-γ, all immune responses that are necessary for a successful response to *Babesia* infection. Thus the inhibition of the splenic immune response is already initiated by the time the protozoa begin infecting red blood cells. The longer the tick feeds during babesial infection, the worse the immune status becomes.

Younger animals, including humans, tend to be more resistant to the babesial induction of IL-10 (or to overcome it more quickly). Their bodies upregulate IL-12, IFN-γ, and NO much more strongly than adults who are infected. Adults, irrespective of species, generally experience a delayed and depressed expression of IL-12, IFN-γ, and NO, resulting in more severe illness of longer duration than the young. In essence, immune senescence contributes significantly to the spread and seriousness of the disease.

Researchers Chauvin et al. (2009) comment that "an inverse relationship, between age and resistance to babesiae, has been reported with young animals being more resistant than adults." This appears to be, they continue, "due to differences in localization and timing of the immune mechanisms." And as they go on to note, "Even in the natural well-adapted host, a delayed, unsuitable or insufficient immune response could lead to clinical manifestations of babesiosis and eventually death of the infected host." The finding that the severity of babesiosis is directly related to differences in immune status means that any treatment of a non-pharmaceutically responsive infection *must* include immune intervention.

Over time, as the body's immune function begins to catch up with the disease, the cytokine profile alters. IL-10 levels begin to decrease with corresponding increases in IL-1β, IL-12, IL-18, TNF-α, IFN-γ, and NO. Both CD4+ and CD13+ cells begin to proliferate.

At this stage in the disease process, the spleen and immune response begin to become effective against the protozoa, whose numbers begin to decrease. Antibodies to the protozoa begin to circulate in the blood, keeping their numbers low, or even eliminating them entirely. At this point, the body then begins to downregulate the immune response. As the disease begins to resolve, IL-10 levels begin to increase (appropriately) and this decreases IL-1β, IL-12, IL-18, TNF-α, IFN-γ, and NO.

During relapsing forms of the disease, the process simply repeats itself. The protozoa release genetic variants from their sequestered niches and produce IL-10 and arginase, once again reducing immune responses. The body figures it out, and once more deals with the infection. The continual creation and release of antigenic variants (and a partially unhealthy immune system) facilitate this relapsing form of the disease.

Note: Pharmaceuticals that repress immune responses such as IFN-γ, TNF-α, IL-12, IL-1β, and so on can aggravate babesial infection, making the infection more severe. It is well recognized that people on immunosuppressive drugs are more at risk during a babesial infection; however, even such pharmaceuticals as etanercept, a TNF inhibitor, used in treating rheumatoid arthritis, have been found to exacerbate babesiosis. Any natural treatment of babesia should be accompanied by detailed questioning regarding pharmaceutical intake.

SEVERE BABESIOSIS VERSUS MILD, MODERATE, AND CHRONIC FORMS

Severe or acute babesiosis can occur with low parasite loads and can lead, under some circumstances, to sepsis, septic shock, multiple organ failure, coma, and death. This condition has much in common with the sepsis and septic shock that occurs in *Ehrlichia* and *Anaplasma* infections. This is dealt with in chapter 8. In general, the more acute forms that do not include sepsis will respond perfectly well to the protocol for mild, moderate, and chronic forms. A few specifics are offered in chapter 8.

4

Natural Healing of Babesia

The advantages of natural compounds are fewer side effects in comparison to orthodox medical drugs, and the production of synergistic effects for a more positive treatment outcome.

K. KITAZATO, Y. WANG, AND N. KOBAYASHI,
"VIRAL INFECTIOUS DISEASE AND NATURAL
PRODUCTS WITH ANTIVIRAL ACTIVITY"

Your body hears everything your mind says.

NAOMI JUDD

Each patient carries his own doctor inside him.

NORMAN COUSINS

To effectively treat babesial infections there are five points to keep in mind about the parasites:

1. They infect red blood cells.

2. They significantly inhibit nitric oxide production in the body (the body's main defense against them).

3. They, during all but severe babesial infections, *lower* inflammation by preventing the inflammatory Th1 response the body would naturally use to counteract them.

4. They infect and distort the endothelial cells that line blood vessels, using them as a niche in which to hide, and they cluster red blood cells around those sites, which causes a number of blood vessel and organ problems from the subsequent coagulation and blockage of the vessels.

5. Studies on the treatment of *Babesia* infections have found that a 7- to 10-day treatment approach is, *in half of all infections,* insufficient; treatment must last 30 days or longer to successfully treat the infection, to prevent recurrence, and to prevent pharmaceutical resistance from developing.

That said, babesial infections are highly responsive to natural protocols. There are many plants that are directly effective against the parasites and to which the organisms do not develop resistance. As well, plants that protect red blood cells, the spleen, and other affected organs and enhance immune function by counteracting the parasite effects on immune response are common.

Treating Babesiosis with Natural Protocols

First, some basics . . . I know this is repetitive, but there seems to be a general confusion that commonly arises among both practitioners and the infected about the following points, hence the continual repetition (I get scores of e-mails about it every month).

*The herbs and supplements in this book are **not** the only ones in the world that will help.* Please use the protocols outlined herein *only* as a starting place, a guideline. Add anything that you feel will help you and delete anything that you feel is not useful. Protozoa, when they enter a human body, find a very unique ecosystem in that particular person. Thus the disease is always slightly different every time it occurs. This means that a pharmaceutical or herb that works for one person may not work or work as well for another. There is no one-size-fits-all treatment that works for all people in all times and places.

Also: *there is no one thing that always has to happen first, that has to be treated first, or that you must always do or must never do in order to get well.* There is no one herb that will always work for everyone; there is no one protocol that contains the solutions to all the infectious organisms that exist or all the forms of infection that the Lyme group can cause.

Again: there is no one-size-fits-all treatment that works for all people in all times and places.

Anyone who says there is, is either trying to sell you something or doesn't really understand the Lyme group of infectious organisms (or has powerful self-image needs involved). *There is not and never has been one single way to health such that in all times and in all places and with all people it will always work.* Life, and disease, and the journey to wellness are much more complex and challenging than that.

All of us, practitioners and the infected alike, of necessity must learn to see what is right in front of us and adapt our interventions to what is actually occurring in the unique ecological system we are encountering. Our interaction with these disease complexes has to occur out of a living communication—with the organism, with the body, with the medicine. Each treatment intervention, as treatment progresses, will become unique to each person. It has to do so for healing to occur.

Thus the protocols in this book should solely be considered as a foundational place to begin. For most people they will help considerably; for some they will clear the infection completely. Nearly everyone (practitioners and the infected alike), however, will find that they will need to add this or subtract that. *Please do so.* Please trust your own feeling sense and pay attention to what your body is telling you. *You* are the best judge of whether something is working for you or not, whether you need to add something else or not, whether you are getting better . . . or not.

Now, about dosages: I will often suggest a dosage or a *range* of dosages for the herbs and supplements that can help. If you have a very healthy immune system, or a very mild case, you will probably need smaller doses; if your immune system is severely depleted or if you are very ill, you may need to use larger doses. If you are *very* sensitive to outside substances, as some people with Lyme and these coinfections are, then you might need to use very tiny doses, that is, from one to five drops of tincture at a time. (This is true for about 1 percent of the people with these infections.) I have seen six-foot-five, 280-pound men be unable to take more than five drops of a tincture and a tiny, 95-pound woman need a tablespoon at a time. *Dosages need to be adjusted for each person's individual ecology.* **Again . . . dosages need to be adjusted for each person's individual ecology.** And now, a few other points that commonly arise:

1. Yes, you *can* combine all the herbs together in the liquid of your choice. You do not have to take them separately.
2. Yes, these herbs *can* be taken along with antibiotics.
3. No, the protozoa do not develop resistance to the herbs.
4. Yes, you *can* take these herbs along with protocols suggested by other practitioners.
5. No, except for a very few herbs (such as the 1:1 form of eleutherococcus tincture), you do not need to pulse the herbs—that is, to take them in an on-again, off-again cycle, such as five days on, two days off. In fact, I have continually heard from people struggling with the Lyme group of infections that they were getting better, were told to pulse by their personal practitioner, and once they did, relapsed.
6. Yes, it is common for about half the people who use an herbal protocol, when they begin to get better, to be so excited about being themselves

again that they do too much, overexert themselves, and relapse. This is extremely common (and very understandable; it's tiring being sick for so long). So, please be very careful once your strength and joy begin to return. It may seem as if you can immediately begin exerting yourself as you used to do; however, your body has been under a long-term stress, and its reserves are low. It will take, if you have been ill for a long time, at least a year to rebuild.

Part of the function of serious chronic illnesses is to increase personal awareness (I know from personal experience). There is the life you had before Lyme, there is the life you have after. It is very rarely possible to go back to being unaware of the impacts of stress on your system, the kind of self-caretaking your body (and spirit) needs, or the dangers of overextending yourself and your energy. Ignorance may be bliss (however short that bliss may be) but awareness is empowering . . . and health enabling.

And, finally, *please be conscious of how you respond to the medicines you are taking. If something disagrees with you, if you feel something is not right in how you are responding to a medicine,* **stop taking it.** Remember: you will always know yourself better than any outside physician.

INITIAL INTERVENTION PROTOCOL

The initial intervention, using a natural protocol, suggested for mild to moderate babesial infection, relapsing or not, entails the following.

1. **Antibabesial herbs.** The use of antibabesial microbials that are broadly systemic (note, as a counter example, that the berberine plants *are* antibabesial, but they are poorly systemic and cannot clear the parasite from the body)
2. **Organ support and protection.** Protecting and enhancing the function of red blood cells, the spleen, the liver, and the endothelial tissues

3. **Immune modulation.** Modulating the immune response and cytokine cascade by decreasing IL-10 and TGF-β levels; inhibiting the generation of arginase; and increasing levels of IL-12, IFN-γ, L-arginine, and NO

4. **Specific symptom treatment.** These protozoa can create a rather broad range of symptoms. Reducing symptoms helps restore quality of life and feelings of joy, which in and of themselves produce potent beneficial effects during healing. These herbs and supplements are covered in the expanded treatment protocol (page 95).

Again, there are thousands of plants that can be, and are, used in the treatment of disease. The herbs below are only the ones I have found effective; this does not mean there are not others just as good.

Antibabesial Herbs

The primary antibabesial herbs and plant-derived compounds I prefer, and believe the most effective, are *Cryptolepis sanguinolenta, Alchornea cordifolia, Sida acuta* (or similar species), *Bidens pilosa* (or similar species), and the *Artemisia* species and their constituents artesunate, artemisinin, and artemisone. (Note: The whole herb can be used very effectively, if you wish. See *Herbal Antibiotics,* second edition, for preparation methods for the plant itself.) Some additionally useful antibabesial herbs and compounds are *Brucea javanica,* the homeopathics China 30C and Chelidonium 30C, and riboflavin (vitamin B₂).

Other herbs and herbal compounds active against babesial parasites are *Camellia sinensis* (or its constituent epigallocatechin gallate, a.k.a. EGCG), *Allium sativum* (and its constituent allicin), *Phyllanthus niruri* (also a very good liver herb), lactoferrin (colostrum), *Calophyllum tetrapterum, Curcuma xanthorrhiza, Curcuma zedoaria, Elaeocarpus parvifolius* (bark), *Elephantorrhiza elephantina, Excoecaria cochinchinensis, Garcinia benthami, Garcinia rigida, Lansium domesticum, Peronema canescens, Sandoricum emarginatum, Shorea balangeran,* the terpene nerolidol (found in neroli, ginger, jasmine, lavender, tea tree, lemongrass, and *Cannabis sativa*), and the berberine-containing plants such as goldenseal. However, please note: Berberine plants are not systemic enough to use as a primary treatment for babesiosis, though they may in certain circumstances work well as supportive therapy. As well, I do not think garlic (*Allium*) is systemic and potent enough to work as a primary treatment for these protozoa.

CDK inhibitors are very helpful in treating babesial infections. They block red blood cell invasion and the subsequent intraerythrocytic development of the parasites, acting in their own way as antibabesial herbs. Some useful CDK inhibitors are artemisinin, licorice (*Glycyrrhiza* spp.), *Scutellaria barbata,* ginger (*Zingiber officinalis*), *Peganum harmala, Eurycoma longifolia, Magnolia officinalis,* and *Dunaliella salina.*

Organ Support and Protection

The most important parts of the body to protect during babesial infection are the red blood cells, the spleen, the liver, and the endothelial lining of the blood vessels. Respectively, here are the four primary supportive herbs or compounds to utilize in treating babesia infection.

1. ***Sida acuta* (or related species).** This plant is specific for protecting red blood cells and for relieving anemia by increasing red blood cell numbers. It is also a strong, very systemic, broad-spectrum antibacterial for babesial parasites.

2. ***Salvia miltiorrhiza* (a.k.a. danshen).** Danshen is a Chinese herb specific for spleen and liver inflammation and malfunction.

   In the past I have relied primarily on red root (*Ceanothus* spp.) for diseases that affect the spleen. I like red root because it is strongly protective of the spleen and to some extent the liver. It acts to reduce inflammation in both of those organs. It also stimulates the immune activity of the spleen, helping to clear the body of infection while optimizing the removal of microorganism and immune system debris during infections. However, *red root is also a blood coagulant.* Because intravascular coagulation is so common during babesial infections, I now prefer the use of *Salvia miltiorrhiza.* (If you do want to keep using red root, then please supplement its use in this disease with anticoagulants such as nattokinase, ginkgo, and aspirin.)

3. **Milk thistle seed (*Silybum marianum*).** The combined compounds known as silymarin that are extracted from milk thistle seed are strongly liver protective and regenerative. There are four main constituents of silymarin: silibinin, isosilibinin, silicristin, and silidianin. Silibinin strongly upregulates the expression of CDK inhibitors that act to suppress CDK2 and CDK4 kinase actions in the body. As such it will act, to some extent, as an antibabesial herb itself.

4. **L-arginine.** There are a number of herbs that protect and support endothelial function and integrity; however, most of them also inhibit inflammation in the body. That is, they move the endothelial cells' response to infection toward a Th2 state and reduce the Th1 reaction. During mild to moderate babesial infection, this may ultimately support the parasites (note: *may*); hence I believe the initial and most important intervention to support the endothelial cells is the use of L-arginine supplementation. L-arginine is potently effective in improving endothelial function during any type of circulatory system disorder. It normalizes endothelial function, inhibits adhesion to endothelial cells (of all blood cell types), inhibits hyperplasia, reduces endothelial activation, stimulates the production of NO from endothelial cells, corrects induced NO deficiency in the body, and generally restores healthy vascular functioning. It is the primary approach to use to protect and restore endothelial function during babesiosis. (*Salvia miltiorrhiza* is also useful here as it upregulates endothelial NOS and NO production by the endothelial cells.)

Of note: *Bidens pilosa,* a systemic antibiotic for babesial parasites, has the added benefit of normalizing endothelial function during infections and activating CDK inhibitors. *Panax ginseng* also acts to normalize endothelial cells and their functioning; it also inhibits arginase. Both are highly useful.

But again, the best supplement for increasing NO production in endothelial cells (and the body) is L-arginine. It is crucial, as it is necessary for NO production (a combination of L-arginine and L-citrulline appears to work well also). Studies have found that simply supplementing the body with L-arginine will reduce or even eliminate babesial infection from the body.

There are a number of foods that will increase arginine levels in the body; they are very helpful to add to the diet during a babesial infection. Some of them, such as the red meats, also help stimulate the production of red blood cells. The best food source of arginine is red meat, most specifically beef. As an example, a sirloin steak contains 6 grams of L-arginine per one-fifth ounce of meat. So, an eight-ounce sirloin will give you 240 grams of L-arginine. Pork is not quite as good, but still high. And beef liver runs 1.2 grams per four-hundredths of an ounce, very high indeed. Other foods rich in L-arginine are (per 100 grams of the food indicated) spinach (3.3 grams), peanuts (3), almonds (2.5), sunflower seeds (2.4), walnuts (2.2), hazelnuts (2.2), Brazil nuts (2.1), cashews (2.1), pistachios (2), pecans (1.1), canned light tuna (1.7), chicken or turkey (1.2), salmon (1.2), shrimp (1.2), egg, including yolk (1.1), and whole wheat (650 mg) and tofu (same as whole wheat).

Immune Modulation

Again, the point here is to modulate immune function in a specific manner during mild to moderate infections. Specifically, to downregulate IL-10, TGF-β, and arginase and upregulate IL-12, IL-18, IFN-γ, TNF-α, and NO, essentially switching the immune response from

Th2 to Th1. The primary herb for this is ashwagandha (*Withania somnifera*). It counteracts, with great specificity, the exact modulation of the immune system that the tick saliva and the protozoa initiate and maintain.

Herbs that inhibit TGF-β are *Artemisia* spp., *Astragalus* spp., *Schisandra chinensis, Salvia miltiorrhiza, Scutellaria* spp., *Ginkgo biloba, Magnolia officinalis,* and *Paeonia lactiflora.* A combination of *Angelica sinensis* and *Astragalus membranaceus* (one part angelica, five parts astraglus) is also highly effective.

Inhibition of arginase is crucial during a babesial infection. The herbs and supplements specific for arginase inhibition are *Panax ginseng, Scutellaria baicalensis, Scutellaria barbata, Saururus chinensis, Cecropia pachystachya,* and EGCG. Arginase inhibitors, by themselves, have been found to restore endothelial cell functioning.

Other herbs and supplements useful for immune modulation are licorice (downregulates IL-10, acting primarily as an immune modulator and tonic), standardized milk thistle (silymarin inhibits IL-10 overexpression and helps support endothelial health), *Cannabis sativa* (ibid), *Scutellaria baicalensis* (downregulates IL-10 and Treg), *Panax ginseng* and *Panax japonicus* (both upregulate Th1 dynamics), *Labisia pumila* (upregulates Th1 response), *Carica papaya* leaves (as a tea; stimulate IL-12, IFN-γ, and TNF-α), grape seed extract (induces IFN-γ upregulation), *Lycium barbarum* fruit (lychii berries), neem leaf, boneset (*Eupatorium perfoliatum,* primarily from its caffeic acid derivatives), and plants containing scopoletin (an IL-10/Th2 downregulator) such as noni, manacá, passionflower (*Passiflora* spp.), stevia, *Artemisia* spp. (especially *A. scoparia* and *A. capillaris*), nettle leaf (*Urtica dioica*), and black haw (*Viburnum prunifolium*). Plants containing daucosterol are also effective in stimulating a Th1 response and downregulating a Th2-dominant dynamic. Among them are *Garcinia parviflora* and *Gardenia jasminoides.*

A BASIC PROTOCOL FOR MILD TO MODERATE BABESIOSIS

Note: Regimen should be followed for 30 to 60 days. (It can be repeated if necessary.)

1. *Cryptolepis sanguinolenta* tincture, ½ teaspoon 3x daily.
2. *Bidens pilosa* tincture, ½ teaspoon 3x daily.
3. Artemisinin (or artesunate or artemisone), 100–200 mg 3x daily.
4. *Sida acuta* tincture, ¼ teaspoon 3x daily. Note: Some people are highly sensitive to this herb; it may, under certain circumstances, increase symptoms. If so, reduce the dose to just under the dosage that increases symptoms.
5. *Salvia miltiorrhiza*, ½ teaspoon 3x daily.
6. Milk thistle seed, standardized (to 80 percent silymarin) capsules, 600–1,200 mg 3x daily.
7. L-arginine, 2,000 mg 3x daily.
8. Ashwagandha (*Withania somnifera*), ½ teaspoon 3x daily. Note: May cause drowsiness.
9. Riboflavin (B$_2$), 30–40 mg 3x daily. (Suggested: Thorne Research Riboflavin 5' phosphate, 36.5 mg capsules.)
10. Tincture combination of *Panax ginseng*, licorice, *Schisandra chinensis* (equal parts of each), ½ teaspoon 3x daily.

This should take care of nearly all types of babesial infections—and reduce most symptoms, irrespective of species or genetic variant. Again: *the protocol can be repeated if necessary.*

Note: I am often asked what herbs and supplements are absolutely necessary—in other words, what can someone leave out if they really don't want to take all that. Well . . . nothing, especially so if you have an intransigent or relapsing form of the disease. However, about half the people with babesiosis, over the years, have experienced clearance by *only* using cryptolepis. Still, there are many others who need an expanded protocol. Nevertheless, if you have an intransigent form and you really insist on a reduced protocol you should at minimum take numbers 1, 3, 4, 5, 7, and 8.

And a comment on Chinese skullcap root (*Scutellaria baicalensis*): This herb appears to act as a fairly strong immune modulator. It seems to have powerful immune adaptogenic actions. If the immune response is too high—irrespective of the direction (Th1 or Th2)—the herb alters the immune response appropriately. It may turn out to be a primary herb for this infection.

ADD TO THE BASIC PROTOCOL, BASED ON SYMPTOMS

If you have systemic babesiosis . . .

With *severe* anemia, use:
1. *Sida acuta* tincture, at an increased dosage of ½ teaspoon 3–6x daily until the condition resolves, plus . . .
2. N-acetylcysteine, 4,000 mg 2x daily until the condition resolves, and add . . .
3. Bidens tincture, ½ teaspoon 6x daily, and . . .
4. *Angelica sinensis* tincture, 1 teaspoon 3x daily.

With *severe* intravascular coagulation, use:
1. Ginkgo standardized tincture, ½ teaspoon 3x daily, plus . . .
2. Nattokinase, 200 mg 3x daily (same as 4,000 FU 3x daily), plus . . .
3. 4 adult aspirins, 3x daily.

With drenching sweats, use:
1. Boneset (*Eupatorium perfoliatum*), strong infusion, 1 cup 3–6x daily.

With jaundice/liver inflammation, use:

1. Milk thistle seed, standardized (to 80 percent silymarin) capsules, at an increased dosage of 1,200 mg 3x daily, minimum.

With spleen inflammation, use:

1. *Salvia miltiorrhiza* tincture, at an increased dosage of 1 teaspoon 6x daily.

With fever, use:

1. Coral root (*Corallorhiza maculata* or equivalent) tincture, 30 drops each hour, or . . .
2. Boneset (*Eupatorium perfoliatum*), strong infusion, 1 cup each hour or two, or . . .
3. Peppermint tea, 1 cup each hour or two, as needed.

With nausea, use:

1. Peppermint tea, 1 cup each hour or two as needed.

With *extreme* nausea, use:

1. Peppermint essential oil, one drop *only*, on the tongue, followed by water, as needed.

With muscle and joint pain, use:

1. *Pedicularis* tincture, 1 teaspoon each hour as needed, or . . .
2. Indian pipe (*Monotropa uniflora*) tincture, ¼–1 teaspoon up to 6x daily.

With severe pain, use:

1. *Salvia miltiorrhiza* tincture, 1 tablespoon (yes, that's right) every 15 minutes, slowly decreasing the dosage as the pain subsides.
2. Theramine can also be of help.

With headache, use:

1. Herbs that relieve intravascular coagulation, plus . . .
2. *Pedicularis* tincture, 1 teaspoon each hour as needed, and/or . . .
3. Indian pipe (*Monotropa uniflora*) tincture, ¼–1 teaspoon up to 6x daily, and/or . . .
4. Kudzu root (*Pueraria lobata*) tincture, ¼–½ teaspoon up to 6x daily.

With anxiety/hysteria, use:

1. Pasqueflower (*Pulsatilla patens*) tincture, 10 drops each hour for as long as necessary, and/or . . .
2. Motherwort (*Leonurus cardiaca*) tincture, ¼–½ teaspoon up to 6x daily, and/or . . .
3. Coral root (*Corallorhiza maculata*) tincture, 30 drops (a full dropper) up to 6x daily.

With extreme fear, use:

1. Vervain (*Verbena officinalis*) tincture, 30 drops up to 6x daily.

With sleep disturbance, use:

1. Melatonin liquid, following the manufacturer's directions, 1 hour before bed, and/or . . .
2. Ashwagandha (*Withania somnifera*), ½ teaspoon of the tincture 1 hour before bed, or 1 gram in powder or capsule form 1 hour before bed, and/or . . .
3. Motherwort (*Leonurus cardiaca*) tincture, ¼ *ounce* (yes, that is right) in liquid just before bed (if the melatonin does not help).

With severe fatigue, use:

1. Eleuthero (*Eleutherococcus senticosus*) tincture (a 1:5 ratio tincture, *not* the 2:1 Herb Pharm brand), ¼ teaspoon 3x daily, plus . . .

2. Rhodiola (*Rhodiola* spp.) tincture, ¼ teaspoon 3x daily, plus . . .

3. Schisandra (*Schisandra chinensis*) tincture, ¼ teaspoon 3x daily, plus . . .

4. Motherwort (*Leonurus cardiaca*) tincture, ½ teaspoon 3x daily, and . . .

5. Fermented wheat germ extract, if you can afford it. All for 6 months.

Note: Severe fatigue is often caused by mitochondrial dysfunction, something that happens when babesia begin infecting endothelial cells. The primary herbs/supplements for treating mitochondrial dysfunction are motherwort, ginkgo, schisandra, rhodiola, luteolin, and fermented wheat germ extract.

With wasting (i.e., severe weight loss), use:

1. Fermented wheat germ extract, 9 grams daily (best choice), or (not as good) . . .

2. Shiitake mushrooms, powdered or as food, 6–16 grams per day. A pure extract of lentinan can also be used, at 1–3 grams per day.

For detoxification and help with Herxheimer reactions, use:

1. Zeolite powder, 2 heaping teaspoons 3x daily (do *not* accidentally inhale), and/or . . .

2. Activated charcoal, 2 capsules 2x daily.

3. Bentonite clay may also be of help. Soak 1 teaspoon in a full glass of water for 30 minutes to 2 hours. Take on an empty stomach, early in the morning or just before bed.

Some comments on epilepsy/seizures:
Coinfections can sometimes cause seizures of various sorts. The best approach to the treatment of epilepsy is a high-fat—that is, a ketogenic—diet. This has been successfully used in Britain for some time, especially in the treatment of childhood epileptic seizures.

There is a lot of good research on it; it does work, basically by altering brain chemistry. Fasting can be used to treat epilepsy as well, but during a mycoplasma infection this can seriously lower nutrients in the body, increasing bacterial scavenging. A ketogenic diet is the best approach in this instance *if the seizures are severe*. The reduction of glucose in the brain and the increase of fats (ketones) stimulates the production of antioxidants, especially glutathione, and detoxifies the enzymes that are breaking down neuronal structures. Inflammation in the brain is sharply reduced, and excitatory neurotransmitters are reduced.

If, however, the seizures are minor and occasional, the best overall herb is Chinese skullcap. It will be most effective if combined with N-acetylcysteine. Bidens and sida can also be of some use.

5

Ehrlichia
and Anaplasma

An Overview

Human monocytotropic ehrlichiosis was first reported in the United States in 1987, but during the ensuing 20 years it has become the most prevalent life-threatening tick born disease in the US.

N. Ismail, K. C. Bloch, and J. W. McBride,
"Human Ehrlichiosis and Anaplasmosis"

The incidence is likely underestimated since active surveillance studies performed in HME-endemic areas in Missouri, Tennessee, and Georgia have revealed an incidence 10–100 times higher than reported by passive surveillance.

Institute of Medicine (U.S.) Committee on
Lyme Disease and Other Tick-Borne Diseases,
*Critical Needs and Gaps in Understanding
Prevention, Amelioration, and Resolution
of Lyme and Other Tick-Borne Diseases*

Not only are these pathogens new to science, but their maintenance in nature requires the complex interactions of tick vectors and vertebrate hosts that are sensitive to environmental influences that can drive epidemics. . . . Reports of severe and fatal ehrlichiosis . . . will increase as an unavoidable consequence of environmental forces that increase the risk of exposure to these pathogens, coupled with dramatic changes in human demography.

C. D. PADDOCK AND J. E. CHILDS,
"EHRLICHIA CHAFFEENSIS"

Ehrlichia and *Anaplasma* spp. are closely related bacteria that are infecting increasing numbers of people each year. Most people haven't heard of them, though, including many physicians. They are still relatively new to our human world . . . and our awareness. Like many organisms in the Lyme group, we have barely begun to learn anything about them. As Christopher Paddock and James Childs (2003) comment:

In April 1986, a medical intern scanning the peripheral blood smear of a severely ill man with an unexplained illness observed peculiar intracytoplasmic inclusions in several of the patient's monocytes. The patient described multiple tick bites sustained approximately 2 weeks earlier during a visit to a rural area in northern Arkansas . . .

It was not until 1991, five years later, that those bacteria were identified as a unique *Ehrlichia* species, a genus believed at the time to be limited to veterinary infections. As Paddock and Childs continue:

During this interval, surveillance efforts identified several hundred cases of moderate to severe, and occasionally fatal, ehrlichiosis in patients with unexplained illnesses following tick exposures. These findings indicated that ehrlichiosis was a widespread and significant public health problem of increasing but undefined magnitude.

Further research found that those early infections were only the first, shy indicators of a substantial problem. It soon became clear that the infections were widespread and were in fact caused by a number of similar organisms, not just one. As Paddock and Childs continue:

> During the 1990s, two additional *Ehrlichia* spp., *Anaplasma* (formerly *Ehrlichia*) *phagocytophila* (the agent of human granulocytic ehrlichiosis [HGE]) and *E. ewingii* (a cause of granulocytic ehrlichiosis in dogs), were identified as human pathogens, and these reports greatly expanded the geographic region and the size of the human population at risk for acquiring one of these potentially lethal infections.

Nor were these infections limited to the United States. As researcher Heather Stevenson (2009) observes, "The incidence of ehrlichial species throughout the world has been increasing with recent identification of cases being reported in Mexico (1999), Brazil (2004), Spain (2004), France (2007), Africa (2005), Netherlands (2006), Russia (2001), and Thailand (1997)."

In fact, the more deeply the diseases were examined, the more pervasive they were found to be. New species and genotypes in the genus continue to emerge and species not formerly thought to infect humans in fact do so. Completely unknown 20 years ago, this group of infections is now one of the most serious worldwide. Treatment failures are common and there are few alternatives (in the medical community) to conventional pharmaceuticals when they fail.

THE ANAPLASMATACEAE

The two most common infectious species among the *Ehrlichia* group of bacteria—and the ones causing the most concern within the Lyme community—are in two different genera, *Ehrlichia* and *Anaplasma*. The one most commonly heard of is *Ehrlichia chaffeensis*, the other is its close cousin *Anaplasma phagocytophilum*.

Both of these organisms are in the family Anaplasmataceae, the members of which are bacteria, not protozoa (thank god). They are part of the Proteobacteria phylum (meaning a tribe or clan—the next level up from a family), all of whom are Gram-negative bacteria. Gram-negative bacteria (so called because they refuse to take a Gram stain—I can't help but like them for that), as opposed to Gram-positive, have a double cell wall, making them less susceptible to antibacterial and environmental damage. Medically, the Gram-negative group tend to be tougher to treat.

Unfortunately, due to the spread of infectious taxonomitis among scientists and researchers, the taxonomy of this family and genera is in flux. (Something that is apparently true for every life form on this planet.) Until 2001, the genus *Ehrlichia* appeared well defined; nevertheless, as taxonomitis spread further among the human population, it, too, suffered meddling. The *Ehrlichia* group has now been split into three closely related but very distinct genera: *Ehrlichia, Anaplasma,* and *Neorickettsia*. All are still in the Anaplasmataceae family. Other genera in that family include *Aegyptianella* (known to *only* infect birds at this point), *Wolbachia* (which does infect people), and a very new (as of 2013), sixth genus, *Neoehrlichia,* that also infects people from time to time.

Neorickettsia, Neoehrlichia, and Wolbachia

Neorickettsia has four species (so far) within it, all transmitted by trematodes in fish. The known species are *N. sennetsu* (infects people, four genotypes of this species exist), *N. risticii* (Potomac horse fever, infects horses), *N. helminthoeca* (salmon poisoning disease, infects dogs), and *N. elokominica* (salmon poisoning disease, infects dogs, bears, racoons, and ferrets). *N. sennetsu* is believed (though not confirmed) to only be carried by trematodes in fish, the usual source of infection. It is generally contracted by eating undercooked fish and is primarily found in Japan and Malaysia. (I am not going to deal with it in this book.)

The new genus, *Neoehrlichia*, contains one member so far, *N. mikurensis* (which I am not going to cover herein). It is considered an emerging pathogen for people in Europe, Asia, and Africa. Similarly to *Ehrlichia ruminantium*, these bacteria tend to infect the endothelium, especially in the liver and spleen.

The *Wolbachia* (and no, I am not going to deal with these either) infect a wide range of insects, including nematodes, mosquitoes, and, occasionally, ticks. Up to 70 percent of all insects are considered to be potential hosts for the organisms. The primary diseases caused by this genus in humans are elephantiasis and river blindness (generally in Africa) and, in dogs, heartworm.

The *Ehrlichia* Genus

The *Ehrlichia,* as of 2014, contains seven species known to researchers: *E. canis, E. ewingii, E. chaffeensis, E. muris, E. ruminantium, E. mineirensis* (a new species found in 2011 in Brazil that blends genome structures from both *E. canis* and *E. chaffeensis*), and a new species with some similarities to *E. muris* (but not yet formally named) that was discovered to be infecting people in the Wisconsin/Minnesota area in 2009. (Hence its temporary designation as *Ehrlichia muris*-like or EML.) Five of the species are known to infect people, the exceptions being *E. muris* and *E. mineirensis*. However (just an FYI), people with antibodies to *E. muris* have been found in Japan, indicating previous infection by that species. Many researchers (and physicians) still insist that *E. ruminantium* does not infect people. However, a number of peer-review journals reveal it to be an emerging pathogen in Africa, especially in children. It is almost invariably fatal. (As is usual in the United States, the CDC information on the organisms, and the diseases they cause, is unreliable.)

Like most of the Lyme group, the *Ehrlichia* genus is undergoing rapid genetic alteration in response to environmental pressures. Each ehrlichial species has been found to generate multiple genotypes; at least 21 different genetic variants of *E. chaffeensis* have been identified to date. This is beginning to alter how the organisms in this genus are referred to. For example, because of the continuing emergence of new and distinct genotypes among *E. muris* and *E. canis,* some researchers now refer to these species as the *E. muris* group and the *E.canis* group. (A new, possibly human-infectious member of the *E. canis* group, for example, is *Ehrlichia* sp. AvBat discovered in France in 2010.) Because of this, it is probably more accurate to refer to *E. chaffeensis,* as well, as the *E. chaffeensis* group.

The genetic recombination that is occurring among these bacteria and the presence of such a large number of distinct genotypes makes pharmaceutical treatment more difficult and failures more common. (There is a reason they call these second-generation or stealth pathogens.) The *Ehrlichia* are, in fact, a potent emerging pathogenic group and more extensive spread throughout the human community is inevitable. Researchers at Columbia University comment:

> Since that [first report of a human infection in 1987], the number of case reports has grown fairly steadily and currently stands at around 500 per year. Although ehrlichiosis is a nationally reportable disease, reporting is passive, and the true incidence of *Ehrlichia* infection is thus assumed to be significantly higher. This suspicion is bolstered by the high rates of background seroprevalence (~12–15%) in endemic areas, a finding that also indicates that many infections are mild and self-limiting or asymptomatic. (Columbia University Medical Center, n.d.)

In fact, in-depth research indicates that the true incidence is anywhere from 10 to 100 times greater than reported infections. In other words, at minimum 5,000 infections are occurring per year and perhaps as many as 50,000. Since the majority of infections are self-limiting, most people just think they are having a bout of the flu.

The *Anaplasma* Genus

The *Anaplasma* group includes at least eight species: *A. marginale, A. centrale, A. mesaeterum, A. ovis, A. platys, A. bovis, A. caudatum,* and *A. phagocytophilum,* though there are probably many more. (Two unnamed species were recently identified in African elands.) Most of these organisms infect red blood cells (though *A. platys* infects platelets). *A. phagocytophilum,* the primary organism that infects people, instead infects white blood cells, not red.

The other *Anaplasma* species can sometimes infect people (*A. ovis* is an example). These infections are (herbally) treated similarly to babesiosis and with the same pharmaceuticals used for ehrlichiosis, i.e., doxycycline. (And, no, I am not going to deal with these other *Anaplasma* here either.)

As with ehrlichial infections, anaplasmosis is relatively new to physicians. The first case of infection by *A. phagocytophilum* was not encountered until 1990 (in Wisconsin . . . again). While thought at first to be a newly emerging *Ehrlichia* species, after examination the bacteria were found to possess distinct differences. A deeper look found them to be very similar to two known veterinary pathogens, *Ehrlichia equi* and *E. phagocytophila.* After a lot of DNA analysis, the three pathogens were eventually determined to be one organism and combined under one rubric as *Anaplasma phagocytophilum.* Despite its later discovery, cases of anaplasmosis now outnumber those of ehrlichiosis in the United States.

Similarly to the *Ehrlichia,* anaplasmal organisms are undergoing tremendous genetic recombination; over 130 genotypes of *A. marginale* have been described so far. *A. phagocytophilum* also shows a massive tendency to create new genotypes; the bacteria possess a high capacity for genetic diversity.

TRANSMISSION

Both *Ehrlichia chaffeensis* and *Anaplasma phagocytophilum* are transmitted by ticks, most commonly hard ticks. Unfortunately, as with most of the Lyme group, little research has been done on soft ticks (or other arthropods) as a vector. This, it turns out, is in fact a problem, since soft-tick transmission does occur in mammals and, in consequence, may occur in people.

Ehrlichia spp. have been found in soft ticks such as *Argas vespertilionis* (as have various *Borrelia* and *Rickettsia*) and transmission to mammals (bats) has been documented. As Socolovschi et al. (2012) note, "The findings from our study have repercussions for public health in many parts of Europe, Asia, and Africa because *A. vespertilionis* ticks have a wide geographic range and may bite humans." In fact, that species of soft tick, as they comment, "can be highly aggressive toward humans" and infections from soft-tick bites (with symptoms similar to those from the Lyme group) have been documented in people—though no analysis of the infectious agents was performed.

There is emerging evidence that *Ehrlichia* and *Anaplasma* may be transmitted by fleas. Both organisms are commonly found in cats and dogs (up to 60 percent of those tested in some studies) and are widespread in foxes and other wild mammals. Testing of fleas from pathogen-positive species has found them to be infected by both types of bacteria. Studies of dogs and their owners in a number of locations has found that some owners are seropositive for the same *Ehrlichia canis* genotype as that of their dogs, indicating that transmission occurred from the pet to the owner. Whether such transmission is via fleas or direct has not yet been determined. Again, the research on these organisms is very new.

Ehrlichia Transmission

Ehrlichia chaffeensis is, most commonly, transmitted by two tick species in the United States. The first, *Amblyomma americanum,* the Lone Star tick, ranges from west-central Texas, north to Iowa, and eastward in a broad range spanning the southeastern United States. It extends, as well, northward along the Atlantic coast through the coastal areas of New England. These particular ticks are relatively nonspecific in their feeding habits (they bite anything at all when they are hungry) and are, as researchers put it, "notorious" for their aggressive behavior when hungry. Studies in 15 states have found that between 5 and 15 percent of all *A. americanum* ticks tested are positive for ehrlichial bacteria.

Ixodes scapularis, the other major vector, has nearly the same range though it extends farther north into Michigan, Wisconsin, Minnesota, and Canada. *Ixodes* ticks such as this one are common carriers of Lyme-group infections. For example, *Ixodes pacificus* (the Western black-legged tick) is responsible for many of the Lyme-group infections in the western United States while *Ixodes ricinus* (the castor bean tick) spreads the group throughout Europe, Iceland, Russia, North Africa, and the Middle East. All members of this genus carry ehrlichial organisms and can spread the disease.

Nevertheless, ehrlichial tranmission is not limited to that genus; many other species of hard ticks are known to carry the organisms. They have been found throughout the various, most common genera of hard ticks: *Amblyomma, Dermacentor, Haemaphysalis, Hyalomma, Ixodes,* and *Rhipicephalus.* These genera are common worldwide; so is ehrlichiosis.

Ehrlichial organisms have also been transmitted through transfusion and organ transplantation. Blood transfusion transmission is considered to be an increasingly serious problem as the organism is not generally (in 2014) tested for. Eleven percent of blood donors in New York State have tested positive for *Ehrlichia,* as have 3.5 percent in Connecticut, and 0.5 percent in Wisconsin.

Previous infection seems to be the norm throughout Lyme-endemic areas as antibodies to ehrlichial organisms are rather common. Studies have found that 0.4 percent of tested adults in northern California have positive antibodies to ehrlichial organisms, as do 3.4 percent in New York State, and 15 percent in Wisconsin. However, even these figures could be too low, as Ismail et al. (2010) note:

The true incidence of human infection with *E. chaffeensis* is likely to be much higher [than current estimates and studies show], as two-thirds of the infections are either asymptomatic or minimally symptomatic. A seroprevalence study found that 20% of the children residing in endemic areas had detectable antibody to *E. chaffeensis,* without prior history of clinical disease.

Anaplasmal bacteria have been transmitted through a wider range of routes (see below) than are currently known for the ehrlichial. Suspicion exists that these other routes of transmission are occurring for the *Ehrlichia* genus as well.

Anaplasma Transmission

Anaplasma phagocytophilum is most commonly transmitted by *Ixodes scapularis* in the northeast United States; however, as with *Ehrlichia chaffeensis* the range of genera (and species) that can, and do, carry the organism is much broader. Specifically: *Ixodes, Dermacentor, Rhipicephalus, Haemaphysalis,* and *Amblyomma* genera have all been found to harbor the bacteria. (As an aside, similarly to the babesial protozoa, the *A. phagocytophilum* bacteria induce the expression of an antifreeze glycoprotein in all ticks infected by them. This enhances the ticks' ability to survive cold winters.)

In Europe the main vector for *A. phagocytophilum* is *Ixodes ricinus.* In southern Europe, northern Africa, and India it is *Rhipicephalus sanguineus.* In eastern Europe and Asia it is *Ixodes persulcatus. Ixodes pacificus* carries it in the western United States and Canada. And still other species in the genus *Haemaphysalis* carry the bacteria in Japan, India, Russia, China, Korea, Thailand, and North America. Anaplasmal organisms can infect Lone Star ticks but appear to do so with much less frequency than *Ehrlichia.*

As with ehrlichial infections, anaplasmosis is often asymptomatic or merely presents as a minor case of the flu. Studies in Europe have found that up to 15 percent of the general populace have antibodies to the bacteria; on the island of Crete it is 24 percent. Seroprevalence studies in the United States show high rates as well, as much as 15 percent in Wisconsin.

Person-to-person transmission of anaplasmal organisms has been documented: 1) to hospital staff via contact with patient blood; 2) through respiratory secretions to family members; and 3) to hospital patients through blood transfusion and bone marrow transfer. Developing infants in the womb have contracted the disease from their mothers and, in one instance, transmission through breast milk is suspected. Transmission to hunters while cleaning carcasses, via deer blood, is strongly suspected in three cases.

HUMAN INFECTION AND SYMPTOMS

Despite the fact that most genera of hard ticks can carry these organisms, infections in the United States tend to congregate in certain geographic locations. Most human infection with *E. chaffeensis* (commonly known as human monocytic ehrlichiosis or HME) occurs in the south, south-central, and southeast states. Infection with *Anaplasma phagocytophilum* (known as human granulocytic anaplasmosis or HGA) occurs primarily in the northeast and north states. *E. ewingii* infection (known as human ewingii ehrlichiosis or HEE) is, at this point, still relatively rare. (Similarly to *A. phagocytophilum, Ehrlichia ewingii* infects neutrophils rather than monocytes. Treatment would be the same as that for anaplasmosis.) The majority of infections tend to be self-limiting, mimicking a bout of the flu. Onset generally occurs within 5 to 21 days after tick bite. Most people do not seek treatment and the disease tends to clear on its own. A few people develop a relapsing form of the disease or can't clear it and seek medical help. HME and HGA, as researchers comment,

> have similar clinical presentations including fever, headache, leukopenia, thrombocytopenia and elevated liver enzymes. Symptoms typically begin a median of 9 days following tick bite, with the majority of patients seeking medical attention within the first 4 days of treatment. (Ismail et al. 2010)

Still, there are some significant differences. HME is more common in the south and southeast, HGA more common in the typical Lyme-endemic areas of the country. HME is generally a bit more serious; some 48 percent of those infected need hospitalization with around 17 percent experiencing life-threatening complications. More people with HME infections have serious neurological symptoms than those with HGA and it is more commonly fatal (about 3 percent total). Around 36 percent of those with anapasmal infections are hospitalized, and less than 1 percent die. While HGA is, in general, a more benign disease, both HGA and HME can, under some circumstances, progress to a fatal septic shock type of infection.

Once the bacteria enter the host tissues, they are spread by the blood and lymph system throughout the body. Infected cells seek out protected niches in fixed macrophages in numerous sites, including the bone marrow, spleen, lymph nodes, and hepatic sinusoids. There are varying populations also to be found in the meninges, brain, lungs, kidneys, GI tract, and heart.

Infections with either organism can be followed by a subclinical phase that lasts months or even years. The subclinical phase can become chronic, with recurrent mild or severe episodes of the initial primary symptoms.

HME

HME infections are more common throughout the South and Southeast and in Texas, Missouri, Kentucky, Tennessee, North Carolina, and Arkansas. The bacteria actively infect several specific white blood cell types, most commonly monocytes and macrophages, hence the infection's designation as human monocytic ehrlichiosis. Still, the bacteria can infect a much wider range of cells if they wish: lymphocytes, atypical lymphocytes, promyelocytes, metamyelocytes, endothelial cells, eosinophils, and neutrophils. The general symptoms accompanying HME (and their relative percentages in those infected) are:

Fever	97%
Headache	81%
Myalgia	68%
Nausea	48%
Arthralgia	41%
Vomiting	37%
Rash	36%
Cough	26%
Pharyngitis	26%
Diarrhea	25%
Lymphadenopathy	25%
Abdominal pain	22%
Confusion	20%

Chills, shaking, night sweats, and low back pain are commonly reported. Skin eruptions occur more frequently in children than in adults, with around 66 percent exhibiting them. Rashes can be maculopapular (a flat red rash with small raised bumps), petechial (pinpoint round spots—red, brown, or purple—on the skin due to bleeding just under the surface), or a diffuse erythroderma (patchy red blotches with scaling); it is rarely on the face, palms, or soles of the feet. Abdominal pain can sometimes be so severe it mimics appendicitis. Men are more often infected than women (no one knows why, but there is a joke in there somewhere), generally by a 2:1 ratio.

The most frequent neurological problems are meningitis and meningoencephalitis. Around 20 percent of those infected have more extensive central nervous system involvement; in severe cases seizures and coma can occur. Cranial nerve palsy is sometimes reported, almost always after antimicrobial therapy (successful or not—this is one of the common side effects of antibiotics with this disease). Long-term problems in children include cognitive delays, fine motor impairment, and persistent foot drop. In adults, self-reported neurocognitive deficits are moderately common. Delays in treatment are associated with more pulmonary complications, transfer to intensive care, and longer duration of treatment.

During severe disease, interstitial pneumonia, hepatic dysfunction, aseptic meningitis, and hemorrhages can occur. This can lead, in fatal disease, to a toxic shock–like syndrome, severe tissue damage, and ultimately multisystem organ failure. The liver is the most impacted of all the organs, though the spleen, lungs, and kidneys can be similarly impacted.

Severe infections occur most readily in those over 50, those with immune disease (HIV), and those on immunosuppressive drugs. Still, the immunocompetent are frequently reported to experience severe HME. As with most of the Lyme group *the severity of infection is directly proportional to the health of the immune system.*

HGA

Anaplasmal organisms generally infect polymorphonuclear leukocytes (neutrophils), a different type of white blood cell than that infected during HME. These white blood cells have granules or secretory vesicles inside them so they are sometimes referred to as neutrophil granulocytes, hence the disease's designation as human granulocytic anaplasmosis or HGA. (However, the bacteria do infect other cells, e.g., neutrophil and monocyte progenitors in bone marrow such as CD34+ and CD14+ cells, endothelial cells, fibroblasts, eosinophils, and mononuclear phagocytes.) Although infection with these bacteria does occur throughout the United States, it is most common in the upper midwestern and northeastern states and northern California. Most infections are reported in New York, Connecticut, New Jersey, Rhode Island, and Wisconsin (again). Nearly all infections are with one specific species, *Anaplasma phagocytophilum* (though other *Anaplasma* species—an *A. ovis* variant, for example—can sometimes infect people). The symptoms of HGA infections, again, are similar to those of HME:

Fever	97%
Headache	81%
Myalgia	68%
Nausea	48%
Arthralgia	41%
Vomiting	37%
Cough	26%
Pharyngitis	26%
Diarrhea	25%
Lymphadenopathy	25%
Abdominal pain	22%
Confusion	20%
Rash	6%

As with HME, men are much more likely to be infected than women (also again, no one knows why) by a ratio (again) of 2:1 (sexism). The usual symptoms of infection are flu-like, nonspecific febrile illness accompanied by high-grade fever, rigors, generalized myalgias, severe headache, chills, dizziness, malaise, and fatigue. As with ehrlichiosis, leukopenia (low white blood cell count), thrombocytopenia (decreased platelet count, blood does not clot properly, easy bruising), and elevations in transaminases are common during HGA infections. Central nervous system involvement is much less common than with HME (less than 1 percent of those infected); however, peripheral nervous system impacts are often reported. Such peripheral manifestations include brachial plexopathy, cranial nerve palsies, demyelinating polyneuropathy, and bilateral facial nerve palsy. It often takes several months for the conditions to improve. Less common symptoms are anorexia, arthralgias, nausea, unproductive cough, and rash.

During severe infections prolonged fever, hepatitis, cholestasis, myocarditis and cardiomegaly (abnormal enlargement of the heart), interstitial pneumonitis, adult respiratory distress syndrome, acute renal failure, gastrointestinal bleeding, rhabdomyolysis (muscle cell destruction), respiratory insufficiency, intravascular coagulation, seizures, and coma have all been noted. In fatal disease a toxic shock–like syndrome occurs, accompanied by severe tissue damage and ultimately multisystem organ failure. The bone marrow, red blood cells, liver, spleen and lymph system, and lungs are the most commonly impacted organs and tissues.

As with HME, severe infections occur most readily in those over 50, those with immune disease (HIV), and those on immunosuppressive drugs. Still, the immunocompetent are frequently reported to experience severe infections of HME. As with most of the Lyme group *the severity of infection is directly proportional to the health of the immune system.*

DIAGNOSIS

Diagnosis of HME and HGA is often difficult due to the relative newness of the organisms to physicians—misdiagnosis is common. Both conditions generally present at early onset with fever, headache, myalgia, and malaise. The usual flu-like symptom picture.

Despite the commonness of misdiagnosis, both HME *and* HGA infections possess a fairly unique, and rather definitive, profile, specifically: 90 percent of infections show elevated AST and 84 percent elevated ALT. Thrombocytopenia occurs in 73 percent, leukopenia in 72 percent, and anemia in 55 percent.

In other words, if a patient presents with flu-like symptoms accompanied by two or more of elevated liver enzymes, thrombocytopenia, leukopenia, and anemia, differential diagnosis indicates either HGA or HME.

Among children a mild hyponatremia (low sodium levels in the blood) occurs in around 50 percent.

Acute infections can be accompanied by a number of abnormalities depending on the organ involved. Specifically: increased creatinine, lactate dehydrogenase, creatine phosphokinase, and amylase levels; electrolyte abnormalities such as hypocalcemia, hypomagnesemia, and hypophosphatemia; prolonged prothrombin times; increased levels of fibrin degradation products; metabolic acidosis; hypotension; disseminated intravascular coagulopathy; adrenal insufficiency; myocardial dysfunction; and hepatic and renal failure.

The clinical symptoms for hospitalization include immune impairment, pain requiring management, confusion, abnormal spinal fluid, infiltrates on chest radiographs, hypotension, shock, or acute organ failure.

As an initial diagnostic finding, history of tick exposure is often inconclusive since many people don't notice the tick bite. And other than initial flu-like symptoms, early infection has few signs. As well, a reliance on residence in an endemic area is inconclusive and should not be definitively relied upon. Infection can occur in nearly every state in the United States. Hence . . .

It is malpractice for a physician to definitively state that a person cannot possibly be infected with a pathogen from the Lyme group because of where they live, especially if this is followed by the physician's refusal to test after testing is specifically requested. Unfortunately, scores of people report having had this experience with their physicians. Most of them subsequently suffered years of progressively worsening illness that could have been avoided by competent medical care.

A note to those who are ill: remember, **you** *are paying them, they are not paying you. In other words, physicians, despite their reluctance to recognize the fact, work for you; you do not work for them. You are not lucky to have gotten an appointment, they are lucky that you made one. You are the one that is ill; they are there to serve you and they need to be reminded of that, every* *day of their careers. Do not allow them to redefine the relationship otherwise.*

TESTING

The most common diagnostic tests are the following.

Blood Smears

Microscopic examination of Wright's, Diff-Quik, or Giemsa stains of peripheral blood smears. These look for dark staining morulae (bacterial inclusions) within either monocytes and neutrophils. Unfortunately, very low bacterial burdens are common during these infections. In many instances only 0.1 to 0.2 percent of cells may be infected, which would demand the inspection of 500 to 1,000 cells to find one containing the bacteria. As Thomas, Dumler, and Carlyon (2009) comment:

> A limitation of this assay is that it requires a well-trained microscopist. For instance, prolonged examination is often required to accurately detect *A. phagocytophilum* morulae, as they can be present in less than 0.1% of neutrophils.

Determination of the presence of infection relies on the microscopist. However, they often miss the inclusions, not only because of low parasite density, but also because the inclusions are similar to many common intracellular inclusions and blood smear artifacts. This can include such things as crystal stain artifacts, bacterial contamination of the stain solutions, Döhle bodies, and toxic granulation and platelets overlying leukocytes. As Dawson et al. (2001) comment, "These obligate intracellular bacteria are extremely difficult to detect upon routine examination of blood smears or hematoxylin and eosin (HE)-stained tissues." As they continue, "We often failed to identify morulae unequivocally in HE-stained sections where antigen, as determined by IHC, was abundant. Therefore, routine HE staining should not be used to exclude a diagnosis."

Sensitivity for this approach to testing is highest during the first week of infection—again a problem, as symptoms may not show for up to three weeks.

PCR Assay

PCR assay runs 60 to 85 percent effective for ehrlichial organisms and 70 to 90 percent accurate for anaplasmal. This is the best test for both HME and HGA. Unfortunately, there is a limited availability of rapid diagnostic tests such as PCR for these diseases so many physicians do not utilize it.

Serological Testing (IFA)

Serological testing (IFA) for antibodies is a common testing approach, but both IgG and IgM are negative in as many as 80 percent of people during the first week of infection. As Dawson et al. (2001) comment, "Many, if not most, *E. chaffeensis*-infected patients who present early in the course of the disease may be missed by serologic methods due to lack of detectable antibody." Additionally, there is a fairly high rate of false positives, usually from cross-reactive antibodies. Failure to seroconvert occurs in a number of instances due to immune impairment. Early treatment with tetracyclines can abrogate the antibody responses.

Immunohistochemistry (IHC)

Immunohistochemistry or IHC is a rarely used test (for these bacteria) that acts to detect antigens in cells in tissue sections. It looks for antibodies that are bound to antigens in tissues. IHC is, in fact, a very good diagnostic test for both anaplasmal and ehrlichial infections. As Dawson et al. (2001) comment,

> All tissue blocks from all cases were positive for IHC, establishing the IHC technique as a sensitive diagnostic tool. Similarly, a recently published IHC study demonstrated that the granulocytotropic ehrlichiosis agent infects many tissues. The greatest number

of [them] were seen in the spleen, lung, and liver [and bone marrow]. . . . *E. chaffeensis* antigens were consistently seen in mononuclear phagocytotic cells in the spleen, lymph nodes, bone marrow, lung, and liver."

Tissue samples from the spleen, lymph nodes, bone marrow, and liver are, as they note, "excellent tissues for confirmation" of infection by these agents.

The most effective diagnostic approach is differential diagnosis accompanied by all four tests.

TREATMENT

Ehrlichial and anaplasmal bacteria are resistant to most antibiotics: aminoglycosides (gentamicin), fluoroquinolones (cipro), beta-lactams (penicillins), macrolides and ketolides (erythromycin and telithromycin), and sulfa-containing drugs (co-trimoxazole). They do respond well to tetracyclines, especially doxycycline (100 mg 2x daily for 10 to 14 days, or 30 days, or for 3 days postfever according to various sources). Note: Ehrlichial bacteria have been reisolated from both blood and tissues in animals after doxycycline treatment that was of too short a duration, i.e., less than 14 days. This is why a number of journal papers now recommend a minimum of 30 days of treatment with at least 3 days of postfever intake.

If doxycycline can't be used, rifampin (300 mg 2x daily for 10 to 14 days, or 30 days, or 3 days postfever, same sources) is an effective alternative. Chloramphenicol has also been used successfully in a few cases despite the fact that in vitro testing appears to show it to be ineffective. Levofloxacin has shown effectiveness in vitro but mixed results in practice. Its use in at least one case merely suppressed the bacteria; it did not clear them. Some evidence exists that a combination of doxycycline and chloroquine stimulates a much more rapid and healthier recovery from infection. Paclitaxel has also been found to be active in preventing monocyte penetration by ehrlichial species.

Note: Corticosteroid treatment during undiagnosed HME or those subsequently infected by the bacteria is associated with a much greater risk of mortality. There is also some evidence that infection with either of these organisms concomitant with statin use may, in some circumstances, stimulate rhabdomyolysis-induced acute kidney injury.

6

Ehrlichia and Anaplasma

A Deeper Look

Ehrlichia are able to repress genes that are critical for induction of host innate immune responses.

H. STEVENSON, "EHRLICHIA"

Ehrlichia and Anaplasma multiply within endosomes ultimately reprogramming host cell defense mechanisms and processes in order to facilitate their survival.

N. ISMAIL, K. C. BLOCH, AND J. W. McBRIDE, "HUMAN EHRLICHIOSIS AND ANAPLASMOSIS"

Ehrlichiosis manifests as an undifferentiated febrile illness that is difficult to diagnose, and delayed treatment can lead to serious complications and poor prognosis. There are no vaccines for human rickettsial diseases including ehrlichiosis, and therapeutic options are limited. The rapid growth in antibiotic resistance among microbes suggests that a potential for ineffective antibiotics for ehrlichial and rickettsial infections exists in the future. The lack of broader therapeutic options is complicated by the fact that there are no effective vaccines available to prevent disease in susceptible populations.

J. W. McBride and D. H. Walker,
"Molecular and Cellular Pathobiology
of *Ehrlichia* Infection: Targets for New
Therapeutics and Immunomodulation Strategies"

A disparity exists between the small number of organisms in tissues and the relatively larger number of pathologic lesions induced, especially in the liver where occasional hepatocytes undergo cell death without evidence for ehrlichial infection or accompanying inflammation. These findings suggest that infected cells that are released into the peripheral circulation adhere to endothelial cell or vascular surfaces, usually in peripheral capillary beds. The presence of ehrlichiae or ehrlichia-mediated modifications to the infected cells induce localized inflammatory responses.

H. Lepidi, J. E. Bunnell, M. E. Martin, et al.,
"Comparative Pathology and Immunohistology
Associated with Clinical Illness after
Ehrlichia phagocytophila-Group Infections"

Ehrlichiosis and anaplasmosis are part of a large group of worldwide emerging diseases that are becoming more prevalent every year, primarily due to ecological dysregulation. New forms, even new species, of the initiating organisms are emerging into the human population and causing disease. Here is a deeper look at what they do in the body.

THE PREFERRED CELLULAR HABITAT OF EHRLICHIA AND ANAPLASMA

These two closely related organisms are small, intracellular Gram-negative bacteria that cannot exist outside host cells, hence their designation as "obligately" intracellular bacteria. In essence, they are "obligated" for their survival to their host cells. While they can, and sometimes do, infect a number of different cell types (lymphocytes, atypical lymphocytes, endothelial cells, hematopoietic stem cells, promyelocytes, metamyelocytes, and neutrophils, as examples) *Ehrlichia* bacteria prefer what are called mononuclear phagocytes while *Anaplasma* prefer neutrophils.

"Mononuclear" is a descriptive for the ehrlichial organisms' cellular habitat because the cells possess one large round nucleus. They are "phagocytes" because they engulf other cells (*phago* being "eat" and *cyte* meaning "vessel" or cell). These particular cells are white blood cells (a.k.a., leukocytes) and are part of the innate immune system. "Innate" here means the capacities of this part of the immune system were already programmed in at our birth.

The innate system, developed over long evolutionary time, is what responds to an organism's initial encounters with pathogens and/or cellular damage. This is a broad-spectrum response; it is not specific. After birth, living beings develop a secondary, or adaptive, form of immune response. Rather than a general response, it is oriented to deal with specific pathogens. When a pathogen is encountered, identified, and analyzed, a very specific molecular response is crafted to deal with it. Every successful response then becomes part of the memory store of immune events that the organism experiences during its life span. It works something like this . . .

When a pathogen enters the body, the innate system uses evolutionarily developed memory patterns to respond. It looks for any expression of a large number of foundational patterns that are common to all pathogens and/or cellular damage (such as trauma). Once a pattern is identified, automatic, general responses to pathogens are initiated. Among these responses is the identification of the exact pathogen involved and the creation of specific chemical strategies to deal with it.

The creation of these specific responses is what is called the adaptive system. This part of our immune response creates specific antibodies to the pathogen. It is a narrow-spectrum, engineered response. This event is then held as memory in the adaptive immune system. If that pathogen is encountered again, the immune response is already programmed with the most effective response. Many times this prevents that particular pathogenic illness from recurring. This is, in fact, the reason that vaccinations work the way they do. They create a memory that the adaptive immune system later uses to prevent illness from specific pathogens. (And yes, some vaccinations are useful, some are not very useful, and some cause terrible side effects, but I am not going to go into that here.)

MONOCYTES AND MACROPHAGES

Monocytes are the largest of the leukocytes and make up anywhere from 2 to 10 percent of all the white blood cells in our bodies. Their primary function, in response to any kind of inflammation stimulus in the body (including bacterial infections), is to translocate to the site of the infection, defend the body, and correct any damage that has occurred.

Monocytes can directly attack pathogens themselves or they can transform into other types of white blood cells such as macrophages and dendritic cells. Macrophages and dendritic cells have expanded capacities, allowing them to counter infection and damage through a number of mechanisms unavailable to monocytes.

Monocytes are created in the bone marrow from precursor cells, a kind of specialized stem cells called monoblasts (hematopoietic stem cells). Once created, monoblasts circulate in the bloodstream for a few days, then sequester themselves in various organs in the body, awaiting immune stimulation in order to act. Half of the body's monocytes, for instance, are stored in the red pulp of the spleen. (This is why the spleen is often inflamed during infections; a substantial number of responses to pathogens occurs there.) Monocytes and their offspring—macrophages and dendritic cells—act as immune agents by utilizing a number of mechanisms: phagocytosis, antigen presentation, and cytokine production.

Phagocytosis is the process of encapsulating or vacuolizing (engulfing) an invading pathogen inside an immune cell. This sequesters the pathogen from the rest of the body, preventing it from doing harm. Once vacuolized, the immune cell can direct any of a number of molecular killing agents (nitric oxide is an important one) into the vacuole to kill the microbe. Once killed, the pathogen is "digested" by the white blood cell. In other words, the pathogen is reduced to simpler cellular and molecular fragments. Many of these fragments possesses molecular signatures unique to the pathogen they came from. So some of these fragments are transferred to the white blood cell's membrane surface, where they are used as antigens. That is, they are used as a kind of cellular memory cue about the pathogen. This stimulates the production and release of T cells (part of the adaptive immune system), which then use that molecular pattern to actively seek out the pathogen in order to destroy it. These T cells act somewhat like predator drones that circulate through the system, seeking out and killing specific invading pathogens.

There are a number of different T cells (a.k.a. T lymphocytes): helper, cytotoxic, memory, regulatory, natural killer (NK), mucosal associated invariant, and gamma delta (for instance). Each performs different functions in a healthy immune system. T cells mature in the thymus (hence "T" cell—the guys in the nineteenth century who named these things . . . they had a limited articulation capacity and a very narrow view). T cells can also be created from precursor stem cells in the bone marrow—the same ones that create monoblasts, i.e., hematopoietic stem cells (cells that *Ehrlichia* and *Anaplasma* can also infect).

The younger the thymus is, the more effective it is at T-cell creation. As people age the thymus decreases in size (about 3 percent a year); this is one of the reasons why older people have poorer immune function—the thymus just gets worn out. One of the terms for this is immune senescence; it's one of the primary factors enabling more serious ehrlichial and anaplasmal infections. It is why these bacteria usually cause more damaging disease in people over 50.

T cells become activated once antigens are presented on the surface of monocytes (or their offspring). This tells the T cells that they are needed and what they are looking for. They then hunt down the pathogens and kill them. (They can't be bargained with; they don't feel pity, or remorse, or fear. And they absolutely will not stop, ever, until what they are looking for is dead. . . . We really shouldn't be artificially programing them in labs—didn't those guys ever see the movie?)

The monocytes (and macrophages and dendritic cells) also release small messenger molecules that stimulate (or inhibit) certain kinds of inflammation in the body in order to regulate bodily infection, damage, and repair.

These messenger molecules are given a variety of names—cytokines, chemokines, and variously named proteins and adhesion molecules, for example—though I think of them all as cytokines. (The rationality police are often upset by this.)

These are the molecules, especially with Lyme-group infections, that cause the troubling symptoms that can occur during many stealth pathogen diseases. They occur because the pathogens have learned to use cytokines for their own purposes; they have learned how to hijack the immune system and to modulate its behavior in very specific ways. Their sophisticated use of cytokines facilitates their entry into the body and enables the breaking apart of host cells. This gives them access to the nutrients they need and facilitates their reproduction.

It is in the interventive re-modulating of these molecules'
behaviors via the sophisticated use of plant medicines
that the most effective treatment for the Lyme group of
infections can occur. Interrupting the cytokine cascade
interferes with pathogen entry into cells and denies the
bacteria the nutrients they need to survive. This reduces,
even eliminates, symptoms, helps the body repair
itself, and, in many instances, also eliminates
the pathogens from the body.

Dendritic cells (DCs) act as what are known as sentinel cells. They mostly concentrate in bodily locations that touch the outside world: GI tract, lungs, skin, and so on. They are also strongly present in the lymph system, especially during infections. Generally, DCs exist in an immature state in the body; they mature or transform only when they encounter a pathogen. Immature DCs are constantly analyzing their surrounding environment, searching for pathogens, using very old evolutionarily developed pattern recognition systems to do so. They look for certain kinds of molecules that nearly all pathogens have incorporated into their cellular membrane. This works well because most microbes, over time, learned to use similar molecules to get inside host tissues. To identify these molecular patterns, DCs use what are called pattern recognition receptors (PRRs). A PRR is a kind of software program that constantly searches for matches to the pattern it is specific for. (One major PRR is what is called a toll-like receptor, or TLR.) Once a PRR recognizes a pathogenic molecule, a unique cascade of immune responses is immediately initiated. Normally, this includes the production of various messenger molecules—cytokines, chemokines, or various proteins and adhesion molecules—all of which have specific actions in the body.

An immature dendritic cell that finds a match to any of its PRRs becomes what is known as an activated or mature DC. Like monocytes, DCs can engulf (or phagocytose) pathogens, destroy them, and upload pathogen cell fragments to their cellular membranes. Activated DCs then migrate to the lymph nodes, where they stimulate (in the spleen and lymph system) T and B immune-cell generation and activity.

> *Rather than being reductively located in one place, the spleen and lymph system (including such organs as the appendix and the bone marrow) are part of a larger organ that is spread throughout the body. It is a form of swarm intelligence that, despite being in multiple locations, makes up one organ, something we call the immune system. The nineteenth-century view of the body that we have inherited is, as is increasingly understood, incorrect. This is why utilizing that model in the training of contemporary healers is creating such poor outcomes. The appendix, for example, is **not** a vestigial organ and never has been. It is a functional and crucial part of the immune system. Because they understand this, Chinese physicians are able to treat most cases of appendicitis without surgery.*

The activation of T cells occurs because activated DCs upregulate certain kinds of molecules to the surface of their cells, e.g., CD80, CD86, and CD40 proteins. These CD proteins, once they emerge onto the surface of a cell, act as powerful stimulants for T-cell activation and production.

> *CD is an acronym for the term "cluster of differentiation" (or "designation" according to some). It refers to the various kinds of surface molecules or proteins that can be found on immune cells. CD57, for instance, is a surface molecule that is upregulated on certain T cells (specifically natural killer or NK cells) during specific kinds of infections. NK cells with that CD protein on their surface are particularly effective*

against Lyme spirochetes. Hence bodily levels of that CD
molecule can be used as a testing marker for immune
strength against Lyme infection. Over 350 CD cells have
been identified in the human immune system so far. All
of them have unique actions.

Macrophages act similarly to dendritic and monocytic cells. They phagocytose pathogens, then present antigens on their cellular surface to stimulate T-cell activation. Macrophages are particularly good at digesting pathogens and dead or dying cells. They can digest more than a hundred of them before they die.

Like monocytes, activated macrophages produce a variety of cytokines, chemokines, and proteins, depending on what has activated them. Among them are the interleukin-1 (IL-1) supergroup, a family of 11 different cytokines. This group of cytokines is strongly involved in creating inflammation in the body (among the symptoms of which is fever); IL-1α and IL-1β are two of the strongest. Other important ones are IL-12 and IL-18. These stimulate natural killer and other T cells to release interferon-gamma (IFN-γ), a powerful element of the immune response.

Macrophages are also unique in that they act to metabolize (or change) the amino acid L-arginine into either nitric oxide (NO) or L-ornithine. (If the NO pathway is suppressed, L-ornithine is automatically generated.) NO is a potent antimicrobial, often expressed as a gaseous burst, that is used to kill pathogens in the body. L-ornithine, on the other hand, is a kind of repair molecule. It stimulates the production of polyamines (and collagen) that the body uses to repair damage to tissues. (Babesial parasites suppress the NO pathway to avoid NO and then utilize the L-ornithine that is subsequently created to help foster their replication.)

Macrophages also act as the body's scavengers, phagocytosing and thus removing dead or dying cells and other debris from the system. During early stages of inflammation, for example, there is a clustering of large numbers of neutrophil granulocytes at the inflamed site.

These have to be removed, usually by macrophages, once their function is accomplished. (It is these white blood cells, the neutrophils, that *Anaplasma* infect. The bacteria activate and utilize neutrophils' innate clustering response to foster continued infection of the body.)

NEUTROPHILS

Neutrophils, comprising 40 to 75 percent of all white blood cells, are the most abundant white blood cells in the body. They are one of the first responders to pathogens or traumatic damage to the body's tissues. They follow chemical signals through the blood, then move through interstitial tissue (if necessary) to the site of the damaged tissues. Pus is primarily composed of dead neutrophils; it is removed from the body by macrophages.

> *Organs that are severely damaged by ehrlichial and anaplasmal infections are filled with pockets of pus that the body is not able to remove. These abscesses in the organs are often accompanied by other, non-neutrophil, immune cells, i.e., inflammatory aggregates, that have infiltrated that location. Healthy cells surrounding these areas often continue to die whether there are bacteria present or not, something called focal necrosis.*

Cytokines—such as IL-8, which is released by various cells in the body during infection and damage—signal neutrophils to translocate to the site where they are needed. Once they arrive, the neutrophils analyze the nature of the problem, then release their own unique spectrum of cytokines designed to respond to that exact kind of problem.

Neutrophils are short lived, lasting between two and five days. Once they reach senescence, whether they were used to fight infection or not, they are ingested by macrophages. At sites of infection, after neutrophil ingestion is completed, the macrophages release growth factors that act in very specific ways to heal the damaged area. The growth factors generate new blood vessels, new endothelial cells, and more of the extracellular matrix that surrounds the cells.

Not only do macrophages move through the blood, but large numbers of them are what are known as fixed macrophages. These remain in specific locations: lungs, liver, kidneys, brain, bone marrow, spleen, and the connective tissues. There, they actively work to protect the organs/locations from pathogens. (When these macrophages are activated by the cytokines that stealth pathogens create, they can cause powerful inflammatory impacts in the organs in which they are located. This is the cause of the severe organ injury that can occur during acute ehrlichial and anaplasmal infections.)

EHRLICHIAL AND ANAPLASMAL PENETRATION OF TARGET CELLS

When these bacteria are first ingested by a tick (during feeding on a host), they immediately travel to the tick midgut. There they alter form and immediately translocate again, infecting the tick's salivary glands. This positions them for insertion into a new host via tick saliva during tick feeding.

The bacteria remain in the ticks during every stage of their development (three stages usually), but unlike babesial parasites they don't appear to infect tick ovaries. This means that they are not passed down through the generations via egg laying. (And yes, despite many medical websites asserting the opposite, some Lyme-group pathogens are present in tick larvae when they hatch from eggs.) Because they are not transovarially transmitted, *Ehrlichia* and *Anaplasma* have to infect new hosts before the ticks die after their final stage of development. (To facilitate this, the organisms create and systemically release a kind of antifreeze that helps the ticks remain active during freezing temperatures. This means that tick bites can occur in the winter and yes, the bacteria have no mercy. They don't even care about Christmas.)

Both *Anaplasma* and *Ehrlichia* bacteria continually alternate between two poles of a biphasic developmental cycle. That is, they transition between two distinct morphological forms (called dense-cored and reticulate) that perform different and distinct roles. Dense-cored organisms possess electron-dense nucleoids, a.k.a. nucleoli (hard to see into—hence their name), which are very small, and have a somewhat ruffled exterior membrane. The reticulate forms have larger nucleiods (this is a funnier word than nucleoli), thus electron microscopes can see within them. They are pleomorphic (can alter their shape and size in response to environmental perturbations), are generally larger than the dense forms, and have outer membranes that are relatively smooth.

The dense-cored forms of these bacteria are strongly adherent to their preferred cells and highly infectious. However, the bacteria cannot replicate when in this form. (The dense-cored form can be thought of as a kind of encysted or seedlike form of the bacteria.) This is the bacterial form that flows into the bloodstream of new hosts along with injected tick saliva.

Again, large numbers of tick salival compounds actively downregulate the normal, innate immune response of the host, allowing the bacteria to more easily find and infect their target cells. This is why infection via tick bite (versus needle injection, for example) results in an infection of longer duration. The Lyme-pathogen modulation of the host immune system is highly synergistic with the tick salival compounds. Infection that occurs in the presence of tick salival compounds, for instance, promotes the growth of significantly more bacterial pathogens in the spleen, and for longer time periods, than that which occurs if the bacteria are needle-injected into a host. As well, host immune responses to tick-injected bacteria are much slower.

The dense-cored ehrlichial organisms predominate during the first 24 hours of infection. They actively search for free monocytes in the blood and, once found, adhere to them using extremely powerful chemical bonding agents. Anaplasmal organisms engage in an identical process, but their dense-cored forms search for neutrophils rather than monocytes.

Once attached to the host cells, the bacteria utilize those cells' natural engulfment or vacuolization processes for their own ends. (They trick them. Like a fisherman, they get their trust, then abuse it.) This allows the bacteria to gain access to the interior of the cell—which is what they need to do in order to reproduce. Once inside the cellular compartment or vacuole

Also, sometimes, referred to as a morula, which comes from the Latin root morum, *meaning mulberry. Why? Because they look like mulberries, of course—at least they did to people in the nineteenth century, though I am not sure anyone else has ever seen a mulberry.*

they deactivate the cells' normal microbial killing processes and, as well, stop the infected cells' natural death (apoptosis) process. By 48 hours postinfection, the dense forms have transitioned into reticulate forms so they can reproduce. (They reproduce by fission, i.e., without intercourse, i.e., taxonomist sex). Reproduction and the subsequent transformation of the offspring back into dense-cored forms takes another 24 hours.

During reproduction, the reticulate forms create new vacuoles for their children in order to protect them from the cell. Each vacuole contains widely varying numbers of bacteria, as few as one bacterium to as many as a hundred. Once the white blood cell is filled with bacteria-containing vacuoles the cell bursts open, releasing the vacuoles into the bloodstream. Once outside the cells, the vacuoles open, releasing the new bacteria into the bloodstream, where they immediately begin to seek out new host cells. (*Only* dense-core forms can be found extracellularly in the bloodstream. The dense-core forms are hardier and can survive the extracellular environment while the reticulate forms cannot.)

An alternative process of bacterial release also occurs simultaneously: a few of the vacuoles exit

the host cell by opening a doorway in the cellular
membrane—exocytosis.

For *Ehrlichia* bacteria, the entire process takes 72 hours. Thus, new waves of infection occur in the host every 72 hours or so in a continual, repeating cycle. This repetitive cycle is why some people experience an oscillation of worsening then lessening then worsening symptoms throughout the course of their illness. Just to make things more difficult, each new generation of bacteria possess differences in their outer membrane proteins. That is, new genetic variants are continually created every time the bacteria reproduce. This interferes with the ability of the host immune system to clear the infection (and reduces the effectiveness of pharmaceuticals). By the time immune cells have uploaded bacterial antigenic markers to their cellular membranes, the bacteria have altered those exact genetic markers on *their* cellular membranes.

Anaplasma bacteria, while nearly identical in their reproductive processes, utilize a shorter timeline. Once inside the white blood cell, the dense forms spend four to eight hours transitioning into reticulate forms to enable reproduction (by taxonomist sex as well). Anaplasmal reproduction takes around 24 hours, then the organisms again alter their form over the next 4 to 12 hours, becoming dense-cored once more. When this process is completed, the bacteria burst open the cell and enter the bloodstream. New waves of anaplasmal infection occur every 32 to 36 hours on a continual cycle, about twice as fast as the ehrlichial.

During early infection, both bacteria actively manipulate host genes involved in three areas of pathogen response. First, they suppress the expression of the cellular cytokines that are normally released during an early innate immune response, specifically IL-12, IL-15, and IL-18. Second, they upregulate NF-κB (nuclear factor kappa-B) and apoptosis inhibitors in order to enhance the infected host cell's survival. Third, they inhibit the transcription of genes in the nucleus of their host cell. This allows them to take over its cellular functions so that they can reproduce. They are very sophisticated at it.

Normally, once bacteria, inside a vacuole, are engulfed by an immune cell, the cell releases antimicrobial agents to kill the encapsulated pathogen. However, these bacteria can inhibit the microbial killing activity of the cell. They then extensively remodel the vacuole within which they exist, making it a perfect habitat for them rather than a holding cell in which they are incarcerated. The bacteria also manipulate the host cell membrane traffic to divert incoming nutrients to the vacuole (keeping it away from the cell) in order to foster replication. They hijack the nutrients the cell needs to live and use them for themselves. Both anaplasmal and ehrlichial bacteria are highly dependent on iron as a nutrient. So they strongly increase ferritin levels via the upregulation of transferrin receptors in the vacuoles. This pulls iron, an essential nutrient, into the vacuoles where they can use it for replication. (One of the ways IFN-γ counteracts infections is to downregulate transferrin receptors, thus reducing the iron pathogens can access during infections. This is also why IFN-γ levels are immediately inhibited by these bacteria as soon as they enter the host body.) The bacteria also alter host cell signaling, in essence interrupting the normal molecular (cytokine) linguistics the cell would use to tell the body what is happening to it. They, in fact, create an entirely different communicatory cascade; they control the conversation.

> *There is nothing wrong with your television set. Do not attempt to adjust the picture. We are controlling transmission. If we wish to make it louder, we will bring up the volume. If we wish to make it softer, we will tune it to a whisper. We will control the horizontal. We will control the vertical. We can roll the image or make it flutter. We can change the focus to a soft blur or sharpen it to crystal clarity.*

They, in fact, alter the entire chemical communication that normally occurs in the body. Increasing some chemical communications to high intensity, lowering others to nearly nothing. This disturbance of the body's chemical linguistics is what causes many of the symptoms of the disease. Through this chemical control, the organisms also delay the death of the infected cell. This allows them their continued habitation within it.

Cell death, a.k.a. apoptosis, is one of the primary ways that host cells kill invading pathogens. Many microbes have, therefore, developed methods to delay or even permanently prevent apoptosis. Over time this can create a number of serious problems; most especially it results in the host body having a large number of what are in essence dead cells within it, cells that are not being allowed to die. This creates a cascade of necrotic events, including, sometimes, the formation of particular kinds of cancers. Decades-long mycoplasma infections, for example, are now known to lead to various forms of cancer. Cancer cells are, after all, cells that do not die when they are supposed to.

Once infection is established in a new host, a variety of bacterial forms can be found inside the white blood cells. Some 42 percent of the infected cells will harbor only dense forms, 38 percent will contain reticulate forms, and 20 percent will contain both. During an ehrlichial infection, about 18 percent of the vacuoles in infected cells will be found inside the nucleus of white blood cells. This gives the bacteria access to the cells' nucleus (through carefully managed portals in the vacuoles), where they can actively control cellular function and processes. Once at the nucleus, the bacteria release compounds that target a variety of specific genes in the DNA structure of the cell. These compounds are powerful DNA-binding proteins such as ankyrin repeat–containing protein p200 and tandem repeat protein 120 (TRP120).

TRP120 switches on certain genes in the DNA structure that cause it to upregulate a specific cascade of inflammatory cytokines, e.g., CCL2, CCL20, and CXCL11. CCL2 (also known as monocyte chemoattractant protein 1, MCP-1) actively recruits monocytes, memory T cells, and dendritic cells to the sites of inflammation. This, in essence, brings monocytes within range of infected cells, allowing easier access to new host cells when bacterial reproduction is complete. CCL20 (also known as macrophage inflammatory protein 3, MIP-3) is strongly attractive for lymphocytes and dendritic cells whenever it appears. When *Ehrlichia* infect macrophages inside organs, the emergence of MIP-3 attracts strongly inflammatory immune cells to that location. This is one of the causes of the necrotic damage that can occur in the organs. This cytokine-initiated inflammation is most strongly impactive on the liver, spleen, appendix, lungs, and to some extent the GI tract. (GI tract impacts are the source of the difficult GI tract pain that these bacteria sometimes cause.) CXCL11 is strongly attractive for activated T cells and is most powerfully expressed in the liver, pancreas, spleen, and lungs, again leading to cytokine inflammatory damage in those organs.

The activation of these cytokines—and their subsequent activation of a variety of other immune cells—stimulates the production of a cascade of very specific cytokines (the bacterial cytokine signature). The bacteria utilize this cascade to modulate the host immune response to infection and to alter host cells in order to facilitate reproduction and gather nutrients. Again, this is the source of many of the symptoms people experience, as well as much of the damage to organ systems in the body by these pathogens. These dynamics are also highly involved in the eventual development of sepsis and septic shock when the infections become acute and self-reinforcing.

The ankyrin repeat–containing protein p200, another DNA-modulating compound, affects genes involved in transcription, apoptosis, ATPase activity, nucleus structural proteins, and membrane-bound organelles. It also activates nuclear genes that strongly upregulate tumor necrosis factor alpha (TNF-α), STAT1, and CD48. TNF-α is a primary inflammatory cytokine in the body and is strongly involved in the regulation of immune cells. It is one of the major cytokines the bacteria dysregulate to produce their effects in the body. STAT1 (a.k.a. signal transducer and activator of transcription 1) is involved in the regulation of the growth, survival, and differentiation of cells. Activation of

STAT1 leads to inhibition of apoptosis, increased blood vessel formation, and specific kinds of immunosuppression. Among other immune
impacts, interferon response in the body becomes dysregulated when
STAT1 is upregulated. CD48, once activated on the surface of monocytes (or other immune cells), stimulates the emergence and activity
of still other immune cells. Importantly, it also is deeply involved in
the modulation of lipids (and lipid rafts) such as cholesterol, which the
ehrlichial pathogens need to survive. The bacteria utilize this to help
them form membrane lipids for their vacuoles, to incorporate the cholesterol into their cell walls, and to subvert the normal vacuole process
that utilizes lipid rafts for cellular engulfment.

Ehrlichia and *Anaplasma* bacteria can't make their own cholesterol.
They have to scavenge it from their hosts. This is why high-cholesterol
diets during these infections have been found to facilitate bacterial
infection and significantly increase parasite density in the spleen, liver,
and blood. Switching to a low-cholesterol diet during infection by either
of these pathogens is a good idea.

Both bacteria also have strong impacts on cellular mitochondria.
Anaplasmal and ehrlichial bacteria are *very* close relatives of mitochondria, which supply much of the power generation in our cells. During
infection, the mitochondria of the invaded cells are drawn to the
bacteria-filled vacuoles and away from the nuclei of the immune cells.
There, they come into direct contact with the vacuole membranes. The
bacteria open portals in vacuoles and begin releasing compounds into
the mitochondria. These serve to stabilize the mitochondria through
a number of mechanisms: upregulation of apoptosis inhibitors BFL-1,
Bcl-2, IER-3, and BIRC-3; inhibition of apoptosis inducers BIK and
BNIP3L; maintenance of mitochondrial membrane potential; and inhibition of caspase-3 activation. (Caspase-3 is highly active in stimulating cell death, i.e. apoptosis.) In essence the Bcl-2 group is upregulated
and Bax is downregulated. (The Bcl-2 protein interferes with apoptosis,
while the closely related Bax protein increases it. Bcl-2 and Bax normally
exist in a modulated balance, annotated as the Bax/Bcl-2 ratio.) This

delays apoptosis of the mitochondria and thus interferes with one of the primary ways host cells generate apoptosis. (Mitochondria in infected cells are strongly motivated to stimulate cellular death as a mechanism to stop pathogenic infections.) Remodulation of Bax/Bcl-2, i.e., upregulating Bax and downregulating Bcl-2, has been found to reverse this process and increase apoptosis in affected cells. (Herbs and supplements useful for this are *Artemisia* spp., *Glycyrrhiza* spp., *Goniothalamus cheliensis, Gynostemma pentaphyllum, Houttuynia* spp., *Leonurus cardiaca, Rhodiola* spp., *Scutellaria* spp., and the isolated constituents arctigenin, beta-sitosterol, and curcumin.)

The bacterially affected mitochondria stop synthesizing DNA, mitochondrial metabolism is inhibited, and the energy they normally produce falls sharply. The mitochondria, in a sense, become dormant and enter a kind of hibernation where they no longer can perform their normal functions. This helps the bacteria because dormant mitochondria cannot initiate apoptosis and cannot compete with the bacteria for nutrients. Unfortunately for us, once the mitochondria begin to be inhibited, cellular energy production lowers. This is one of the main causes of the severe fatigue that can accompany these infections.

Bone marrow effects from infection by these pathogens are also common and pervasive. The diagnostic symptoms of thrombocytopenia and leukopenia occur, in part, from the bacteria-initiated damage to (and infection of) precursors in the bone marrow. While the bone marrow at testing may run from normal to hypercellular, hematopoiesis is always strongly affected. There is a subsequent lack of differentiation and proliferation of immature hematopoietic precursors, which leads to many fewer healthy immune cells. Examination of bone marrow, as Johns et al. (2009) comment, has found

> rapid and profound multilineage deficits in hematopoietic progenitor proliferation or differentiation. This quantitative effect in hematopoiesis was accompanied by induction of myelosuppressive chemokines within the BM [bone marrow], shifts in BM hematopoietic

subsets, including B-lymphocyte depletion, erythroid depletion, and granulocytic hyperplasia, and significant downregulation of CXCL12 in BM cells. Changes were independent of the pathogen burden or the route of pathogen inoculation.

The effects on bone marrow are cumulative. By 10 days postinfection there is a striking decrease in myeloid and erythroid progenitors. There is an increase in the frequency of immature granulocytes in the bone marrow with, again, substantial B-lymphocyte decreases.

Because blood cell precursors are damaged, thrombocytopenia (a deficiency of platelets, up to 50 percent), leukopenia (a reduction of white blood cells in the blood), and anemia (low red blood cell count) are common during infection. Bone marrow colony formation is markedly reduced by up to 50 percent and reductions can last for up to four months after infection.

The bone marrow cells are stimulated to upregulate a number of cytokines such as CXCL1, MIP-2α (CXCL2), MCP-1, TNF-α, and IL-6. CXCL1, MIP-2α (CXCL2), and MCP-1 (CCL2) are all strongly myelosuppressive chemokines. TNF-α expression is elevated twofold. CXCL12 expression is decreased five- to ninefold early in the infection and decreases as much as 20-fold as the disease progresses. The CXCL12 decreases are accompanied by B-lymphocyte depletion in the bone marrow (up to tenfold) and increased granulopoiesis (two- to fourfold). Ter119+ cells (erythroblasts, the precursors to red blood cells), which normally comprise between 20 and 30 percent of cells in the bone marrow, decrease to between 5 and 11 percent during infection.

The bone marrow impacts are accompanied by a compensating infection-induced augmentation of hematopoietic progenitor cell production in the spleen. There is a 66-fold increase in the level of Ter119+ erythroid cells, indicating that splenic erythropoiesis (or red blood cell production) is occurring. These Ter119+ cells will ultimately comprise half the total cells in the spleen during infection.

Despite this, anemia often remains; the splenic attempt to replace lost red blood cells during infection is ultimately unsuccessful due to further actions by the bacteria that inhibit the spleen from releasing the new cells into circulation. Total granulocytes in the spleen also increase tenfold; there is a twofold increase in B lymphocytes. This increase in cellular populations causes a buildup of cells in the spleen with a concomitant enlargement of the spleen; spleen weight significantly increases. (It continues to remain so for four months, or longer, after infection.) There is a marked hypercellularity of the tissues, expansion of the lymphoid follicles (lymphoid hyperplasia), an expanded and disorganized marginal zone, and extramedullary hematopoiesis in the red pulp. NK cell numbers increase substantially, so that they comprise a much greater proportion of the splenocytes. As MacNamara et al. (2009) comment, "These studies demonstrate that the cytopenias observed during ehrlichia infection are associated with marked changes in the numbers of cells in the spleen and bone marrow."

The NK cells are, eventually, disproportionally distributed to the liver, where they produce dramatic local inflammatory effects (hepatitis), including apoptosis of liver cells. Kupffer cell hyperplasia (and apoptosis) is common and the liver can experience a wide range of lesions, from focal hepatic necrosis to inflammatory cell aggregates. Cholestasis is relatively common, sometimes accompanied by bile duct epithelial injury. This spectrum of impacts is what produces the increased AST and ALT levels that are diagnostically indicative of infection. This substantial increase in NK cells in the liver is a major factor in the severe liver damage that can occur during these infections.

As studies have continually found, the inflammation that occurs in the liver is significantly disproportionate to the numbers of bacteria in infected cells. The sites of inflammation are, as well, far removed from the cells that are infected (so-called bystander hepatic injury). As researcher Trevor Waner (2008) comments, " A striking feature of Ehrlichial infections is the small to negligible number of organisms found in blood or other tissues in contrast to the sometimes severe damage that the infection can incur."

Both anaplasmal and ehrlichial bacteria actively inhibit NADPH (nicotinamide adenine dinucleotide phosphate) production during infections. The NADPH system has a number of functions, among which is the generation of free radical oxygen species that the immune system uses to destroy pathogens. This bacteria-initiated inhibition protects the pathogens but also has other, system-wide, impacts. Lipid synthesis, cholesterol synthesis, fatty acid chain elongation, the cytochrome P450 hydroxylation of numerous compounds, and the regeneration of glutathione are all inhibited. (Upregulating glutathione can help reduce the impacts of infection. *Andrographis paniculata, Cordyceps* spp., *Nigella sativa, Salvia miltiorrhiza,* and *Scutellaria baicalensis* are some of the herbs that act to upregulate glutathione.)

During anaplasmosis, the *Anaplasma*-infected neutrophils increase their expression of CD11b and CD66b and stimulate MMP-9 activity in the body. Neutrophil gelatinase granules liberate matrix metalloproteinases (MMPs) that degrade basement membranes and interstitium. (Because neutrophil apoptosis is significantly inhibited, this prolongs the impacts of MMP-9 release.) The MMP production facilitates bacterial and immune cell penetration deeper into the body. Infected neutrophils are commonly found, not only in the blood, but in the hepatic sinusoids, spleen red pulp, lungs, bone marrow, kidney glomeruli, heart capillaries, meningeal vessels, cerebral capillaries, and adrenals. Ninety percent of the infected neutrophils locate within the vessel lumens. The bone marrow, spleen, liver, and lymph nodes are the most commonly damaged areas of the body. Lymphoid depletion is common in the lymph nodes, which often show foamy macrophage infiltrates and erythrophagocytosis.

Monocytes, which naturally cross endothelial barriers more easily than neutrophils, once infected, are even more able to do so. This is the reason for more brain and central nervous system problems during ehrlichial infections than during anaplasmal ones.

THE EHRLICHIAL / ANAPLASMAL CYTOKINE CASCADES

Specifically, the bacteria upregulate the pro-inflammatory cytokines IL-1α, IL-1β, IL-4, IL-6, IL-8, NF-κB, p38 MAPK, TNF-α, CCL2 (MCP-1), CCL3 (MIP-1α), CCL4 (MCP-1b), CCL5 (RANTES), CCL20 (MIP-3), MMP-9, CXCL1, CXCL2 (MIP-2α), and CXCL11. TNF receptor expression is high (and very high in fatal conditions). TNF-α is low at initial infection but increases 30-fold by day five.

The bacteria also immediately upregulate unique *anti-inflammatory* cytokines such as IL-10 and IL-13. These latter two cytokines inhibit the body's normal Th1 adaptive immune response, which is needed to clear these particular organisms from the host body. The upregulation of IL-10 and IL-13 inhibits the immune system's production of IL-2, IL-12, IL-15, IL-18, and IFN-γ. These are normally needed to clear the infection; however, later induction of IFN-γ does not help because the bacteria are generating iron through IFN-γ-independent mechanisms. (When using plant medicines, the most important cytokines to downregulate are TNF-α, MMP-9, IL-1, IL-6, IL-8, IL-10, IL-13, CCL2, CCL3, CCL4, CXCL1, CXCL2, and CXCL11. The most important to upregulate are IL-12, IL-18, IL-2, and phospholipase C gamma-2, PLCG2.)

Protein kinase A (PKA), during ehrlichial infections, is upregulated 25-fold, primarily through the inhibition of JAK/STAT. PKA plays a number of crucial roles in the body. As with other protein kinases it is involved in the regulation of cellular pathways, especially those involved in signal transduction, cellular growth and movement, and apoptosis. PKA is also strongly involved in the regulation of glycogen, sugar, and lipid metabolism in the body and cellular tissues. PKA is especially active in fat (adipose) tissues, the heart, the liver, and the kidneys (and to some extent in the central nervous system). The upregulation of PKA to such extreme levels is one of the factors involved in the damage to the heart, liver, and kidneys that can occur during these particular bacterial infections. The upregulation of PKA has several other crucial impacts during anaplasmal/ehrlichial infections. It downregulates arginine production (thus reducing one of the major antimicrobial actors for infections); impairs prefrontal cortical functioning and working memory performance; inhibits the JAK/STAT pathway; and, most especially, inhibits the body's production of IFN-γ. Reducing PKA levels inhibits survival of these bacteria in their host cells. Herbs and supplements useful for this are *Aphanamixis polystachya* (stem and root bark), *Brosimum acutifolium* (bark), *Cinnamomum zeylanicum* (cinnamon), *Empetrum nigrum* (crowberry), *Punica granatum* (pomegranate), *Syzygium aromaticum* (clove), and the isolated constituent EGCG.

The JAK/STAT pathway transmits information into the gene promoters on DNA in the cell nucleus, stimulating gene expression or suppression. It is crucial for, among other things, the activation of macrophages by interferons (especially IFN-γ) and interleukins. Dysregulation of this pathway activates STAT1, which leads, again, to inhibition of apoptosis, increased blood vessel formation, and specific kinds of immunosuppression. Dysregulation also allows the bacteria to control a range of DNA gene promoters in the nucleus. Remodulation of the JAK/STAT pathway will inhibit the bacterial subversion of cellular DNA, increase apoptosis, and reduce bacterial ability to survive in host cells. Herbs good for this include *Andrographis* spp., *Bletilla striata, Salvia miltiorrhiza, Silybum marianum* (seed, standardized), and *Withania somnifera* (ashwagandha).

The upregulation of p38 MAPK is another mechanism the bacteria use to inhibit apoptosis. Inhibitors of p38 MAPK reverse apoptosis inhibition and reduce bacterial survival during infection. *Cordyceps* spp. and *Scutellaria baicalensis* are very good for this.

Phospholipase C gamma-2 (PLCG2) is also strongly downregulated. This enzyme is a critical regulator of innate immune cells; it plays crucial roles in the activation of B lymphocytes and their upregulation of antigen markers. This is part of the mechanism that the bacteria utilize to inhibit adaptive immunity responses. Upregulation of PLCG2 strongly inhibits the entry of these pathogens into host cells. Herbs useful for this are *Euphorbia kansui* (gan sui), *Houttuynia* spp. (houttuynia), *Peganum harmala* (Syrian rue), and *Salvia miltiorrhiza* (red sage, danshen).

The bacteria also inhibit the induction of caspase-3, stopping cellular apoptosis and thus allowing infection to continue. They inhibit the proapoptotic translocation of Bax to mitochondria, upregulate the antiapoptotic Bcl-2, inhibit both caspase-9 and caspase-3 activation, and stop the cellular activation of caspase promoters. Both bacteria strongly stimulate histidine kinases within their host cells. Caspase-3 promoters and normalization of Bax/Bcl-2 activity via plant medicines can reduce levels of infection by both these bacteria. Herbs useful for this are *Aphanamixis polystachya* (stem and root bark), *Cynomorium songaricum, Dalbergia odorifera, Eucommia ulmoides, Glycyrrhiza* spp. (licorice), *Goniothalamus cheliensis, Gynostemma pentaphyllum, Houttuynia* spp. (also upregulates caspase-9), *Magnolia officinalis, Paeonia lactiflora, Panax ginseng, Phellodendron amurense, Salvia miltiorrhiza* (a potent modulator, raising or reducing caspase-3 as needed), *Scutellaria* spp. (baikal skullcap, Chinese skullcap; also upregulates caspase-9), *Tinospora cordifolia,* and the isolated constituents apigenin (strongly so; also upregulates caspase-9), arctigenin, beta-sitosterol, butein, curcumin, and emodin (caspase-9 only).

Histidine kinases (HKs) are proteins that play crucial roles in signal transduction across the cellular membrane. They exist along an axis that crosses the cellular membrane; part of them are outside the cell, part of them span the cellular membrane, and other portions are inside the cell. When an HK encounters certain molecules, it is activated, sending a signal into the cell. Once the signal is received, molecules within the cell are altered, and a response from the cell is generated. *Ehrlichia* and *Anaplasma* bacteria modulate HKs when they infect a cell. They interrupt the signal that tells the cell that a bacteria is inside a vacuole and inhibit what is called lysosomal fusion with the vacuole. Lysomal fusion is what allows antimicrobial compounds to be injected into the vacuole, killing invading pathogens. The use of HK inhibitors (the pharmaceutical closantel or various plant medicines) stops the lysomal inhibition, induces lysomal fusion, and kills the bacteria. Some useful ones are *Aphanamixis polystachya* (stem and root bark), *Pueraria* spp. (kudzu root), and the isolated constituents genistein (strongly so but needs higher dosages) and quercetin.

The bacteria also inhibit the induction of what are called major histocompatibility complex (MHC) class II genes, causing a downregulation of MHC-II. MHCs are a set of cellular surface molecules that mediate the interaction of leukocytes with the rest of the body's cells. The MHC-II group, when activated, is what interacts with the CD4+ T-cell group of the immune system. It mediates the establishment of adaptive immunity to specific pathogens. When the gene expression of MHC-II is repressed, the adaptive immune system is prevented from successfully combating the infection. The suppression of MHC-II produces infections of much longer duration with concomitant low CD4+ T-cell/high CD8+ T-cell activity. (There is some speculation that the bacteria actually enhance MHC-I gene expression, which increases CD8+ T-cell activity, which is generally high during these infections.) The worse that MHC-II expression is during infection, the poorer the outcome. Fatal infection, accompanied by severe organ damage, is much more common when MHC-II activity is impaired. Upregulating the gene expression of MHC-II (through the use of plant medicines) helps reduce the severity and length of infection. Some useful herbs for that are *Achyranthes bidentata, Astragalus membranaceus, Astragalus mongholicus, Cordyceps* spp., *Morus* spp. (mulberry fruit), *Panax ginseng, Phellinus linteus,* and *Plantago asiatica.*

Pattern recognition receptors TLR-2 and TLR-4 are also strongly downregulated; this inhibits the antimicrobial activation of macrophages against the bacteria. However, during acute episodes, TLR-2 and TLR-4 are strongly *upregulated*. (Enhancing TLR-4 during moderate infections can help clear the infection, but it must be *suppressed* during acute conditions.) The more serious the disease, the more strongly they are upregulated. The increased level of TLR-4 stimulates the production of HMGB1, which, in sufficient quantities, is enough to induce septic shock and death. (See page 183 for more on HMGB1.) In all cases of fatal infections, the levels of TLR-4 and HMGB1 are extremely high (see chapter 8). IL-8, granulocyte colony-stimulating factor (G-CSF), and TNF-α are extremely high in seriously acute and fatal infections. G-CSF is produced in high levels in the spleen and lymph in compensation for bone marrow suppression. This should increase neutrophil counts but does not. The neutrophils instead actively migrate to the organs, where they participate in the inflammatory damage that occurs. CD4+ T-cell numbers decline significantly, IFN-γ is reduced 40-fold, and IL-12 levels are very low. Tissue injury is also accompanied by a significant increase in NK T cells and antigen-specific CD8+ T cells. Reducing CD8+ and NK T-cell levels enhances resistance to lethal infection, increases CD4+ T-cell levels, and reduces inflammatory impacts on organs. (Again, see chapter 8.)

Interference in any of a number of these processes can significantly reduce symptoms and even clear the infection. There are many plants that are highly effective for this. The next chapter looks at some of them.

7

Natural Healing of Ehrlichia and Anaplasma

A class of herbal medicines, known as immunomodulators, alters the activity of immune function through the dynamic regulation of information molecules such as cytokines.

K. SPELMAN, J. J. BURNS, D. NICHOLS, ET AL.,
"MODULATION OF CYTOKINE EXPRESSION
BY TRADITIONAL MEDICINES:
A REVIEW OF HERBAL IMMUNOMODULATORS"

The effects of plant based remedies may be due to one active compound with a single mechanism of action, to compound(s) that possess multiple modes of action, . . . to the combined activity of more than one active ingredient in a single species, . . . or the synergic interactions of different active ingredients from several plant species processed as a medicinal formula.

E. ELISABETSKY, "PHYTOTHERAPY AND THE
NEW PARADIGM OF DRUGS MODE OF ACTION"

Despite the sophisticated modulation of the immune system that these bacteria are capable of, it is quite possible to reverse it. Plant medicines are very good at subtle remodulations of immune function, in fact much better than pharmaceuticals. They are excellent for reducing the levels of cytokines that cause inflammatory damage in the body while simultaneously upregulating immune-supporting cytokines that the bacteria have inhibited. Plant medicines are also very effective at protecting the various organ and cellular systems that have been adversely affected, helping them heal any damage that has occurred, and stimulating the organs to work more efficiently. And finally, they are excellent for reducing or eliminating many of the symptoms that infection causes.

Treating Ehrlichiosis and Anaplasmosis with Natural Protocols

First, some basics . . . I know this is repetitive, but there seems to be a general confusion that commonly arises among both practitioners and the infected about the following points, hence the continual repetition (I get scores of communications about these points every month).

The herbs and supplements in this book are **not** the only ones in the world that will help. Please use the protocols outlined herein only as a starting place, a guideline. Add anything that you feel will help you and delete anything that you feel is not useful. Bacteria, when they enter a human body, find a very unique ecosystem in that particular person. Thus the disease is always slightly different every time it occurs. This means that a pharmaceutical or herb that works for one person may not work or work as well for another. There is no one-size-fits-all treatment that works for all people in all times and places.

Also: there is no one thing that always has to happen first, that has to be treated first, or that you must always do or must never do in order to get well. There is no one herb that will always work for everyone;

there is no one protocol that contains the solutions to all the infectious organisms that exist or all the forms of infection that the Lyme group can cause.

Again: there is no one-size-fits-all treatment that works for all people in all times and places.

Anyone who says there is, is either trying to sell you something or doesn't really understand the Lyme group of infectious organisms (or has powerful self-image needs involved). *There is not and never has been one single way to health such that in all times and in all places and with all people it will always work.* Life, and disease, and the journey to wellness are much more complex and challenging than that.

All of us, practitioners and the infected alike, of necessity must learn to see what is right in front of us and adapt our interventions to what is actually occurring in the unique ecological system we are encountering. Our interaction with these disease complexes has to occur out of a living communication—with the organism, with the body, with the medicine. Each treatment intervention, as treatment progresses, will become unique to each person. It has to do so for healing to occur.

Thus the protocols in this book should solely be considered as a foundational place to begin. For most people they will help considerably; for some they will clear the infection completely. Nearly everyone (practitioners and the infected alike), however, will find that they will need to add this or subtract that. *Please do so.* Please trust your own feeling sense and pay attention to what your body is telling you. *You* are the best judge of whether something is working for you or not, whether you need to add something else or not, whether you are getting better . . . or not.

Now, about dosages: I will often suggest a dosage or a *range* of dosages for the herbs and supplements that can help. If you have a very healthy immune system, or a very mild case, you will probably need smaller doses; if your immune system is severely depleted or if you are very ill, you may need to use larger doses. If you are *very* sensitive to outside substances, as some people with Lyme and these coinfections are, then you might need to use very tiny doses, that is from one to five drops of tincture at a time. (This is true for about one percent of the people with these infections.) I have seen six-foot-five-inch, 280-pound men be unable to take more than five drops of a tincture and a tiny, 95-pound woman need a tablespoon at a time. *Dosages need to be adjusted for each person's individual ecology.* **Again . . . dosages need to be adjusted for each person's individual ecology. And now, a few other points that commonly arise:**

1. Yes, you *can* combine all the herbs together in the liquid of your choice. You do not have to take them separately.
2. Yes, these herbs can be taken along with antibiotics.
3. No, the bacteria do not develop resistance to the herbs.
4. Yes, you *can* take these herbs along with protocols suggested by other practitioners.
5. No, except for a very few herbs (such as the 1:1 form of eleutherococcus tincture), you do not need to pulse the herbs—that is, to take them in an on-again, off-again cycle, such as five days on and two days off. In fact, I have continually heard from people struggling with the Lyme group of infections that they were getting better, were told to pulse by their personal practitioner, and once they did, relapsed.
6. Yes, it is common for about half the people who use an herbal protocol, when they begin to get better, to be so excited about being themselves again, that they do too much, overexert themselves, and relapse. This is extremely common (and very understandable; it's tiring being sick for so long). So, please be very careful once your strength and joy begin to return. It may seem as if you can immediately begin exerting yourself as you used to do; however, your body has been under a long-term stress, and its reserves are low. It will take, if you have been ill for a long time, at least a year to rebuild.

Part of the function of serious chronic illnesses is to increase personal awareness (I know from personal experience). There is the life you had before Lyme, there is the life you have after. It is very rarely possible to go back to being unaware of the impacts of stress on your system, the kind of self-caretaking your body (and spirit) needs, or the dangers of overextending yourself and your energy. Ignorance may be bliss (however short that bliss may be) but awareness is empowering . . . and health enabling.

And, finally, *please be conscious of how you respond to the medicines you are taking. If something disagrees with you, if you feel something is not right in how you are responding to a medicine,* **stop taking it.** Remember: you will always know yourself better than any outside physician.

INITIAL INTERVENTION PROTOCOL

The initial intervention, using a natural protocol, suggested for mild to moderate anaplasmal and ehrlichial infections, relapsing or not, entails: 1) the use of herbs that interfere with the organisms' ability to invade their target cells; 2) organ-protective herbs; 3) immune modulators to restructure the immune response; 4) cytokine disruptors to remodulate the bacteria-controlled cytokine cascade; and 5) herbs for reducing specific symptoms. To be a bit more specific:

1. **Antibacterial herbs.** A caveat: please note that there has been very little study on herbs that are *directly* antibacterial for these organisms. Specifically, "directly" means testing for plants that kill these bacteria upon contact with the plants. Hence, I approach this category of intervention through the use of herbs that interfere with or interrupt the mechanisms used by the bacteria to infect their host cells, control those cells' DNA, prevent host cell apoptosis, or reproduce inside those cells. Plants that have these kinds of effects *are* antibacterial; they just don't directly kill the invading organisms.

(Because similar organisms cause so much illness in domestic animals, primarily livestock, especially in Africa, there is a fairly broad range of plants that have been used to treat them. I include an extensive list at the end of this chapter; please consider exploring them in treatment.)

2. **Organ support and protection.** These bacteria create powerful impacts on a number of the body's organs, including the spleen and lymph system, liver, and bone marrow. Supporting and strengthening those systems reduces infection impacts and enables those organs to better combat the infection.

3. **Immune modulation.** These bacteria restructure the architecture and response of the immune system to meet their own needs. Counteracting the pathogen restructuring restores immune integrity and supports the clearance of the organisms from the body.

4. **Cytokine disruptors.** Herbs that are specific for interfering with the cytokine cascade that the organisms initiate will stop most inflammation in the body and interfere with the pathogens' abilities to find and enter target cells, gather nutrients, and reproduce.

5. **Specific symptom treatment.** These bacteria can create a rather broad range of symptoms. Reducing symptoms helps restore quality of life and feelings of joy, which in and of themselves produce potent beneficial effects during healing. These herbs and supplements are covered in the expanded treatment protocol (page 161).

Again, there are thousands of plants that can be, and are, used in the treatment of disease. While I include a wide range of plants that are active in the categories I just outlined, the following list contains the ones that, based on use, analysis of the organisms and the herbs, exhaustive journal research, and the experiences of both practitioners and those with the diseases, I think are the most effective. (This includes some that *may* be very good, which I have not used, and which I think show promise.) This does not mean there are not others, not listed herein, that are just as effective.

Antibacterial Herbs

As discussed in the previous chapter, the following categories of herbs are effective at counteracting the unique mechanisms the bacteria utilize to enter and control their host cells and their cellular function. If you are using antibiotics, these herbs can be used at the same time; they will help potentiate the antibiotics' actions.

- PLCG2 inhibitors: *Euphorbia kansui* (gan sui), *Houttuynia* spp. (houttuynia), *Peganum harmala* (Syrian rue), *Salvia miltiorrhiza* (red sage, danshen).
- Caspase-3 (and caspase-9) upregulators: *Aphanamixis polystachya* (stem and root bark), *Cynomorium songaricum, Dalbergia odorifera, Eucommia ulmoides, Glycyrrhiza* spp. (licorice), *Goniothalamus cheliensis, Gynostemma pentaphyllum, Houttuynia* spp. (also upregulates caspase-9), *Magnolia officinalis, Paeonia lactiflora, Panax ginseng, Phellodendron amurense, Salvia miltiorrhiza* (a potent modulator, raising or reducing it as needed), *Scutellaria* spp. (baikal skullcap, Chinese skullcap; also upregulates caspase-9), *Tinospora cordifolia,* and the isolated constituents apigenin (strongly so; also upregulates caspase-9), arctigenin, beta-sitosterol, butein, curcumin, and emodin (caspase-9 only).
- Bax/Bcl-2 apoptosis pathway remodulators (which specifically increase Bax and reduce Bcl-2): *Artemisia* spp., *Glycyrrhiza* spp., *Goniothalamus cheliensis, Gynostemma pentaphyllum, Houttuynia* spp., *Leonurus cardiaca* (motherwort), *Rhodiola* spp., *Scutellaria* spp., and the isolated constituents arctigenin, beta-sitosterol, and curcumin.

    Note: *Salvia miltiorrhiza* is an apoptosis modulator. It modulates the actions of Bax/Bcl-2, decreasing or increasing the ratio as needed during inflammatory episodes, e.g., it increases apoptosis of cancer cells but decreases apoptosis of hypoxia-damaged cells.

- JAK/STAT remodulators (which counteract bacterial apoptosis inhibition): *Andrographis* spp., *Bletilla striata, Salvia miltiorrhiza, Silybum marianum* (seed, standardized), and *Withania somnifera* (ashwagandha).
- Histidine kinase inhibitors: *Aphanamixis polystachya* (stem and root bark), *Pueraria* spp. (kudzu root), and the isolated constituents genistein (strongly so but needs higher dosages) and quercetin.
- PKA inhibitors: *Aphanamixis polystachya* (stem and root bark), *Brosimum acutifolium* (bark), *Cinnamomum zeylanicum* (cinnamon), *Empetrum nigrum* (crowberry), *Punica granatum* (pomegranate), *Syzygium aromaticum* (clove), and the isolated constituent EGCG.

Note: *Aphanamixis* is a traditional herb in Asia and in Ayurveda. It has a fairly broad antimicrobial activity against Gram-negative bacteria and is also liver protective, reduces spleen inflammation, regulates thymus action, normalizes lymph function, stimulates apoptosis, and acts to inhibit PKA and histidine kinase while upregulating caspase-3. It has a broad range of actions for the systemic effects of both ehrlichia and anaplasma bacteria; it should be explored as a primary antibacterial for these organisms. (As of 2014, I have not yet used it.)

Organ Support and Protection

The most important parts of the body to protect during these infections are the spleen, lymph nodes and lymph system, liver, bone marrow function—specifically the bone marrow's stem cells—and mitochondria. Secondary systems to protect are the heart (see the expanded treatment protocol on page 161, as well as the profiles of hawthorn and *Salvia miltiorrhiza* in chapter 9) and lungs (see the expanded treatment protocol, page 161). Other important specifics are lowering ALT and AST levels and increasing red blood cell and platelet counts. Here are the primary supportive herbs and compounds to utilize in supporting organ function during ehrlichial or anaplasmal infection.

1. *Salvia miltiorrhiza* (a.k.a. danshen). Danshen is a Chinese herb specific for spleen and liver inflammation and malfunction.

   In the past I have relied primarily on red root (*Ceanothus* spp.) for diseases that affect the spleen. I like red root because it is strongly protective of the spleen and to some extent the liver. It acts to reduce inflammation in both of those organs. It also stimulates the immune activity of the spleen, helping to clear the body of infection while optimizing the removal of microorganism and immune system debris during infections. However, *red root is also a blood coagulant*. Because intravascular coagulation is so common during some Lyme coinfections, I now prefer the use of *Salvia miltiorrhiza*. (If you do want to keep using red root, then please supplement its use in this disease with anticoagulants such as nattokinase, ginkgo, and aspirin.)

2. *Silybum marianum* (milk thistle) seed. The combined compounds known as silymarin that are extracted from milk thistle seed are strongly liver protective and regenerative. There are four main constituents of silymarin: silibinin, isosilibinin, silicristin, and silidianin. This herb, if standardized, will strongly protect the liver from inflammatory damage, reduce inflammatory infiltrates, protect the Kupffer cells, reduce ALT and AST levels, and help remodulate the JAK/STAT pathway. (*Salvia miltiorrhiza* is also strongly liver protective and may be used instead, though I do strongly suggest the use of milk thistle seed given the considerable damage that these bacteria can do to the liver.)

3. **Herbs to support bone marrow.** The most active herbs for the bone marrow's stem cells (reducing myelosuppression and

stimulating hematopoiesis) are *Agaricus blazei, Angelica sinensis, Astragalus* spp., *Bidens* spp., *Cordyceps* spp., *Ganoderma lucidum* (reishi), *Glycyrrhiza* spp., *Paeonica lactiflora* (peony root), *Panax ginseng, Salvia miltiorrhiza, Tinospora cordifolia, Tricholoma matsutake, Zataria multiflora,* and the supplement carnosine. The strongest are astragalus, angelica, *Salvia miltiorrhiza, Panax ginseng,* and cordyceps. All reverse anemia, leukopenia, and thrombocytopenia. All counteract hematopoiesis suppression in the bone marrow.

Note: *Salvia miltiorrhiza* increases white blood cell counts, reduces neutrophil adhesion (inhibits intercellular adhesion molecule 1, or ICAM-1), inhibits MCP-1 (CCL2, a myelosuppressive cytokine), reduces ALT and AST, improves liver, spleen, thymus, and lymph node function, and stimulates the production of bone marrow progenitor cells.

4. **Herbs to support mitochondria.** The mitochondria are best protected by *Leonurus cardiaca* (motherwort), *Rhodiola* spp., *Salvia miltiorrhiza, Schisandra chinensis,* and the supplements luteolin, coenzyme Q10, and fermented wheat germ extract.

Immune Modulation

Again, the point here is to modulate immune function in a specific manner during mild to moderate infections. Of initial importance is the downregulation of IL-10 and the upregulation of IL-2, IL-12, IL-18, and IFN-γ, essentially switching the immune response from Th2 to Th1. The primary herb for this is ashwagandha (*Withania somnifera*). It counteracts, with great specificity, the exact modulation of the immune system that the tick saliva and the bacteria initiate and maintain.

Other herbs and supplements useful for this kind of immune modulation are (in no special order) licorice, i.e., *Glycyrrhiza* spp. (downregulates IL-10, acting primarily as an immune modulator and tonic); standardized milk thistle (silymarin inhibits IL-10 overexpression and helps support endothelial health); *Cannabis sativa* (inhibits IL-10 overexpression); *Scutellaria* spp. (downregulates IL-10 and Treg); *Panax ginseng* and *Panax japonicus* (both upregulate Th1 dynamics); *Labisia pumila* (upregulates Th1 response); *Carica papaya* leaves (as a tea; stimulate IL-12, IFN-γ, and TNF-α); *Lycium barbarum* fruit (lychii berries); neem leaf; boneset (*Eupatorium perfoliatum*, primarily via its caffeic acid derivatives); and any plants containing scopoletin (an IL-10/Th2 downregulator) such as noni, manacá, passion flower (*Passiflora* spp.), stevia, *Artemisia* spp. (especially *A. scoparia* and *A. capillaris*), nettle leaf (*Urtica dioica*), and black haw (*Viburnum prunifolium*). Plants containing daucosterol are also effective in stimulating a Th1 response and downregulating a Th2-dominant dynamic; among them are *Garcinia parviflora* and *Gardenia jasminoides*.

Cytokines Disruptors

In addition to IL-10, the primary inflammatory cytokines that need downregulation are TNF-α, MMP-9, IL-1β, IL-6, IL-8, IL-13, CCL2, CCL3, CCL4, CXCL1, CXCL2, and CXCL11. Here is a list of plants active for downregulating those cytokines:

TNF-α inhibitors: *Andrographis paniculata*, *Cannabis* spp., *Cordyceps* spp., *Eupatorium perfoliatum* (boneset), *Glycyrrhiza* spp. (licorice), *Houttuynia* spp, *Panax ginseng*, *Polygala tenuifolia* (Chinese senega) root, *Pueraria lobata* (kudzu), *Salvia miltiorrhiza*, *Sambucus* spp. (elder), *Scutellaria baicalensis*, *Tanacetum parthenium* (feverfew), *Zingiber officinalis* (ginger).

MMP-9 inhibitors: *Polygonum cuspidatum* (Japanese knotweed), *Salvia miltiorrhiza*.

IL-1β inhibitors: *Cordyceps* spp., *Eupatorium perfoliatum*, *Polygala tenuifolia* (Chinese senega) root, *Polygonum cuspidatum*, *Pueraria lobata*, *Salvia miltiorrhiza*, *Scutellaria baicalensis*.

IL-6 inhibitors: *Andrographis paniculata*, *Isatis* spp., *Pueraria lobata*, *Salvia miltiorrhiza*, *Scutellaria baicalensis*.

IL-8 inhibitors: *Cordyceps* spp., *Isatis* spp., *Polygonum cuspidatum.*

IL-13 inhibitors: Unknown at this time.

CCL2 (MCP-1) inhibitors: *Coptis chinensis, Lonicera japonica, Salvia miltiorrhiza* (strongly so), *Scutellaria baicalensis, Sophora flavescens, Tanacetum parthenium.*

CCL3/CCL4 inhibitors: *Panax ginseng, Scutellaria baicalensis.*

CXCL1 (GRO-KC) inhibitors: *Curcuma longa* (turmeric), *Euterpe oleracea* (acai) berry, *Lonicera japonica, Panax ginseng, Rhododendron brachycarpum, Uncaria* spp. (cat's claw).

CXCL2 (MIP-2) inhibitors: *Andrographis paniculata, Angelica sinensis, Lithospermum erythrorhizon, Scutellaria baicalensis, Tanacetum parthenium,* and the isolated constituent quercetin.

CXCL11 inhibitors: *Andrographis paniculata, Panax ginseng.*

Cytokines to upregulate include the following:

IL-2: *Angelica sinensis, Bidens pilosa, Cordyceps* spp., *Ganoderma lucidum, Lycium barbarum, Salvia miltiorrhiza, Smilax* spp., *Tylophora asthmatica, Withania somnifera.*

IL-12: *Astragalus* spp., *Cannabis* spp., *Cordyceps* spp., *Ganoderma lucidum, Grifola frondosa, Lycium barbarum, Panax ginseng, Tinospora cordifolia,* and the kampo formulation juzentaihoto.

IL-18: *Cordyceps* spp., *Tinospora cordifolia* (also restores thymus function), *Salvia miltiorrhiza,* and the kampo formulation juzentaihoto.

MHC-II: *Achyranthes bidentata, Astragalus membranaceus, Astragalus mongholicus, Cordyceps* spp., *Morus* spp. (mulberry fruit), *Panax ginseng, Phellinus linteus, Plantago asiatica.*

Primary Herbs Suggested for Treating Ehrlichial/ Anaplasmal Infections

The following are the herbs that possess the strongest actions and/ or cross over into the most categories of action. *Salvia miltiorrhiza* is the foundational herb for treating these bacteria, closely followed by *Withania somnifera* (ashwagandha) because of its modulation of the specific immune dysregulation that is occuring.

Antibacterial actors: *Glycyrrhiza* spp., *Houttuynia* spp., *Pueraria lobata*, *Salvia miltiorrhiza*, *Scutellaria baicalensis*, and the supplement genistein.

Immune modulators: *Angelica sinensis*, *Astragalus* spp., *Cordyceps* spp., *Glycyrrhiza* spp., *Houttuynia* spp., *Panax ginseng*, *Salvia miltiorrhiza*, *Scutellaria baicalensis*, *Withania somnifera* (primary).

Bone marrow protectors/modulators: *Angelica sinensis*, *Astragalus* spp., *Cordyceps* spp., *Glycyrrhiza* spp., *Panax ginseng*, *Salvia miltiorrhiza*.

Liver protectors/modulators: *Salvia miltiorrhiza*, *Silybum marianum*.

Spleen/lymph node protectors/modulators: *Salvia miltiorrhiza*, *Ceanothus* spp.

A BASIC PROTOCOL FOR EHRLICHIOSIS AND ANAPLASMOSIS

Note: Regimen will likely need to be followed for about 12 months (or until infection resolves).

1. Tincture combination of *Salvia miltiorrhiza* and *Houttuynia* spp. (equal parts of each), ½ teaspoon 6x daily. (This can be increased substantially in more severe or recalcitrant infections, from 1 teaspoon to 1 tablespoon 6x daily.)

2. Genistein, 250 mg 2–3x daily (Note: Please see contraindications in chapter 9). Quercetin is a decent substitute; take 1,000 mg 2x daily.

3. Tincture combination of *Scutellaria baicalensis, Cordyceps* spp., *Pueraria lobata* (equal parts of each), ½ teaspoon 3–6x daily.

4. Tincture combination of *Astragalus* spp., *Angelica sinensis, Glycyrrhiza* spp. (equal parts of each), ½ teaspoon 6x daily.

5. Tincture of *Withania somnifera*, ½ teaspoon 3x daily. (Note: May cause drowsiness.)

6. Tincture of *Panax ginseng,* ¼ teaspoon 3x daily.

7. *Silybum marianum* (milk thistle) seed, standardized, 1,200–2,400 mg daily, depending on severity of condition (function: protection of liver).

ADD TO THE BASIC PROTOCOL, BASED ON SYMPTOMS

If you have ehrlichiosis or anaplasmosis . . .

With severe anemia, use:

1. *Sida acuta* tincture, ¼ teaspoon 3–6x daily until condition resolves, plus . . .

2. N-acetylcysteine, 4,000 mg 2x daily until condition resolves, and add . . .

3. *Angelica sinensis* tincture, 1 teaspoon 3x daily.

With severe intravascular coagulation, use:

1. Ginkgo, standardized tincture, ½ teaspoon 3x daily, plus . . .

2. Nattokinase, 200 mg 3x daily (same as 4,000 FU 3x daily), plus . . .

3. 4 adult aspirins, 3x daily, or . . .

4. *Salvia miltiorrhiza,* at an increased dosage of 1 teaspoon up to 6x daily.

With drenching sweats, use:

1. Boneset (*Eupatorium perfoliatum*), strong infusion, 1 cup 3–6x daily.

With fever, use:

1. Coral root (*Corallorhiza maculata* or equivalent) tincture, 30 drops each hour, or . . .

2. Boneset (*Eupatorium perfoliatum*), strong infusion, 1 cup each hour or two, or . . .

3. Peppermint tea, 1 cup each hour or two, as needed.

With nausea, use:

1. Peppermint tea, 1 cup each hour or two as needed.

With extreme nausea, use:

1. Peppermint essential oil, one drop *only,* on the tongue, followed by water, as needed.

With muscle and joint pain, use:

1. *Pedicularis* spp. tincture, 1 teaspoon each hour as needed, or . . .
2. *Monotropa uniflora* (Indian pipe) tincture , ¼–1 teaspoon up to 6x daily.

With severe pain, use:

1. *Salvia miltiorrhiza,* 1 tablespoon (yes, that's right) every 15 minutes, slowly lowering dosage as the pain subsides.

With headache, use:

1. *Pedicularis* tincture, 1 teaspoon each hour as needed, and/or . . .
2. Indian pipe (*Monotropa uniflora*) tincture, ¼–1 teaspoon up to 6x daily, and/or . . .
3. *Pueraria lobata* (kudzu) root tincture, ¼–½ teaspoon up to 6x daily.

With anxiety/hysteria, use:

1. *Pulsatilla* spp. (pasqueflower) tincture, 10 drops each hour as long as necessary, and/or . . .
2. Motherwort (*Leonurus cardiaca*) tincture, ¼ to ½ teaspoon to 6x daily, and/or . . .
3. Coral root tincture, 30 drops (full dropper) to 6x daily.

With extreme fear, use:

1. *Verbena officinalis* (vervain) tincture, 30 drops to 6x daily.

With sleep disturbance, use:

1. Melatonin liquid, manufacturer's directions, one hour before bed, and/or. . .

2. Ashwagandha (*Withania somnifera*) tincture, ½ teaspoon one hour before bed or powder or capsules, 1 gram an hour before bed, and/or . . .

3. Motherwort (*Leonurus cardiaca*) tincture, ¼ *ounce* (yes, that is right) in liquid just before bed (if the melatonin does not help).

With severe fatigue, use:

1. Eleuthero (*Eleutherococcus senticosus*) tincture (a 1:5 ratio, *not* the 2:1 Herb Pharm brand), ¼ teaspoon 3x daily, plus . . .

2. Rhodiola (*Rhodiola* spp.) tincture, ¼ teaspoon 3x daily, plus . . .

3. Schisandra (*Schisandra chinensis*) tincture, ¼ teaspoon 3x daily, plus . . .

4. Motherwort (*Corallorhiza maculata*) tincture, ½ teaspoon 3x daily, and . . .

5. Fermented wheat germ extract, if you can afford it. All for 6 months.

With wasting (i.e., severe weight loss), use:

1. Fermented wheat germ extract, 9 grams daily (best choice), or (not as good) . . .

2. Shiitake mushrooms (*Lentinula edodes*), powdered or as food, 6–16 grams per day. A pure extract of lentinan can also be used: 1–3 grams per day.

For detoxification and help with Herxheimer reactions, use:

1. Zeolite powder, 2 heaping teaspoons daily (do *not* accidentally inhale), or 3 capsules 3x daily.

2. Activated charcoal, 2 capsules 2x daily.

3. Bentonite clay may also be of help. Soak 1 teaspoon in a full glass of water for 30 minutes to 2 hours. Take on an empty stomach, early in the morning or just before bed.

SEVERE HME AND HGA VERSUS MILD, MODERATE, AND CHRONIC FORMS

Severe or acute infections with either of these bacteria can occur, often accompanied by extremely low parasite loads. Despite the low loads, under certain circumstances, this can lead to sepsis, septic shock, multiple organ failure, coma, and death. In general, the more acute forms that do not include sepsis will respond perfectly well to the protocol for mild, moderate, and chronic forms. A few specifics are offered in chapter 8.

ETHNOVETERINARY APPROACHES

Plants used in ethnoveterinary practice in Africa for treatment of *Anaplasma* and *Ehrlichia* infections in domestic animals include the following:

Allium cepa root, water extract with sedimentary rock, salt, and ampicillin; *Aloe dawei* leaf, water extract; *Aloe ferox* sap, decoction; *Aloe tweediae* exudate, water extract; *Aspilia mossambicensi* root, water extract combined with *Solanum* spp. fruit; *Capparis fascicularis* var. *elaeagnoides* bark, water extract; *Capparis* spp. root or branch, water extract; *Capparis sepiaria* var. *citrifolia* root, decoction; *Capsicum annum* fruit, water extract; *Carissa spinarum* root, infusion; *Chasmanthera dependens* root, water extract; *Cissus quadrangularis* leaf, water extract; *Coccinia adoensis* root, infusion; *Croton megalocarpus* root bark, decoction; *Cucumis* spp. fruit, water extract combined with *Warburgia salutaris* and sedimentary rock ($CaCO_3$); *Cussonia spicata* bark, decoction; *Euphorbia bongensis* whole plant, water extract; *Euphorbia candelabrum* stem, water extract with sedimentary rock ($CaCO_3$); *Fagaropsis angolensis* bark, water extract; *Grewia occidentalis* leaf combined with *Olea europaea* ssp. *africana* leaf, *Zanthoxylum capense* leaf, and *Aloe ferox* sap, soaked in cold water (water extraction); *Ledebouria revoluta* leaf, decoction; *Leucas capensis* leaf mixed with *Brachylaena ilicifolia* leaf, decoction; *Leucas deflexa* plant, macerate; *Marrubium vulgare* leaf, decoction; *Pentarrhinum insipidum* leaf, hot decoction; *Podocarpus latifolius* bark, decoction; *Sideroxylon inerme* bark, decoction; *Solanum aculeatissimum* and *S. incanum* fruit, water extract; *Tephrosia* spp. whole plant, paste; *Terminalia brownii* bark, paste; *Teucrium africanum* leaf, decoction; *Tinospora caffra* root, water extract; *Trichilia prieuriana* bark, water extract; *Warburgia salutaris* bark, decoction and decoction combined with sedimentary rock ($CaCO_3$); *Zanthoxylum chalybeum* bark or root, water extract.

And *Urginea sanguinea, Aloe marlothii, Elephantorrhiza elephantina,* and *Rhoicissus tridentata* have been found, during in vitro tests, to be active against *Ehrlichia ruminantium*.

8

Acute Infections, Sepsis, and Septic Shock

In the USA, sepsis is the second leading cause of death within noncoronary intensive care units, with increased mortality rates of between 20% for sepsis and 60% for septic shock.

S. DENK, M. PERL, AND M. HUBER-LANG,
"DAMAGE- AND PATHOGEN-ASSOCIATED
MOLECULAR PATTERNS AND ALARMINS"

A point is reached at which the severity of the disease increases. . . . Unfortunately, this critical point does not immediately appear to lend itself to definition in the individual patient. . . . These changes [in the cytokine profile] have the characteristics of a self-perpetuating and amplifying system of functional derangement.

I. A. CLARK, L. M. ALLEVA, A. C. MILLS, ET AL.,
"PATHOGENESIS OF MALARIA AND
CLINICALLY SIMILAR CONDITIONS"

In fatal disease in the form of toxic shock-like syndrome, uninfected hepatocytes undergo apoptosis without evidence of ehrlichial infection.

N. ISMAIL, K. C. BLOCH, AND J. W. MCBRIDE,
"HUMAN EHRLICHIOSIS AND ANAPLASMOSIS"

Whether the presence of a particular cytokine is beneficial or detrimental to the host's protective immune response depends on several factors, such as the time during infection when it is produced, the concentration of the cytokine, and whether it is present at high levels systemically in the serum or locally in the foci of infection.

H. STEVENSON, J. M. JORDAN, Z. PEERWANI, ET AL.,
"AN INTRADERMAL ENVIRONMENT PROMOTES A
PROTECTIVE TYPE-1 RESPONSE AGAINST LETHAL
SYSTEMIC MONOCYTOTROPIC EHRLICHIAL INFECTION"

Infections with *Babesia, Anaplasma,* and *Ehrlichia* can, under some circumstances, shift into a more acute form. Sometimes this can lead to what is called sepsis or even further into septic shock. This is caused by an extreme shift in the immune system's cytokine response to the infections. During mild and moderate infections, and during the initial stages of all infections, the bacteria shift the body's immune response to Th2 rather than the more effective Th1. During these more extreme infections the immune system suddenly shifts into an overreactive Th1 response.

It's almost as if the body, in response to being artificially suppressed for so long, has slowly built up a counterresponse that, as the suppression goes on, increasingly grows in strength. Then, suddenly, the suppression of Th1 responses just ceases. What

> *remains is a powerful, overreactive, inflammatory Th1*
> *response that, without a counteracting downregulation,*
> *overwhelms the body.*

A positive feedback process begins; inflammation spirals out of control. This is sepsis. If it deepens, the body and its organs will begin to shut down. This is what is known as septic shock.

No one knows exactly why it happens in these diseases, but there are a number of factors that have been identified as being essential to its happening.

SEPSIS

The term *sepsis* has been around for nearly three millennia, but until the 1990s, a concrete clinical definition of the term was hard to find. The root of the word comes from the ancient Greek and means putrefaction or decay (hence "septic" tank). Prior to its redefinition, the term was applied to any serious illness accompanied by decay or putrefaction (such as gangrene). *Septicemia*, a related word (theoretically no longer used), also from the Greek, means putrefied blood, in other words a serious blood infection. Sepsis (and its related conditions) now has a specific meaning (despite its etymology), which is . . .

> *systemic inflammation (specifically, systemic*
> *inflammatory response syndrome, SIRS) that occurs*
> *simultaneously with suspected or proven microorganism*
> *infection. Severe sepsis includes accompanying organ*
> *dysfunction while septic shock is a sepsis-induced*
> *hypotension that persists despite all interventives*
> *(such as fluid resuscitation).*

It specifically refers to a small subset of those who contract microbial infections (with a variety of different organisms, including *Babesia,*

Anaplasma, and *Ehrlichia*) and, despite the microbial element of the definition, it also refers to those who suffer such things as acute trauma (e.g., burns) accompanied by a hyper immune response. For these people the infection (or bodily damage) turns into sepsis, which, in some cases, leads to septic shock. It can, under some circumstances, lead to coma and death.

The sepsis process has identifiably similar dynamics whenever it occurs. This is true no matter which organism is involved or even where no organism is involved at all. In other words, sepsis and septic shock in malaria, babesiosis, ehrlichiosis, severe tissue injury, severe blood loss, and so on are nearly identical in nature. There is something occurring that is, at root, identical in all those circumstances.

Counterintuitively, during pathogen-initiated sepsis there does not seem to be any relation to parasite density and the onset of the sepsis. In other words, in some people who experience sepsis the causative organisms exist in high density throughout the body; in others the parasites, unbelievably enough, have already been eliminated from the body (usually with antibiotics); and in others the parasite density is so low as to be undetectable. As Bitsaktsis et al. (2007) comment, "Susceptibility to fatal IOE [*Ixodes ovatus Ehrlichia*] infection occurs within a narrow range of infectious doses, between 500 and 1000 bacteria."

This is why death from sepsis, when it occurs, can be sudden and inexplicable to medical technicians. Routine testing shows the person clear of parasites. While for some the symptoms are clearly life-threatening, for others medical examination finds few, and fairly minor, symptoms. To illustrate, in one instance, a 44-year-old man, an outdoor worker, from Minnesota, after experiencing a week of fever, chills, myalgia, and severe pain in his jaw, sought medical help from his physician. The physical examination revealed little; a low-grade fever was the only abnormal sign. The heart, lungs, abdomen, lymph, liver, and spleen all appeared normal. The man's physician did not perform a blood test but rather, based on geographical area, type of work, and symptoms, diagnosed Lyme disease. He prescribed amoxicillin and sent the man home. The symptoms did not worsen, but persisted, and 19 days later death occurred. The man's only complaint the night before was a slight shortness of breath.

At autopsy, both lungs were congested with mild to moderate hemorrhagic edema, and the pleura were inflamed. The spleen was found to be enlarged and interior examination found numerous polymorphonuclear leukocytes infiltrating septic foci in its tissue. The heart showed widespread transmural myocarditis with endocardial involvement. There were numerous areas of neutrophilic and lymphocytic infiltrates as well as scattered areas of myocardial necrosis. Cellular infiltrates were found throughout the heart's tissue. Despite the lack of symptoms, the widespread inflammation in the organs caused the man's body to just shut down.

ACUTE BABESIOSIS, ANAPLASMOSIS, AND EHRLICHIOSIS: THE INITIAL STAGE OF SEPSIS

During acute episodes of these coinfections, the immune response and cytokine profiles are quite different than during milder forms of the disease. Such episodes, while they can occur in younger, immunocompetent people (usually children), most often occur in those without a spleen, those on immunosuppressive drugs, those with diseases affecting immune function (such as HIV), or the old (usually over 50) who are experiencing age-related low immune function. There is also some evidence, at least in babesiosis, that less common forms of the protozoa may lead more easily to septic conditions. *Babesia duncani*, formerly *B.* WA1, is an example.

During the initial stages of infection the process is not unlike the milder forms of the diseases: IL-10 is upregulated and suppresses the Th1 immune response. However, at a certain point, the infection, rather than resolving or becoming intermittent, moves rather rapidly into an acute phase in which the immune system suddenly, and inexplicably, shifts to a very strong Th1 response. The cytokine profile alters accordingly. As Shaio and Lin (1998) comment about babesiosis:

> Of the cytokines tested, levels of TNF-α, IFN-γ, IL-2, and IL-6
> were high in the acute phase. . . . Neither IL-4 nor IL-10 were
> detectable throughout the course of the illness. Concentrations of
> E-selectin, VCAM-1, and ICAM-1 were also markedly increased as
> much as six-fold. . . . This study has demonstrated systemic elevation
> of levels of TNF-α, IFN-γ, and IL-2, but not of IL-4 or IL-10 in the
> acute phase of human babesiosis. In addition to the increase in NK
> cells, CD8+ T cells were predominant over CD4+ T cells during
> the acute phase.

This same cytokine profile is identical with that found in other mammals (cows, sheep, mice, and so on) that have developed acute forms of babesiosis. It is also very similar to that which occurs during acute anaplasmosis and ehrlichiosis.

The spleen appears to be the initial site of the Th1 cytokine shift but once the inflammatory cascade reaches a certain point, many of the body's organs also begin producing the same cytokines in copious amounts. The spleen, liver, lungs, heart, kidneys, and brain are generally the most strongly involved.

The immune movement into a powerful Th1 dynamic is often enough to, finally, eliminate the organisms and their effects from the body. Once the infection is dealt with, the body begins producing more IL-10, the inflammation begins to subside, the body returns to normal. However, in some circumstances, the immune system dysregulates. A hyper immune response with unusual qualities occurs. Sepsis begins. As *Anaplasma* researcher Stephen Dumler (2012) observes:

> When the typical homeostatic mechanism of inflammatory damp-
> ening occurs after the inflammatory stimulus has been controlled
> and reduced in quantity, inflammatory signaling ceases and the
> underlying pathologic processes are altered to that of repair and

reconstitution of function. However, significant and unremitting inflammatory injury occurs [under certain circumstances. This] . . . permits an unrestrained amplifying proinflammtory response without benefit of cytolytic homeostatic resolution. The result is a poorly controlled, in cases, relentless downward spiral of inflammatory injury and severe or fatal disease.

Treating Acute Babesiosis, Ehrlichiosis, and Anaplasmosis

Treatment of acute forms of these coinfections would be identical to treatment for the mild to moderate forms of the diseases with one exception: the substitution of *Scutellaria baicalensis* tincture for *Withania somnifera*. Dosage would be ½–1 teaspoon of the tincture 3–6x daily. Rather than downregulating IL-10, this would *modulate* its levels, that is, normalize its actions, lowering it if it is too high, raising if it is too low. There are a number of other herbs good for this, many of which are already in the protocols: *Cordyceps, Glycyrrhiza, Houttuynia, Poria cocos* (a.k.a. *Wolfiporia extensa*, a.k.a. fu ling), and *Sambucus. Withania* itself *does* act as a modulator (though I tend to think of it more as a dampening agent) but in this instance, I prefer the *Scutellaria*. Dosages for the other herbs and supplements in the protocol might have to be increased depending on how acute the conditions become.

COINFECTION-INITIATED SEPSIS AND ITS CYTOKINE CASCADE

Examination of tissues after septic shock episodes has found that the affected organs experience a range of impacts. Hypertrophy of the organs' endothelial cells as well as intravascular aggregates of large mononuclear inflammatory cells are common. This can lead to occlusion of medium veins, thrombosis, and multifocal coagulative necrosis. Again, these impacts have been reported even when levels of peripheral parasitemia remain very low; research commonly finds no relation between parasite density and the hyper immune response that occurs. In the liver, acute inflammation is present in the complete absence of babesial parasites in the affected locations.

During sepsis, the liver's production of cytochrome P450 3A (CYP3A) is significantly inhibited by the high levels of IFN-γ, TNF-α, nuclear factor kappa-B (NF-κB), and nitric oxide (NO) that are being produced by the liver's macrophages and Kupffer cells. (CYP3A, by the way, is responsible for the metabolism of some 50 percent of pharmaceutical drugs including chindamycin and quinine, one of two primary treatments for babesiosis. In consequence the drugs may never reach the levels necessary for successful treatment of babesial infection.) Under the impact of the continual, massive cytokine production the liver's tissue structure alters. The hepatic sinusoids dilate and begin to fill with macrophages and infected red blood cells. There is an increase in inflammatory cellular infiltrations, glutathione and catalase levels fall, nitric oxide and malondialdehyde levels significantly increase; there are increased levels of lactate dehydrogenase and protein carbonyl content. Hypertrophy of the endothelial cells occurs with accompanying occlusion in the veins. Necrosis develops and the tissue begins to crumble.

In the lungs pulmonary edema and phlebitis are common with reduced oxygenation of the blood and resultant shortness of breath. Endothelial cell activation is high with accompanying hypertropy of the endothelial cells. Intercellular adhesion molecule 1 (ICAM-1) is strongly upregulated. Intravascular margination of leukocytes accompanied by prominent lesions occurs in the lung tissue. Generally, there is reduced oxygen saturation and pH along with increased carbonic acid and accompanying hypoxia and respiratory acidosis.

In the spleen significant red pulp hyperplasia may occur. The splenic tissue contains large numbers of plasma cells, lymphocytes, and immunoblasts and large numbers of histiocytes exhibiting erythrophagocytic activity (that is, they consume red blood cells). The parenchyma is highly abnormal with severe integrity degradation. There are large multiple infarcts in the tissue, sometimes leading to rupture. (Again, because babesial infection can recur in endemic areas, procedures to salvage the spleen, if at all possible, should be pursued. There are cases, in the medical literature, where spontaneous splenic rupture has been successfully treated by physicians without splenectomy.)

Increasingly sophisticated examination of the cytokine cascade that occurs during sepsis has found it to be very unusual. IL-10 levels begin to substantially rise, just as should occur during the final stages of acute episodes. However, instead of lowering the inflammation in the body, counterintuitively the inflammation becomes worse, significantly so. Deeper analysis of the interleukin-10 molecules in play have found that the IL-10 itself dysregulates and these dysregulated forms, once circulating in the body, begin to substantially *increase* inflammation. They downregulate some cytokines but increase the presence of others. A very unusual cytokine cascade develops.

During HME-initiated sepsis and septic shock, for example, the cytokine profile finds increased levels of IL-10 and IL-13 (both *anti-inflammatory* cytokines) as well as increased levels of pro-inflammatory mediators TNF-α, IL-1α, IL-1β, IL-6, IL-8, MCP-1, MIP-1α, MIP-1β, G-CSF, TLR-2, and TLR-4, as well as increased levels of macrophages, neutrophils, T cells, and NK cells throughout the affected organs. IFN-γ and IL-2 levels are low, as are CD4+ T cell counts. CD4+ T cells are in fact stimulated to die by the unique cytokine cascade in play. There are accompanying high levels of CD8+ T cells as well as increased ferritin. The cytokine dynamics in play cause massive inflammation throughout the organs, leading to massive cellular infiltration and damage.

The organs' production of granulocyte colony-stimulating factor (G-CSF), for instance, leads to massive neutrophil infiltration. IL-8, also in high levels, stimulates similarly, recruiting neutrophils and T cells to the site of its production. During septic episodes, neutrophil levels in the blood remain low despite the massive increase in neutrophil production. These additional neutrophils instead cluster in the organs, at the sites of cytokine production, where they begin to destroy organ integrity.

MCP-1 (a.k.a. CCL2) recruits monocytes, T cells, and dendritic cells to specific sites where they stimulate massive inflammation. MIP-1α (a.k.a. CCL3) is strongly involved in acute inflammatory states and recruits and activates polymorphonuclear leukocytes (neutrophils, eosinophils, and basophils) at the sites of its expression. MIP-1β (a.k.a. CCL4) is a chemoattractant for NK cells, monocytes, as well as polymorphonuclear leukocytes. Once activated, CCL3 and 4 induce the expression of IL-1α and IL-1β, IL-6, and TNF-α. TNF-α levels become extremely high during sepsis and especially so during septic shock.

TNF-α induces fever, apoptotic cell death, widespread inflammation, loss of weight, muscle atrophy, fatigue, weakness, loss of appetite. TNF-α stimulates the production of NF-κB, which is involved in inflammatory and immune responses, cytokine production, cell survival, dysregulation of Bax/Bcl-2, and initiation of septic shock. It also upregulates p38 MAPK, which stimulates cellular death among other things.

Again, all this leads to massive inflammation and cellular infiltration in the organs expressing these mediators. Local pockets of cellular death (focal necrosis) in the organs begin to occur. As the condition continues, these spread, leading to organ failure.

The increased IL-10 levels should, under normal circumstances, act to reduce the inflammation but they do not; they make it worse. As Shu et al. (2003) observe:

> In critically ill patients, including those with sepsis, IL-10 is increased in circulation and the raised plasma levels of IL-10 have been reported to correlate with the severity and mortality in the pathological inflammatory response.

Studies have found that IL-10 undergoes polymorphic alterations just prior to sepsis. In other words a slightly different molecular form of IL-10 is generated than is usually present in the body. This unique IL-10 still downregulates some cytokines, specifically IFN-γ and IL-2, but it upregulates others that it normally downregulates, TNF-α for example. In every instance of severe sepsis and septic shock caused by these coinfections IL-10 has been found to be excessively high. The higher the levels, the more serious the condition.

However, studies have found that reducing sepsis by inhibiting IL-10 requires very sophisticated timing. Done too soon, it allows acute conditions to continue unabated. In other words, at the end of *healthy and normal* acute episodes, IL-10 production rises and reduces inflammation, and the healing process moves into repair and regeneration. Inhibiting IL-10 in these situations stops that progression. In situations progressing from acute to septic, IL-10 needs to be inhibited *after* sepsis has begun. Speficially, just after the hyperinflammatory process has begun. Studies have found that the inhibition of IL-10 during the hyperinflammatory stage reverses sepsis and septic shock. (It also has a significant and important inhibiting impact on myeloperoxidase levels, discussed in the next section.) This is where the use of *Withania somnifera* and other herbs such as *Glycyrrhiza* are exceptionally useful.

In addition to IL-10, importantly, during septic shock the levels of TLR-2 and TLR-4 increase as well. They rise to a minimum of two times higher than during non-shock infections. Toll-like receptors are a special form of pattern recognition receptor (PRR) molecules that are essential in innate immune responses to pathogens. Normally they respond to certain compounds (lipopolysaccharides) in the cellular walls of Gram-negative bacteria. However, *Ehrlichia* and *Anaplasma* bacteria don't have lipopolysaccharides in their membranes. Upregulation occurs through another mechanism entirely: they are responding to the production of another substance called HMGB1. And HMGB1 is a very potent cytokine indeed. We'll talk more about it in a moment.

THE CAUSES OF SEPSIS AND SEPTIC SHOCK

A cytokine cascade occurs in all people during these types of infections, but for some this progresses to what is more properly called a cytokine storm. It is this storm that leads to sepsis. While it is not known why certain people (and not others) develop sepsis, the initiating factor in all circumstances is the release of what are called damage-associated molecular pattern (DAMP) molecules.

Though, of course, to make things more difficult, they are sometimes also called alarmins or even pathogen-associated molecular pattern (PAMP) molecules.

PAMPs, to get a bit deeper into it, tend to be molecules located on the cellular surface of invading pathogens. DAMPs tend to be molecules that the body's cells release when they are damaged. Both activate an immune response once they are detected by pattern recognition receptors (PRRs) on the surface of immune cells. (TLRs are a specific form of PRRs.)

The innate immune system, over long evolutionary time, developed, and programmed in, an awareness and memory of certain molecular patterns that are potentially dangerous when they are found in the body. The various parts of the circulating innate immune system, whenever they encounter one of those patterns, initiate specific kinds of immune responses. Because both PAMPs and DAMPs activate the innate immune response some authors refer to both of these molecular signals as alarmins (as in burglar alarm, which, in this instance, calls the immune police). Other researchers insist that alarmins are *only* those signals that occur from damage and are never from those initiated by pathogens. (Others say, well, it involves their opponents' mothers somehow; feelings run rather high.) It makes more sense I think (I will probably be attacked on the playground for this) to consider them all as alarmins—PAMPs as exogenous (outside the body) alarmins and DAMPs as endogenous (inside) alarmins. (For reasons that will be clear in a moment, the inside/outside split may not ultimately be useful.)

ENDOGENOUS ALARMINS

There are a number of endogenous alarmins that have been associated with acute conditions leading to sepsis and septic shock, specifically: nucleophosmin, mitochondria, adenosine triphosphate (ATP), DNA, histones, neutrophil extracellular traps (NETs), and HMGB1. These are generally released in the body during nonprogrammed cell death (trauma or infection) and by immune cells using specialized secretion processes during damage or infection.

(As an initial note, the inhibition of NETs, HMGB1, and macrophage migration inhibitory factor, a.k.a. MIF, has been found to negate the cytokine dynamics that create sepsis and septic shock. This can reverse the conditions.)

Nucleophosmin (NPM)

NPM is a phosphoprotein primarily localized in a part of the nucleus of cells called the nucleolus. When cells are broken apart by invading pathogens or when the immune system is stimulated in certain ways, nucleophosmin can be released extracellularly, into the body. NPM release triggers a response release of a number of molecularly active compounds including intercellular adhesion molecule 1 (ICAM-1), TNF-α, IL-6, and monocyte chemoattractant protein 1 (MCP-1, a.k.a. CCL2).

ICAM-1, once produced in enough quantities, can act via a positive feedback loop, creating even more ICAM-1, with deleterious effects on tissues. It acts as a proinflammatory protein on the body's tissues when released. ICAM-1 initiates leukocyte binding to endothelial cells, more porous junctions between the cells, and transmigration of leukocytes into tissues.

TNF-α is a major proinflammatory cytokine that is closely linked with many autoimmune diseases. High levels of TNF-α can, by themselves, induce septic shock–like symptoms.

MCP-1 recruits monocytes, T cells, and dendritic cells to sites of inflammation in the body. MCP-1 is involved in conditions accompanied by monocytic infiltrates, neuroinflammatory conditions in the central nervous system and brain, and a number of autoimmune conditions. (IL-6 is covered in the DNA section; see page 180.)

Mitochondria

Mitochondria are also released into circulation when cells are killed or are broken apart by pathogens. Mitochondria are formerly free-living bacteria that, billions of years ago, were incorporated into cells through symbiogenesis. They act as the power factories of our cells. Mitochondria that are released into the body are identified by pattern receptors on innate immune cells as foreign bodies, as bacteria, because they aren't supposed to be free in the body. They are supposed to be sequestered inside other cells. In consequence, mitochondrial release is accompanied by systemic inflammation. People with major trauma to their body accompanied by severe inflammation have plasma levels of mitochondrial DNA at concentrations several thousand times higher than in people who are healthy.

Adenosine Triphosphate (ATP)

ATP transports chemical energy within cells, powering metabolism. It is used by cells as a coenzyme for a wide variety of processes. During cellular damage, ATP is released from cells into the extracellular environment. Further, a number of secretory organelles in cells store large amounts of ATP that they release as a danger or alarm signal. The release of ATP triggers neutrophils, macrophages, and dendritic cells to activate IL-1β and IL-18 (and the subsequent release of IL-1α). All are involved in the production of inflammation processes in the body.

DNA

DNA is normally held inside cells; it is not (generally) supposed to exist free in the body. In consequence, when it is, the innate immune system experiences it as an alarmin, signaling damage to cellular tissues (hence DAMP). (DNA can, of course, be an exogenous alarmin or PAMP when it is released from killed microorganisms such as babesial protozoa.) Immune mononuclear cells, when they encounter free DNA, immediately bind with it. This stimulates the release of significant amounts of IL-6 in the body, from both bound mononuclear cells and the spleen. The more free DNA in the serum, the more IL-6 that is produced. Overproduction of IL-6 is involved in a number of pathologic conditions in the body such as autoimmune, inflammatory, and lymphoproliferative disorders. Some of the conditions that occur are plasmacytosis, rheumatoid arthritis, encephalomyelitis, glomerulonephritis, dysregulation of new blood cell formation, and general inflammation and cellular dysregulation of bodily tissues, including the organs. Among the severely ill, those in whom sepsis occurs have been found to have significantly higher levels of free DNA (and IL-6) in their serum than those who did not develop sepsis.

Histones

Histones are highly alkaline proteins that exist inside the nuclei of cells. They package and order the DNA into specific structural units (nucleosomes). In essence they are a kind of spool around which DNA winds.

> *As an aside, each cell contains nearly six feet (two meters) of DNA. Wound around a histone protein spool this length is reduced significantly, to around 90 micrometers (0.09 μm), allowing it to fit inside the cell.*

When cells are damaged, for whatever reason, histones, like the DNA that winds around them, are released into the body. Extracellular histones stimulate abnormal endothelial cell activity, neutrophil margination and accumulation, and intra-alveolar hemorrhage.

All these molecules, when released from cells, significantly contribute to inflammation processes in the body and a number of autoimmune conditions; all are involved to differing extents in sepsis. However none are more potent stimulators of sepsis than NETs and HMGB1.

Neutrophil Extracellular Traps (NETs)

Neutrophils freely circulate in the blood vessels and are called to sites of inflammation during microbial infections. For a very long time, neutrophils were viewed through a fairly simplistic (i.e., stupid) lens as being nothing more than dumb killers of pathogens. Specifically, they simply enveloped (phagocytosed) pathogens and killed them. However, this view, in the past decade or so, has come under increasing scrutiny; it is in fact wrong. Neutrophils orchestrate an extremely complex response to microbial pathogens. Among them is the recently discovered capacity to create neutrophil extracellular traps or NETs for trapping and killing microbes.

NETs are formed by neutrophils on contact with many microbes (including a large variety of protozoa), as well as activated platelets and a number of inflammatory stimuli. Once stimulated by this contact a major alteration in the structure of the neutrophil cells occurs. The cells begin to unwind and then extrude their DNA and histones (and a few other substances) to form a kind of net or spiderweb or cage that traps pathogens within it. In essence, the DNA is unspooled and used, along with the histones, to create a webwork to entrap pathogens. NETs are able to trap nearly all types of pathogens, including those too large to phagocytose, among them Gram-negative and Gram-positive bacteria, viruses, protozoa, and yeasts.

To generate NET formation, a number of enzymes, held in special granules in the neutrophils, are, at the moment of contact with a pathogen, released. Neutrophil elastase (NE) and myeloperoxidase (MPO) are two of the most crucial. They break apart the DNA/histone formation and initiate their extrusion into the extracellular space. Once the NET forms, a number of compounds—NE, MPO, cathepsin G, proteinase 3, lactoferrin, calprotectin, and numerous antimicrobial peptides—are also released into the extracellular space. These act to kill the pathogens held inside the NETs. The histones integrated into the NET webs disintegrate the pathogen cell wall membranes, making them more susceptible to these microbial-killing compounds. Unfortunately, once stimulated, under some circumstances NETs continue to form throughout the body and organs, despite microbial clearance.

The continued presence of NETs creates an ongoing inflammation process in the body. Much of this comes from the massive amounts of DNA and histones that remain in circulation. This has been linked to a number of chronic inflammatory and autoimmune diseases such as vasculitis, thrombosis, acute lung injury, and even cancer. DNA, histones, MPO, NE, and cathepsin G are strongly involved in the tissue destruction that occurs in various organs and tissue types, especially endothelial and epithelial cells. NETs are a major factor in the acute conditions that can occur during coinfections, and are participants in both sepsis and septic shock.

Neutrophils that accumulate in specific locations, such as the lungs or brain, can cause serious damage when NET formation becomes self-generating. IFN-γ levels increase substantially in those locations (not in serum) and can cause, as an example, the kinds of problems seen in the neurological manifestations of malaria and babesiosis.

Inhibitors of NET formation can significantly reduce the impacts on organs and cellular tissues. (Some general NET inhibitors found to be effective are EGCG, rutin, vitamin C, and N-acetylcysteine). Inhibiting NE and MPO will stop NET formation entirely. There are a number of plants and isolated constituents/supplements that are very good for this.

Neutrophil Elastase (NE) Inhibitors

The seeds of *Caesalpinia echinata* (brazilwood) inhibit NE (as well as cathepsin G, proteinase 3, and NF-κB). They have been found to directly reduce organ injury caused by NETs, especially in the lungs.

(This herb is not generally available, nevertheless it is specific for this.)

Other NE inhibitors, in no particular order, include the traditional Chinese herb *Spatholobus suberectus* (millettia) stems, *Erythrina velutina* seeds (a.k.a. mulungu, which also inhibits TNF-α and leukocyte migration and stimulates IFN-α and IL-12), *Semiaquilegia adoxoides* (tiankuizi), *Thymus vulgaris* (thyme), *Tamarindus indica* (tamarind) seeds, *Galium aparine* (cleavers), *Arctium lappa* (burdock) root, *Fucus vesiculosus* (bladderwrack), *Pimpinella anisum* (anise) seed, *Angelica sinensis, Harpagophytum procumbens* (devil's claw) root, *Actaea racemosa* (black cohosh) root, *Oenothera biennis* (evening primrose) oil, *Nigella sativa* (black cumin) seed, oleic acid (olive leaf–infused oil), quercetin (also inhibits lactoferrin), heparin, resveratrol (from *Polygonum cuspidatum*), and genistein. The research on natural inhibitors of NE is fairly deep; this is just a look at some of the more prominent ones.

The strongest inhibitors, in my opinion, are *Angelica sinensis, Caesalpinia echinata* seeds, *Erythrina velutina* seeds, *Nigella sativa, Spatholobus subererectus,* and the constituents/supplements oleic acid (olive leaf–infused oil), resveratrol, quercetin, EGCG, rutin, N-acetylcysteine, and genistein.

Myeloperoxidase (MPO) Inhibitors

The research on MPO inhibitors is much less deep than for NE; nevertheless the inhibitors include *Amburana cearensis, Baccharis* spp., *Bauhinia forficata, Cissus sicyoides, Glycyrrhiza* spp., *Oenothera paradoxa* (evening primrose) oil, *Paeonia lactiflora, Punica granatum* (pomegranate), *Scutellaria baicalensis,* and the isolated constituents/supplements myricitrin, quercetin, resveratrol, and silymarin (milk thistle seed). The strongest appear to be *Scutellaria baicalensis, Oenothera paradoxa* (evening primrose) oil, quercetin, rutin, resveratrol, and silymarin.

HMGBI

High-mobility group protein B1 (HMGB1) is a nuclear binding protein. It works to facilitate gene transcription, stabilizing nucleosome formation in the cell. In essence, it is a guardian of the genome, protecting it from oxidant injury while promoting healthy genome formation and function. It is commonly found inside the nucleus and in the cytosol—the fluid inside the cell. It is also secreted from mature dendritic cells, leukocytes, and natural killer cells when they encounter alarmins. Damaged or necrotic cells (including red blood cells) release massive quantities of HMGB1 as they break apart.

HMGB1 is one of the most potent cytokine inducers known. During the early stages of infection, HMGB1 is a powerful, and benign, part of the innate immune response. The cytokines it induces do clear infections. Because it is so potent, HMGB1 stimulates the immune system to respond to and detect extremely low levels of parasite infestation. It also calls stem cells to damaged cellular sites, simulating tissue regeneration. The problem occurs when the immune system dysregulates, a postive feedback loop is generated, and HMGB1 levels do not subsequently decrease.

Interestingly, the molecular form of released HMGB1 is somewhat different depending on the site that releases it. Immune cells release one form, damaged or necrotic cells another. Each type of HMGB1 stimulates slightly different cytokine cascades. During inflammatory episodes as well as bacterial infestations of cells the more cells that are damaged, killed, and broken apart, the more HMGB1 they release. This initiates a powerful storm of cytokines throughout the body.

HMGB1 evokes an extremely potent innate immune response when it interacts with cellular surface receptors. Once HMGB1 is released from damaged cells it binds to specific cell surface receptors such as RAGE (receptor for advanced glycation end-products) and TLR-4. This combination stimulates the production of NF-κB (and its pathway), which then stimulates the production of TNF-α, IL-1β, and IL-6.

Most cytokines have a short life span. TNF-α, for example, only lasts around 90 minutes once its production is stimulated. HMGB1, on the other hand, lasts some 18 hours. During its life span it continues to stimulate the production of other cytokines. It is also a delayed immune stimulant; it generally begins to be released much later than other immune cytokines, anywhere from 8 to 48 hours later, depending on circumstances. This is why sepsis occurs later during infections. (HMGB1 is released more quickly—within two hours—during burns or trauma, but during infections it is slower.) Once initiated, HMGB1 levels tend to remain high. A reduced form with high chemoattractant properties occurs during the first three weeks of infection, then a strongly inflammatory form presents for the next four to eight weeks. And levels remain high, for up to two months after the septic condition appears to have passed.

HMGB1 tends to be much more potent in its effects if there is extracellular DNA present. Thus the more cellular debris there is, the more potent its impacts on the body. Once HMGB1 encounters DNA, it strongly binds to it, producing synergistic impacts throughout the body.

HMGB1 strongly suppresses normal IL-10 production but is involved in the expression of the altered IL-10 that is present during septic episodes. As well, HMGB1 activates specific pattern recognition receptors called toll-like receptors (TLRs) that exist on the surface of sentinel immune cells. It specifically activates TLR-2, TLR-4, and TLR-9 as well as RAGE. (TLR-4 on the other hand, once upregulated, itself stimulates the release of HMGB1, creating a self-reinforcing pattern.) The TLRs strongly upregulate a number of other, very potent cytokines, contributing to the cytokine storm. To make things worse, HMGB1 is strongly synergistic with these cytokines—that is, it amplifies their effects.

Levels of NF-κB, TNF-α, RANTES, IL-6, MIF, IL-12, and IFN-γ, in pretty much that order, are stimulated. The amount of cytokine production is directly proportional to the amount of HMGB1 being produced. The more that is released, the higher cytokine levels go. (And these HMGB1 levels are *tiny*; only microgram quantities are necessary to produce extremely potent effects.) The levels of IL-6, for example, are four times higher, IL-8 three times higher, and IFN-γ two times higher during severe, HMGB1-accompanied infections than the levels in milder cases. The higher the cytokine levels go, the more cells that are damaged by inflammation. As damaged and necrotic cells proliferate, more HMGB1 is released. A positive feedback loop is created. The inflammation becomes self-sustaining. Other cytokines (chemokines) begin to be produced, such as CXCL12, IL-8, MCP-1, and MIP-1 and MIP-2. And still other actors come into play.

Platelets can also express HMGB1; they export it to their cellular surfaces when activated by cytokines. (And the specific spectrum of cytokines we're talking about here does in fact cause them to express HMGB1.) The upregulation of HMGB1 on platelets stimulates the production of RAGE, a.k.a. the receptor for advanced glycation endproducts, by endothelial cells. Once RAGE is upregulated, the endothelial cells increase their expression of vascular cell adhesion molecule 1 (VCAM-1) and intercellular adhesion molecule 1 (ICAM-1). These compounds increase the permeability of the endothelial cells and inhibit their binding to each other, permitting infiltrate movement through the endothelium deeper into the body. Infiltrates can include microbial pathogens, immune cells, and cytokines. This is a source of the infiltrates that occur in damaged organs and the increased inflammation and edema that they experience.

HMGB1 levels tend to be very high in the serum of the acutely ill, especially those with sepsis and septic shock. The higher the levels are, the worse the prognosis. Anemia is common and worsens the higher the levels become. Cytokines such as TNF-α, MIF, IL-12, and IL-10 and babesial protozoal factors such as lysate and hemozin inhibit effective red blood cell production (erythropoiesis), creating anemia.

HMGB1 and NE are, unsurprisingly, synergistic with each other. HMGB1 stimulates the release of myeloperoxidase (MPO), leading to more production of NETs, while neutrophil elastase (NE) stimulates the release of HMGB1, leading to more production of MPO, which leads to more production of NETs, which leads to . . .

HMGB1 also stimulates NET formation because it inhibits the

macrophage engulfment of dying neutrophils. NETs formation is a kind of cellular death (called NETosis by some). At a certain point in time, to reduce their presence and impacts on the body, NETs are engulfed (phagocytosed) by macrophages, removing them from the system. HMGB1 inhibits this process, thus the NETs remain in circulation longer and continue to generate more impacts, more HMGB1, and so on.

Increased levels of HMGB1 cause many of the symptoms of sepsis including fever, dysregulation of intestinal barrier function, tissue injury, massive accumulation of infiltrates in organs such as the liver and kidneys, accumulation of proinflammatory cytokines in the brain, and neutrophil infiltration and acute injury in the lungs.

The spleen's splenocytes are particularly activated by HMGB1 and show strongly enhanced cytokine release. In other words they become hyperactive in their release of inflammatory cytokines. The spleen becomes enlarged, leukocyte numbers substantially increase (leukocytosis), and the spleen tissue begins to experience inflammatory damage accompanied by large numbers of infiltrates. Anti-HMGB1 compounds reverse this and reverse splenomegaly.

The impacts of HMGB1 on the liver are similar, producing the physiological alterations in its tissue that have been found during septic events. Again, anti-HMGB1 reduces all those parameters, protecting the liver's cellular structures and restoring it to normal functioning.

If the infections do affect the brain, the damaged astrocytes and microglia begin to synthesize and release HMGB1 and IL-1β. A rapid release of HMGB1 from the neurons occurs. This process tends to be self-maintaining. Extracellular HMGB1 initiates inflammation through cytokine production and release and the inflammatory mediators then act on the neurocytes, causing more release of HMGB1. At best there is cognitive impairment, at worst epileptic seizures begin to occur. If the brain is subjected to increased levels of HMGB1 over time, cognitive impairment can take a year or more to correct. Again, anti-HMGB1 compounds reverse the process, reducing impairment and alleviating epileptic episodes. Anti-TLR-4 compounds are also effective; reducing IL-1β helps as well. Inhibiting TLR-4 significantly reduces the impacts of HMGB1 on the body as HMGB1 impacts that TLR directly, stimulating cytokine release. (Some useful TLR-4 inhibitors, in no particular order, are resveratrol, artesenuate, guggul, *Panax ginseng,* curcumin, *Astragalus* spp., *Zingiber officinalis, Polygonum cuspidatum, Lycium chinese* root bark, *Glycyrrhiza* spp., *Codonopsis lanceolata, Ginkgo biloba, Scutellaria baicalensis, Salvia miltiorrhiza,* and *Sparganium stoloniferum.*)

Interestingly, both malarial and babesial protozoa contain HMGB-like proteins that they release during infection. They use this, along with other interventions, to stimulate the particular cytokine response they need in order to facilitate infection. During acute infections with either organism, blood levels of HMGB1 are very high. Part of this occurs from the organisms' damage to red blood cells, which release large quantities of HMGB1.

A number of pharmaceuticals have been found useful for reducing both NETs and HMGB1 levels. Of specific note are minocycline (reduces HMGB1), sivelestat (reduces NE and HMGB1 expression and levels), cisplatin (reduces HMGB1), and heparin. Heparin is a rather potent anti-inflammatory, reducing a number of inflammatory cytokines and processes, including HMGB1.

Of note: Corticosteroids (e.g., dexamethasone and cortisone) as well as aspirin, ibuprofen, and indomethacin, even at superpharmacological concentrations, have no effect on HMGB1 levels. They can exacerbate the condition by delaying appropriate intervention. They do **not** provide *any* useful anti-inflammatory actions during sepsis or septic shock.

There are a number of plants and natural substances that have been found to reduce HMGB1 levels and subsequently reduce or eliminate the acute symptoms of infection, sepsis, and septic shock. Aqueous extracts of green tea (*Camellia sinensis*), *Angelica sinensis,* and *Salvia miltiorrhiza* are all effective. All are dose dependent. The compounds EGCG, choline, and nicotine are also effective.

Angelica, dose-dependently, inhibits HMGB1 release and stops the progression of lethal sepsis. Both green tea and EGCG act similarly. They prevent HMGB1 release, attenuate HMGB1-mediated NO (nitric oxide) release, stop the accumulation of exogenous HMGB1 on macrophage cell surfaces, and provide a dose-dependent protection against lethal sepsis, even 24 hours after onset. Circulating levels of HMGB1 are reduced, as are levels of IL-6. Angelica shows similar activity while also inhibiting the endothelial cell permeability that HMGB1 causes.

Both *Salvia miltiorrhiza* and its tanshinone constituents dose-dependently reduce circulating HMGB1 levels and protect against lethal sepsis. The herb/compound also reduces levels of RAGE, TLR-4, and NF-κB. Neurological deficits in the brain (for instance) are alleviated, inflammation decreases, function is normalized. Claudin-5, a protein, is strongly upregulated. Claudin-5 is an integral membrane protein that serves to create tight junction strands in epithelial and endothelial cell sheets. This prevents the migration of infiltrates through the epithelial and endothelial barriers deeper into organ tissues.

Licorice (*Glycyrrhiza glabra*) and its constituent glycyrrhizin are important adjuncts in treating HMGB1-related sepsis. The plant and its compound reduce the release of HMGB1 and, at the same time, through a number of mechanisms, strongly bind to the HMGB1 molecule. Thus, through two mechanisms, they reduce the amount of circulating HMGB1 in the system. Licorice (and glycyrrhizin) has been found to inhibit SIRS, the systemic inflammatory response syndrome, which is an essential component of sepsis. It also normalizes splenocyte function in the spleen, reducing its hyperactivity, primarily from its effects on HMGB1 and a number of the involved cytokines. Licorice (and glycyrrhizin) has similar impacts on the liver if used during sepsis. It attenuates histological hepatic alterations, significantly reducing ALT and AST levels as well as lactate dehydrogenase. Hepatocyte apoptosis, a major element in organ failure and death in severe sepsis, is significantly inhibited by the herb/compound. This is partly due to its impacts on the mitochondria in liver cells; it inhibits the release of the proapoptotic mitochondrial cytochrome C from those cells, especially the Kupffer cells, the primary cells that experience massive die-offs during sepsis. The herb/compound also upregulates expression of proliferating cell nuclear antigen, promoting regeneration of the liver, and confers neuroprotection, reducing HMGB1 levels in the brain and reducing inflammatory damage and epileptic episodes. In addition to its impacts on HMGB1, the herb/compound stimulates the production of normal IL-10 molecules and inhibits a wide range of inflammatory cytokines, chemokines, and adhesion molecules, specifically IFN-γ, TNF-α, CCL2, VCAM-1, E-selectin, caspase-3, MPO, and NF-κB.

Three other important plants that have been found to reduce HMGB1 levels are *Forsythia suspensa* (one of the 50 fundamental herbs in Chinese medicine; it also downregulates TNF-α, IL-6, MPO, and NF-κB and reduces infiltration of leukocytes), *Withania somnifera* (which also reduces leukocyte migration and infiltration, reduces endothelial cell permeability, and inhibits ICAM-1, VCAM-1, IL-6, TNF-α, and NF-κB), and *Paeonia lactiflora* (white peony root, which also downregulates MPO and inhibits RAGE and TLRs 2 and 4).

Others plants of note are *Cannabis* and its constituent cannabidiol, *Rosmarinus officinalis* (rosemary, which also reduces endothelial permeability and leukocyte migration), *Prunella vulgaris* (self-heal), *Cyperus rotundus,* and oleanolic acid (from olive oil/leaf, which also inhibits NF-κB and TNF-α).

Other effective compounds are choline, acetylcholine, nicotine, quercetin (and quercitrin), lycopene, rutin (which also inhibits TNF-α, NF-κB, ICAM-1, VCAM-1, vascular permeability, and the adhesion and migration of leukocytes), emodin, curcumin, berberine (note: plants containing berberine are not systemic enough to counter HMGB1 in sepsis or acute conditions), ethyl pyruvate, and ethyl caffeate.

All are dose dependent.

NATURAL TREATMENT OF SEPSIS
DURING COINFECTIONS

The treatment rationale for sepsis during acute infection with babesia, ehrlichia, or anaplasma is as follows:

1. Inhibit the release and production of HMGB1 while binding free HMGB1 to reduce levels already in the system.
2. Inhibit and reduce NETs formation by inhibiting NE and MPO.
3. Downregulate IFN-γ, NO, TNF-α, NF-κB, IL-1β, IL-2, IL-6, IL-12, ICAM-1, VCAM-1, and E-selectin.
4. Protect and enhance the function of the organs affected by the specific organisms. Specifically, protection of the spleen and liver is crucial.

Specific Herbs and Isolated Constituents

The specific herbs and isolated constituents (some of which have been detailed earlier in this chapter) are as follows:

HMGB1-inhibitors (primary): *Angelica sinensis, Astragalus* spp., *Camellia sinensis, Forsythia suspensa, Glycyrrhiza* spp., *Paeonia lactiflora, Salvia miltiorrhiza, Withania somnifera,* and the constituents acetylcholine, berberine, choline, curcumin, EGCG, emodin, ethyl caffeate, ethyl pyruvate, lycopene, nicotine, quercetin, quercitrin, and rutin. Note: Plants containing berberine are not systemic enough to counter HMGB1 in sepsis or acute conditions.

TLR-4 inhibitors: *Astragalus* spp., *Codonopsis lanceolata, Ginkgo biloba, Glycyrrhiza* spp., *Lycium chinense* root bark, *Panax ginseng, Salvia miltiorrhiza, Scutellaria baicalensis, Sparganium stoloniferum, Zingiber officinale,* and the isolated constituents artesenuate, curcumin, guggul, and resveratrol.

NE inhibitors: *Actaea racemosa* (black cohosh) root, *Angelica sinensis, Arctium lappa* (burdock) root, *Caesalpinia echinata* (brazilwood) seeds, *Erythrina velutina* (mulungu) seeds, *Fucus vesiculosus* (bladderwrack), *Galium aparine* (cleavers), *Harpagophytum procumbens* (devil's claw) root, *Nigella sativa* (black cumin) seed, *Oenothera biennis* (evening primrose) oil, *Pimpinella anisum* (anise) seed, *Semiaquilegia adoxoides* (tiankuizi), *Spatholobus suberectus* (millettia) stems, *Tamarindus indica* (tamarind) seeds, *Thymus vulgaris* (thyme), the isolated constituents genistein, quercetin, oleic acid (olive leaf–infused oil), and resveratrol, and the pharmaceutical heparin. The research on natural inhibitors of NE is fairly deep; this is just a look at some of the more prominent inhibitors.

The strongest inhibitors, in my opinion, are *Angelica sinensis, Caesalpinia echinata* seeds, *Erythrina velutina* seeds, *Nigella sativa, Spatholobus subererectus,* and the constituents/supplements oleic acid (olive leaf–infused oil), resveratrol, quercetin, EGCG, rutin, NAC, and genistein.

MPO inhibitors: *Amburana cearensis, Baccharis* spp., *Bauhinia forficata, Cissus sicyoides, Forsythia suspensa, Glycyrrhiza* spp., *Oenothera paradoxa* (evening primrose) oil, *Paeonia lactiflora, Punica granatum* (pomegranate), *Scutellaria baicalensis,* and the isolated constituents/supplements myricitrin, quercetin, resveratrol, rutin, and silymarin (milk thistle seed). The strongest appear to be *Scutellaria baicalensis, Oenothera paradoxa* (evening primrose) oil, *Paeonia lactiflora,* quercetin, rutin, resveratrol, and silymarin.

IL-12 inhibitors: *Cordyceps* spp., *Salvia miltiorrhiza.*

IFN-γ inhibitors: *Chelidonium majus* (greater celandine), *Cordyceps* spp., *Glycyrrhiza* spp. (licorice), *Morinda citrifolia* (noni), *Paeonia lactiflora, Sambucus* spp. (elder), *Scutellaria baicalensis* root. Note: Elder and licorice are IFN-γ modulators—they raise it if necessary, lower it when needed.

Nitric oxide inhibitors: *Cordyceps* spp., *Eupatorium perfoliatum* (boneset), *Hericium erinaceus* (lion's mane mushroom), *Houttuynia* spp., *Morinda citrifolia* (noni), *Polygala tenuifolia* (Chinese senega) root, *Scutellaria baicalensis* root.

TNF-α inhibitors: *Angelica sinensis, Cordyceps* spp., *Erythrina velutina* (mulungu) seeds, *Eupatorium perfoliatum* (boneset), *Forsythia suspensa, Ginkgo biloba, Glycyrrhiza* spp., *Houttuynia* spp., *Paeonia lactiflora, Polygala tenuifolia* (Chinese senega) root, *Pueraria lobata, Sambucus* spp., *Scutellaria baicalensis* root, *Withania somnifera, Zingiber officinalis,* and the constituents quercetin and EGCG.

IL-1β inhibitors: *Astragalus* spp., *Cordyceps* spp., *Eupatorium perfoliatum* (boneset), *Polygala tenuifolia* (Chinese senega) root, *Polygonum cuspidatum* (Japanese knotweed) root, *Pueraria lobata* (kudzu), *Scutellaria baicalensis* root.

IL-6 inhibitors: *Forsythia suspensa, Isatis* spp., *Paeonia lactiflora, Pueraria lobata* (kudzu), *Scutellaria baicalensis* root, *Withania somnifera.*

ICAM-1 inhibitors: *Cordyceps* spp., *Paeonia lactiflora, Polygonum cuspidatum* (Japanese knotweed), *Sambucus* spp., *Withania somnifera.*

VCAM-1 inhibitors: *Glycyrrhiza* spp., *Polygonum cuspidatum, Pueraria lobata* (kudzu), *Sambucus* spp., *Scutellaria baicalensis* root, *Withania somnifera.*

E-selectin inhibitors: *Glycyrrhiza* spp., *Paeonia lactiflora, Polygonum cuspidatum, Pueraria lobata* (kudzu).

IL-2 inhibitors: *Commiphora mukul* (myrrh), *Scutellaria baicalensis* root.

NF-κB inhibitors: *Astragalus* spp., *Eupatorium perfoliatum* (boneset), *Forsythia suspensa, Glycyrrhiza* spp., *Houttuynia* spp., *Paeonia lactiflora, Polygala tenuifolia* (Chinese senega) root, *Pueraria lobata, Salvia miltiorrhiza, Scutellaria baicalensis* root, *Withania somnifera, Zingiber officinalis.*

Suggested Pharmaceutical Support

Heparin: Because heparin has been found so effective across such a wide range in septic conditions, in truly serious conditions it makes sense to use it. It specifically inhibits neutrophil elastase–induced HMGB1 release and inhibits NE activity in the body. (If its anticoagulant properties are a problem a desulfated heparin can be used instead.) Its actions are particularly effective in alleviating HMGB1-related lung injury.

SUGGESTED PROTOCOL FOR SEPSIS

As you can see from a review of the active herbs, the ones that cover the most areas are *Angelica sinensis, Astragalus* spp., *Cordyceps* spp., *Forsythia suspensa, Glycyrrhiza* spp., *Pueraria lobata, Salvia miltior-rhiza, Scutellaria baicalensis,* and *Withania somnifera.* Thus . . .

1. Tincture combination of *Angelica sinensis* and *Astragalus* spp. (equal parts of each), 1 tablespoon each hour.
2. Tincture of *Salvia miltiorrhiza,* 1 tablespoon each hour.
3. Tincture combination of *Pueraria lobata* and *Cordyceps* spp. (equal parts of each), 1 tablespoon each hour.
4. Tincture combination of *Glycyrrhiza* spp. and *Scutellaria baicalensis* (equal parts of each), 1 tablespoon each hour.
5. Spleen protection is provided by the *Salvia miltiorrhiza.* This will also protect the liver to some extent, as will the licorice. The use of high-dose standardized silymarin compounds is highly suggested to protect the liver's Kupffer cells from apoptosis. (Dosage: milk thistle, standardized tincture, 1 teaspoon 6x daily.)

The tinctures may be mixed together in any liquid (pomegranate suggested) and should be taken until sepsis ameliorates. Note: Such high doses of licorice (*Glycyrrhiza* spp.) are strongly contraindicated for long-term use. This is a short-term, acute condition intervention only.

9

The Materia Medica

The advantages of natural compounds are fewer side effects in comparison to orthodox medical drugs, and the production of synergistic effects for a more positive treatment outcome.

K. KITAZATO, Y. WANG, AND N. KOBAYASHI,
"VIRAL INFECTIOUS DISEASE AND NATURAL
PRODUCTS WITH ANTIVIRAL ACTIVITY"

An illness is like a journey to a far country; it sifts all one's experience and removes it to a point so remote that it appears like a vision.

SHOLEM ASCH

They do not know very good Latin, these botanists.

ALBERT HOFMANN

I have done extensive monographs, in other works, on many of the herbs suggested in this book. Time and space limitations prohibit repeating them here. I will cover the most important ones (to varying extents) in this volume, including the addition of new material not to be found in the longer monographs (there are always new things I am learning, I am not yet at the point where I put up "keep off the grass" signs and yell at clouds . . . though some of my more prominent herbal friends . . . well, I guess I should skip that part).

The only new, in-depth monograph in this book is on *Salvia miltiorrhiza*. It is a crucial, foundational herb for these conditions and, as I am discovering, quite a wonderful plant medicine in its own right. I have become very fond of it the last few years. (It's always this way—some herb begins demanding attention and after a while you listen and find that it is just the new medicine that you needed to learn about.)

If you wish to see the in-depth monographs for the herbs not covered as completely in this volume, here is where you can find them: *Polygonum cuspidatum* (Japanese knotweed) and *Andrographis paniculata* are in *Healing Lyme* (Raven Press, 2005). In *Herbal Antibiotics*, second edition (Storey Publishing, 2012), you can find *Alchornea cordifolia*, *Artemisia* spp. (including the constituents artemisinin, artesenuate, and artemisone), *Bidens pilosa*, *Cryptolepis sanguinolenta*, *Eleutherococcus senticosus*, *Eupatorium perfoliatum* (boneset), *Ganoderma lucidum* (reishi), *Glycyrrhiza* spp. (licorice), *Rhodiola* spp., and *Sida acuta*. In *Herbal Antivirals* (Storey Publishing, 2013), you can find *Houttuynia* spp. and *Scutellaria baicalensis* (Chinese skullcap) root, as well as *Sambucus* spp. (elder), *Isatis* spp., and *Zingiber officinalis* (ginger) if you want to. (These latter three can be useful but neither essential nor primary in treating babesiosis, anaplasmosis, and ehrlichiosis.) *Olea europa* (olive leaf and oil) including the constituents oleic and oleanolic acid (also not essential but nevertheless useful) are covered in depth in *Healing Lyme Disease Coinfections: Complementary and Holistic Treatments for Bartonella and Mycoplasma* (Healing Arts Press, 2013).

MAKING YOUR OWN MEDICINES

I strongly suggest, if you have any inclination at all to do so, that you make your own herbal medicines. There are a number of reasons for this, the most obvious being cost; making your own will lower your cost significantly.

Although herbal medicines are extremely inexpensive compared to pharmaceuticals (and often more effective), treating a long-term, chronic condition can be expensive, especially if you buy them already prepared. This has become especially true as the FDA has begun to exert more control over herbal medicines via its Good Manufacturing Practices regulations, a.k.a. the GMP (not necessarily a good thing), and as the larger herbal companies begin to consolidate their control over the marketplace (very much not a good thing). Those particular marketplace shifts are causing price increases in nearly every area. A small rant . . .

||||||||||||||||||||||||||||||||||||||||||||||||||

Tiny Rant
The Irrational GMP Rationale

The common and oft-repeated rationale for the GMP is that it will make herbal products safer for the public. This is not actually accurate. The main safety problems that occur with herbal products come, and always have come, from two sources: 1) manufacturing errors by a large company (usually product contamination of one sort or another, always inadvertent) and 2) unscrupulous product creation (specifically: herbal energy pills, weight loss products, and muscle development formulations) by corporations of one sort or another. The small, herbalist-owned companies have never had these kinds of problems; their products are almost always better than those produced by the large companies, they are less expensive, and, based on the public record, they are much safer.

The GMP was developed, and supported, by the big herbal companies (as well as a number of large pharmaceutical companies) in order to control the marketplace . . . and as a response to the FDA looking askance at those two problem areas within the natural products world. It wasn't really necessary to put the same restrictions on manufacturing on both the large and small companies—these are two different kinds of companies, with entirely different functions and behaviors—yet, they did. Unfortunately, over time, this will lead to the majority of the smaller companies going out of business. When that occurs, fewer herbal formulations will be available and those at a much higher price. Nevertheless, there are still many good small companies in business (the consolidation will take a few years); I recommend my favorites in a section at the end of the book.

||||||||||||||||||||||||||||||||||||||||||||||||||||||

Fortunately, neither the GMP or anything else prevents you, nor will prevent you, from making your own medicines. Not only will it be much cheaper for you, but there is something exceptionally wonderful that happens when you work directly with a plant for your healing, when you find it in a field, or grow it in your yard (it may already be there, if you just look around), or even if you buy the plant from a grower (several really good ones in "Sources of Supply," page 333). When your life is saved by a plant, nothing is ever the same again. This is most especially true if you have developed a personal relationship with the plant from making it into medicine for yourself.

There are a number of good books on making plant medicines. I generally suggest my own in-depth look at it (inevitably), which is included in the second edition of *Herbal Antibiotics* (it contains, as well, an extensive formulary of over 200 herbs), or Richo Cech's *Making Plant Medicine,* third edition (Horizon Herbs, 2000), or James Green's *Herbal Medicine-Maker's Handbook* (Crossing Press, 2000). All are very good.

If you obtain a resale license from your state (easy and inexpensive) and give yourself a business name (e.g., The Get Rich Very Slowly Herb Company) you will be able to buy herbs wholesale from nearly all wholesalers. This will lower your purchase cost of the herbs by anywhere from half to nine-tenths of their retail price.

THE MATERIA MEDICA

I consider the most important herbs/supplements for the conditions discussed in this book (whether primary, foundational herbs or supportive ones) to be *Angelica sinensis, Astragalus* spp., *Bidens pilosa, Ceanothus* spp., *Chelidonium majus, Cordyceps* spp., *Crataegus oxyacantha* (hawthorn), *Cryptolepis sanguinolenta, Eupatorium perfoliatum, Forsythia suspensa, Glycyrrhiza* spp., *Houttuynia* spp., *Leonurus cardiaca, Paeonia lactiflora, Panax ginseng, Polygala tenuifolia, Polygonum cuspidatum, Pueraria lobata, Rhodiola* spp., *Salvia miltiorrhiza, Scutellaria baicalensis, Sida acuta, Silybum marianum* (milk thistle seed), *Withania somnifera,* and the isolated constituents EGCG, genistein, L-arginine, N-acetylcysteine, and quercetin.

The foundational herbs/supplements, essential for either *Babesia* or *Ehrlichia/Anaplasma* infections, are *Angelica sinensis, Astragalus* spp., *Bidens pilosa, Ceanothus* spp., *Cordyceps* spp., *Cryptolepis sanguinolenta, Glycyrrhiza* spp., *Houttuynia* spp., *Pueraria lobata, Salvia miltiorrhiza* (danshen), *Scutellaria baicalensis, Withania somnifera,* and the isolated constituents L-arginine, genistein, and N-acetylcysteine.

We'll begin with the in-depth look at *Salvia miltiorrhiza,* followed by briefer looks, in alphabetical order, of the remaining herbs and supplements.

Salvia miltiorrhiza (Danshen)

Family: Lamiaceae

Genus

Salvia (mostly but there is a subgenus involved here as well; see the species section for further obfuscation).

Salvia comes from the ancient Latin word *salvus,* meaning "safe," essentially a reference to the extensive and very broad healing properties of this genus. (The word *sage* is a later derivation. It is Middle English, derived from the Old French term *sauge,* which was derived from the

Latin *salvia,* meaning "healing plant," which was derived from, way back there in time, *salvus* again.)

The salvias are a big genus and after a look at the work of numerous well-degreed taxonomists, I can definitively state that the genus contains 700, or 900, or 1,000 species. So, now you know.

Common Names

Red sage, Chinese sage, danshen (or tanshen), as the case may be. Its pharmaceutical name (sometimes encountered) is radix salviae miltiorrhizae.

Species Used

Well, *miltiorrhiza* obviously, however . . . there are 36 species of *Salvia* (and the *Salvia* subgenus *Sclarea*) used by Chinese practitioners; all are considered to be, and are, in common parlance, danshen. In traditional Chinese practice (i.e., in China, *not* in the United States) they are generally considered interchangeable. This has caused much conflict, soul-searching, chemical nitpicking (and fisticuffs) among the Chinese researchers, similar to the DNA-based rearrangement of plants conflicts caused by taxonomists in the West.

There are, according to DNA analysis, three distinct clades of *Salvia* in the world, each roughly distinguished by geography. Species in Clade I are indigenous to China/Asia; those in Clade II are indigenous to the Mediterranean region; and those in Clade III are specific to the Americas (this is the oldest, most isolated group and includes what many consider the most unusual of the salvias, *Salvia divinorum*). There are, of course, just to make things more difficult, subcategories called subclades, i.e., subclades A, B, and C. The problem seems to be that the salvias love to interbreed with each other so unique genotypes abound. (Sex, making life difficult for taxonomists everywhere.)

Clade III in the Americas contains the most species, at well over 500. However, in Clade I, which is what we are interested in here, there are 78 (or maybe 84) species, 24 (or maybe 26) varieties, and 8 (or perhaps 10) forma of salvia. (Taxonomists are really sure about those figures.)

Here is how all that classification stuff goes . . . genus then subgenus, species then subspecies, varietas (varieties) then subvarietas, forma and finally subforma. (This is another reason why no one likes taxonomists.)

Of those 78 (or 84) species, 70 (or maybe 75) are endemic to China and, again, 36 (or 23) of those are used as danshen in Chinese medicine.

And because things are not complicated enough, there is a subgenus of *Salvia* called *Sclarea* and a number of species within the *Sclarea* are used interchangeably for *Salvia* danshens in many Chinese regions. The Chinese *Sclarea* are clustered together in subclade A (of Clade I), which also contains a number of true salvias, including *Salvia przewalskii,* a rather medicinally potent member of the group. Clade I, subclade B is generally considered the most medicinally active of the danshens. It contains what are considered to be the most powerful danshens used in herbal practice, specifically *Salvia miltiorrhiza, S. miltiorrhiza* forma *alba,*

which is identical to Salvia miltiorrhiza *except that it has white flowers (*alba *means white). Other than that one difference, they are pretty much the same plant when it comes to medicinal actions and usage.*

and their very close relatives *S. bowleyana, S. cavaleriei* varietas *simplicifolia,* and *S. yunnanensis.* These five plants are considered to be the strongest interchangeable species of danshen. The other major plant in the danshen group is *S. przewalskii,* which contains more tanshinone IIA (see rant in appendix) than *S. miltiorrhiza,* as well as a number of other compounds unique to itself. A number of Chinese researchers and practitioners believe that the plant is a major and rather unique medicinal within the danshens.

Because more than 176 million pounds of danshen are used in Chinese medicine every year, agricultural production cannot keep up with demand and adulteration is a constant problem. *S. przewalskii*, it turns out, is the most common adulterant of *S. miltiorrhiza*. Although the Chinese are spending more time analyzing the exact identity of the herbs they sell before they ship them out of the country, the best way to avoid this problem is to grow the plant yourself.

Most of the salvias used as danshen in traditional Chinese medicine do contain the same chemical constituents; the amounts just differ a bit. *S. miltiorrhiza* is usually considered to be the strongest of the species used and is the one upon which most research has been done. However, a caveat . . . exhaustive analysis of the chemical constituents of *S. miltiorrhiza* shows a wide variation in those constituents depending on where the plant is grown and when it is harvested. Once again, there is no definitive, final, quantitative analysis of constituents that can be said to be the norm for any plant medicine. (Again, see the rant in appendix.) Things change depending on the ecological scenario in which the plant emerges.

So . . . short answer to species used? The strongest are considered to be *Salvia miltiorrhiza, S. miltiorrhiza* forma *alba, S. bowleyana, S. cavaleriei* varietas *simplicifolia, S. yunnanensis,* and finally *S. przewalskii,* in that order.

This monograph will focus on *S. miltiorrhiza* with minor side trips here and there. Please note that the long isolation of the American salvias produced very different compounds over time than those in the Clade I salvias; they are not interchangeable with the Chinese danshens.

Part Used

The root or rhizome depending on who you ask. The species name *miltiorrhiza* comes from the ancient Greek *miltos,* meaning "red earth," and *rhiza,* meaning "root." The root of the plant, when harvested, is indeed quite a remarkable and beautiful brilliant red, as are the tincture and the tea.

Habitat and Appearance

Salvia miltiorrhiza grows wild in China on sunny mountainsides, in meadows, on forest margins, and along stream beds, generally up to an altitude of 4,000 feet. It is a perennial growing up to two feet in height and flowers from June to September. The flowers truly are beautiful.

Cultivation

The seeds of the plant tend to be viable for at least three years if not a bit longer. They are, as Richo Cech at Horizon Herbs puts it, a "gratifyingly easy germinator." Sow in relatively moist, rich, sandy, moderate- to fast-draining soil; germination usually occurs within 10 to 21 days. (Root transplantation will also work if you want to go that way; just dig up the plant, separate the root into two to three pieces, and replant.) Space the plants 9 to 12 inches apart. The plant likes full sun with a bit of dappled shade; it's heat and drought tolerant (so they say) and likes a bit of regular watering. The herb is hardy to somewhere between 0 and 10 degrees Fahrenheit though there is a bit of controversy around this. I have seen it listed as hardy in USDA zones 5 to 9, and in zones 6 to 10, and in zones 8 to 11; fisticuffs between gardeners, I am sure, occur all the time. It should be heavily mulched to help it overwinter if your area gets colder than 0 or 10 or 15 degrees Fahrenheit, whatever.

Collection and Root Preparation

The root constituents, similarly to red root (*Ceanothus* spp.), reach their potency after the first good frost. Harvesting in China typically occurs in the fall, usually in the first 10 days of November. Harvesting continues, if necessary, until the beginning of spring. After being harvested, the plants are normally covered with a damp cloth until the roots are uniformly moist, then cut into sections, and allowed to dry in the sun (usually for 30 days). However, there are certain drying dynamics necessary for this root prior to its being made into medicine—that is, if you want it to work as a medicinal. Another rant (the long one is still in the appendix) is in order . . .

|||||||||||||||||||||||||||||||||||||||||||||||||||||||||||

Tiny Rant
Irremovable Ignorance

One of the points I have tried to make to new herbalists, herbal schools, and manufacturers over the years is the degree of irremovable ignorance we all possess, and will always possess, when it comes to the natural world. Specifically, every time we think we have a handle on the foundational reality of herbal medicines, we are generally proved wrong. Plants are not linear, mechanical contrivances. They are living entities and what little we learn of them is itself subject to change as the environment in which we are embedded alters itself under pressure—for the plants alter themselves, and their chemical structure, considerably in response to environmental perturbations.

> *We engage the unknown that surrounds us, attempting to understand the nature of the scenario in which we are enmeshed, but the more we learn about it, as Aldous Huxley once put it, the greater the surrounding darkness.*

Despite the fact that I know this, I am continually surprised by my own ignorance as well as my continual inability to reason, often about the most obvious of things. For example: 1) It took 10 years of hearing about estrogenic plants before the thought occurred to me that there might be androgenic plants that contained testosterone (e.g., pine pollen); 2) It took 25 years before I realized that the word *alkaloid* meant "alkaline-like." This means, by definition, that the alkaloids in plants do not extract well in alkaline solutions; it takes an acidic liquid to most efficiently extract them. Thus, competent extraction during tincturing needs either water that is slightly acidic or the addition of a teaspoon of vinegar to the water prior to tincturing. This rather elementary fact was not present in any of the herbal texts

I had ever read, and none of my teachers mentioned it, nor did any herbal lecturer over a nearly 30-year period.

The subject of the current rant concerns the dynamics that occur when drying herbal medicines. It is a neglected area of awareness, improperly so, and possesses ramifications, obvious ones, that affect the quality of our medicines. (It especially affects the production and effectiveness of this salvia.)

Despite the fact that historical use indicates a wide range of harvesting and drying techniques for medicinal plants, very little work has been done on the constituent alterations that occur in herbal medicines when they are dried or how that alters during various drying approaches. This is a serious oversight. Xiao-Bing Li and his colleagues, in a rather remarkable paper ("Production of Salvianolic Acid B in Roots of *Salvia miltiorrhiza* [Danshen] during the Post-Harvest Drying Process"), are the first I am aware of to address this oversight with the sophistication it deserves.

They make an obvious observation (I hate it when I miss something this obvious) and articulate an inherent hypothesis lurking within the observation, which they then test. They begin by stating a very common belief about the drying of medicinal plants:

> The general belief is that levels of bioactive components in medicinal plants were a pre-harvest accumulation and were decreased in the post-harvest drying process [the decrease worsening] as the temperature increased and the duration was prolonged. Therefore, the fundamental target of research on drying processes for medicinal plants up to now was how to best retain the initial levels of bioactive ingredients, and hence the freeze-drying protocol was recommended as the most suitable method.

They then make the obvious point that . . .

> from the point of view of plant physiology, the newly harvested

fresh plant materials, especially roots, are still physiologically active organs. . . .

Incredible that none of us recognized this decades ago. They continue . . .

. . . and the drying process is a bona fide dehydration stress to these organs. Thus, the post-harvest drying process, especially at its early stage, could induce a series of anti-dehydration mechanisms including the production or increase of related secondary metabolites of these organs. That is to say, pharmacologically important ingredients of medicinal plants might emerge or increase during a certain period of drying in post-harvest processing. The drying-induced increase of bioactive components might especially be true for some root materials and some types of secondary metabolites with important ecological functions. This physiological peculiarity of the post-harvest plant materials has not been documented aside from the mention of its role in preventing water loss in the drying of fresh ginseng.

So, they test their hypothesis, that is, that some of the active constituents in medicinal plants might just be occurring in response to dehydration stress. Their focus is on the roots of *Salvia miltiorrhiza,* which, contrary to the normal drying processes of herbalists in the United States, in China are dried in the sun (sun-cured) for a month prior to storage or sale. (There is a reason that the Chinese herbalists have done things a certain way for thousands of years.) They found their hypothesis to be correct, specifically . . .

Salvianolic acid B (SaB), considered one of the major active constituents of danshen, is present in only trace amounts in fresh roots. However, during the drying process there is a surge of that compound within root tissues. As Li et al. note,

"Higher temperatures tended to result in a higher yield of SaB." They tested fairly high temperatures, up to 160 degrees Celsius (322 degrees Fahrenheit). They found that maximal values of SaB occurred between 120 and 130 degrees Celsius (250–270 degrees Fahrenheit). The accumulation of SaB in the roots began to be pronounced at temperatures above 70 degrees Celsius (160 degrees Fahrenheit). As they comment:

> SaB has been revealed to be the most abundant ingredient of [dried] Danshen in most research publications up to now. Our result demonstrated for the first time that this compound was actually not an essential ingredient accumulated in the growing and pre-harvest stage in roots of *S. miltiorrhiza,* but instead was a post-harvest product of the drying process. . . . A significant negative correlation between production of SaB and levels of moisture meant that this compound might be an important anti-dehydration ingredient of the plant, and the mechanism might be closely related to its effective abilities in scavenging the oxygen free radicals. (Li et al. 2012)

Tanshinones, especially tanshinone IIA, for many researchers, are considered to be *the* most pharmacologically active of the compounds in the roots (again, see appendix). They are also the most prevalent active constituent in the fresh roots at harvesting; however, they, too, increase substantially when dried at heat. Tanshinone IIA increased 50 to 60 percent when the roots were dried at heat; total tanshinones increased 3.5 times.

The researchers dried the roots for 11.5 hours: 6 hours at 50 to 60 degrees Celsius (testing the roots every hour for constituent amounts), 3.5 hours at 70 to 90 degrees Celsius (testing the roots every 30 minutes for constituents), and 2 hours at 90 to 160 degrees Celsius (testing every 20 minutes).

So, in short . . . these roots need to be dried in the sun, preferably inside a house (since it is November), behind glass, where the heat can concentrate in the roots, but not in a covered container (the moisture needs to evaporate), for 30 days. Once the roots are dry, store them whole in plastic bags, in covered plastic tubs, in a dark and cool location. They will last for several years.

Plant Chemistry

There are perhaps a hundred constituents that have been identified in this species so far but that number seems to be increasing daily.

Over 40 tanshinones and their analogs have currently been found in the plant, including the three most commonly used by reductionists as activity markers: tanshinone I, tanshinone IIA, and cryptotanshinone.

A general listing of compounds in this plant includes the abietane diterpenoids: 1,2,5,6-tetrahydrotanshinone I; 1,2-didehydrotanshinone II; 1,2-dihydro-1,6-dimethylfuro[3,2-c]-naptha[2,1-e]oxepine-10,12-dione; 3-hydroxytanshinone IIA; 4-methylenemiltirone; 6,7,8,9-tetrahydro-1, 6,6-trimethylfuro[3,2-c]naptha-[2,1-e]oxepine-10,12-dione; 7beta-hydroxy-8,13,abietadien-11,12-dione; acetyl danshenxinkun A; abietatriene; arucadiol; cryptoacetalide; cryptotanshinone; danshenol A and B; danshenspiroketallactone; danshenxinkun A through D; dehydromiltirone; dihydrotanshinone I; epicryptoacetalide; epidanshenspiroketallactone; formytanshinone I; hydroxytanshinone; isocryptotanshinone; isotanshinone I, IIA, and IIB; ketoisocryptotanshinone; methyl tanshinonate; methylene tanshiquinone; methylenedihydrotanshinquinone; miltiodiol; miltionone I and II; miltipolone; miltirone; neocryptotanshinone; neocryptotanshinone II; nortanshinone; oleoyl danshenxinkun A; oleoyl neocryptotanshinone; przewalskin; przewaquinone; salvinone; salviol; salviolone; secodialdialdehyde; sugiol; tanshinaldehyde; tanshindiol A, B, and C; tanshinketolactone; tanshinlactone; tanshinone I, IIA, IIB, and VI; trijuganone A, B, and C . . .

and the caffeic acid derivatives: 2-(3-methoxy-4-hydroxyphenyl)-5-(3-hydroxypropyl)-methoxybenzofuran-3-carbaldehyde; 9"-methyl lithospermate; ammonium potassium; caffeic acid; danshensu; dimethyl lithospermate; ethyl salvialolic acid B; lithospermic acid; lithospermic acid B; magnesium salvianolic acid B; methyl rosmarinate; rosmarinic acid; salviaflaside; and salvianolic acids A, B, C, D, E, F, G, and K.

Other compounds include: protocatechuic acid; protocatechuic aldehyde; ferulic acid; isoferulic acid; yunnanin A; ferruginol; normilt-ioane; baicalin; beta-sitosterol; isoferulic acid; ursolic acid; lactic acid; genipin, umbelliferone, tormentic acid, and so on.

The medicinal actions of the plant are considered, by reductionists, to be primarily provided by tanshinone IIA, total tanshinone content (despite the more than 40 tanshinones and their analogs, the only markers used are tanshinone I, tanshinone IIA, and cryptotanshinone), and salvianolic acid B. And, in fact, a concerted push for standardization is occurring with this herb—not the tincture or capsules, rather it is for the plant itself. As usual, this perspective is seriously flawed. Again, a rant is in order here and it has been written: see appendix.

Actions

Anticoagulant, antihypertensive, anti-inflammatory, antibacterial (Gram-positive and Gram-negative, broadly so against Gram-positive), antimicrobial, antifibrotic, antioxidant, antianaphylactic, antiathero-sclerotic, antineoplastic, analgesic, apoptosis normalizer, vasodilating, sedative, hepatosplenic tonic, cardiotonic, organ protectant (central nervous system, liver, spleen, lungs, heart, bones, red blood cells) and normalizer, immunomodulant.

Uses

I consider this plant specific for liver and spleen enlargement, for normalizing cytokine dysregulation, as a potent anticoagulant and vascular normalizer, and as a generalized full-body organ tonic. It is specifically indicated for use with stealth pathogens and in any condition where sepsis might occur. In cases where intravascular coagulation is a possibility, it is the indicated alternative to *Ceanothus* spp. (red root). A number of people consider it specific for cancer but I have never used it for that purpose.

Traditional Chinese Medicine (TCM)

Salvia miltiorrhiza (and all the other danshens) have been used in Chinese medicine for two millennia (at least). It was first recorded in the classic Chinese text *Shen Nong Ben Cao Jing* in the second century CE. The herb is considered to be bitter and cool in the TCM system.

Its TCM functions are: promoting blood circulation and removing blood stasis, clearing heat from the blood, resolving swelling, tranquilizing the mind, regulating menstruation to relieve pain, cooling the blood to relieve carbuncle, and clearing heat and toxic substances.

Indications for use are: irregular menstruation, dysmenorrhea, amenorrhea, postpartum tormina, arthalgia syndrome due to wind-dampness, heat invasion of nutrient yin and blood divisions in epidemic febrile disease, restlessness with disturbance of the mind, pyogenic toxin, enlargement of the liver and spleen.

It is commonly used for: irregular menstruation, amenorrhea, postpartum abdominal pain, pain and stifling sensations in the chest, masses in the abdomen (from blood stagnation), inflamed liver and/ or spleen, pancreatitis, arthritis, traumatic injury, broken bones, pain and bruising, redness, swelling, delirium, high fever, unconsciousness, irritability, insomnia, purpura and petechiae and ecchymosis, vasculitis, endometriosis, fibroids, cysts.

The Chinese have conducted a large number of clinical trials with the herb; see the scientific research section below.

Ayurveda

Not known as far as I can tell.

Western Botanic Practice

Unknown until its recent introduction from China during the past few decades. It is still rarely used in Western practice.

Scientific Research

There are around 2,000 journal articles listed on PubMed, the U.S. National Library of Medicine's online database of research in the life sciences and biomedical fields. The Chinese database CNKI (Chinese National Knowledge Infrastructure), similar to PubMed, lists over 10,000 journal entries. Google Scholar lists 22,000 or so, which includes another 10,000 entries beyond PubMed and CNKI. All of these articles have been produced in the past 35 years. The following material just catches a few of the highlights. First, however, a crucial comment on the actions of this herb . . .

The herb tends to act as a cytokine normalizer, that is, it modulates cytokine expression during abnormal states. If cytokine activity is inappropriately high, it lowers it, if inappropriately low, it raises it. Thus, studies show that in some circumstances the herb lowers nitric oxide production, in others it raises it. In some circumstances it inhibits caspase activity, in others it raises it. In some instances it stimulates apoptosis, in others it inhibits it.

Salvia miltiorrhiza appears then to be an immune-response adaptogen, specifically for use during altered, and unhealthy, cytokine responses to infection. Comparison of the herb's pharmacokinetic actions in both disease and non-disease states finds that during disease conditions, the herb's constituents localize to the sites of damage, where they initiate modulation of the specific types of inflammation that is occurring there. Whereas in non-disease states they don't seem to produce any cytokine modulating action at all.

For example, in-depth studies in mice found that the cytokine profile was unaltered in healthy mice when the herb was added (in various amounts) to their diets. However, when the mice were intentionally infected with *Listeria* bacteria the herb modulated the exact cytokine alterations the organisms caused. Thus, again, the herb appears to work as a cytokine-response adaptogen, that is, it normalizes cytokine responses to adverse events, such as microbial infection. With that in mind, here is a look at its cytokine actions from various journal papers.

In Vitro Studies

Salvia miltiorrhiza root inhibits caspase-3 (and caspase-9) activity (thus inducing apoptosis in apoptosis-inhibited cells); inhibits microbial-induced NF-κB signaling in epithelial and endothelial cells (by inhibiting IκB kinase, an enzyme complex that is involved in propagating the body's cellular response to inflammation); inhibits ICAM-1 (intercellular adhesion molecule 1, present in low concentrations in the cell membranes of leukocytes and endothelial cells, and activated by pathogens to stimulate clustering of leukocytes on endothelial cells); inhibits mast cell degranulation by inhibiting PLCG2 and MAPK; inhibits NADPH oxidase (nicotinamide adenine dinucleotide phosphate oxidase, which produces reactive oxygen species, ROS, which activate an enzyme that stimulates macrophages to adhere to endothelial cells); inhibits the overproduction of IL-12 during acute microbial infection–induced inflammation (thus reducing IFN-γ production as well); inhibits TNF-α and its expression of VCAM-1 (vascular cell adhesion molecule 1, which stimulates the adhesion of various white blood cells to the vascular endothelium; inhibition of VCAM-1 suppresses the adhesion rate of neutrophils to endothelial cells *and* erythrocyte aggregation as well, thus lowering intravascular coagulation); inhibits E-selectin (which also stimulates the accumulation and adhesion of leukocytes to endothelial cells and their penetration deeper into tissues); inhibits the proinflammatory cytokines IL-1β and IL-6; and inhibits MMP-2 and MMP-9 (matrix metalloproteinases 2 and 9 are enzymes that actively break down collagen, leading to inflammation and damage in the joints), but it also upregulates MMP-2 when necessary to normalize function.

The herb inhibits MCP-1 (monocyte chemoattractant protein 1, a.k.a. CCL2, which recruits immune cells to sites of microbial infection); inhibits ROS production; modulates Bax/Bcl-2 expression (thus normalizing apoptosis dynamics in cells, increasing it where suppressed, decreasing it where stimulated); inhibits overexpression of angiotensin II (which affects both blood pressure and apoptosis); inhibits levels of hydrogen peroxide (H_2O_2) in damaged cells, thus reducing white blood cell clustering and over-inflammatory responses; stimulates endothelial nitric oxide synthase (eNOS) production (thus creating more nitric oxide production by endothelial cells as well as more L-citrulline); modulates p38 MAPK/JNK activity; inhibits TLR-4 expression (thus reducing hyper immune responses during sepsis); inhibits expression of IL-2, IL-4, and IFN-γ; stimulates production of IL-10 (except when it is dysregulated as in sepsis, in which case it normalizes IL-10 functioning); inhibits PGE2 (prostaglandin E2, which stimulates osteoblasts to increase bone resorption by osteoclasts, thus increasing osteoporosis; it also softens the cervix and stimulates uterine contractions, and induces fever during infections); both increases and decreases inducible nitric oxide synthase (iNOS) and subsequent NO production (depending on which is needed during disease conditions); decreases RANTES (a.k.a. CCL5, which is chemotactic for T cells, eosinophils, and basophils and recruits leukocytes to inflammatory sites; it induces the proliferation and activation of NK cells to inflammatory sites); inhibits CX3CL1 (which potently attracts T cells and monocytes when expressed and promotes adhesion of leukocytes to endothelial cells); inhibits IL-18 and increases IL-13; modulates IL-4 and TGF-β expression (inhibiting or increasing as the case may be); inhibits VEGF (vascular endothelial growth factor); inhibits ERK-1 and ERK-2; inhibits HMGB1 production; and stimulates HMGB1 clearance from the body, making the herb specific for sepsis.

Other in vitro activity includes: strong inhibition of the proliferation of keratinocytes (thus reducing the tendency to psoriasis in the skin); stabilization of mitochondria during microbial assault; inhibition of mitochondrial apoptosis during hypoxia events; inhibition of cancer cell proliferation and stimulation of apoptosis of cancer cells; repression of the accumulation of collagen in damaged organs, thus preventing the development of fibrosis in various diseases of the internal organs (kidneys, liver, lungs, and so on); inhibition of apoptosis in damaged liver cells, protecting from organ failure; decrease in malondialdehyde levels (a marker of oxidative stress); decrease in lactate dehydrogenase and creatine phosphokinase levels; amelioration of reperfusion injury in liver cell mitochondria; inhibition of tyrosinase; stimulation of red blood cell apoptosis during red blood cell infections.

In Vivo Studies

Healthy mice given the herb in their diet as a regular additive did not show any toxic responses, even at high levels of the herb. Nor did the mouse cytokine levels alter. However, when the mice were infected with *Listeria* bacteria, the herb acted as a very specific immune modulator. The herb inhibited the induction of the particular cytokines the bacteria (tried to) initiate. Host defenses and immune function increased in just the optimum manner to counteract infection. Spleen and liver organs were protected from damage. NO production in the liver was inhibited, thus protecting the liver's Kupffer cells from damage. (NO production in the spleen was unaffected.) HMGB1 levels remained low in the treated mice but increased four- to tenfold in the untreated mice. Bacterial clearance in the treated group was enhanced; sepsis was significantly reduced. The effects were dose dependent; the higher the dose, the better the outcome.

Rats suffering severe acute pancreatitis or obstructive jaundice, when treated with *Salvia miltiorrhiza,* experienced decreased mortality, less movement of endotoxins and bacteria through the GI tract membrane into the body, and much less pathological damage to the spleen and thymus than rats who were not given the herb. Plasma levels of endotoxins were considerably lower than in the untreated group. Damaged Kupffer cells in the liver were cleared more quickly, liver function increased, and the liver was protected from damage. The mesenteric lymph nodes in the intestinal tract suffered much less pathological damage; their function was enhanced.

The herb significantly reduces the impacts of ischemia-reperfusion injury in rats. It reduces levels of ALT and AST and increases SOD (superoxide dismutase, an antioxidant defense mechanism). It acts similarly in mice. In response to microbial infection the herb decreases both

ALT and AST, decreases NO levels, and reduces the degree of liver injury. In other studies the herb protected mice from potentially lethal microbe-induced liver injury. The CD4:CD8 ratio improved.

The herb plays an important role in protecting and reestablishing the mucosal integrity of the GI tract during infections. Liver injury, for example, is often associated with a significant alteration in the intestinal microflora. Enterococci and enterobacteria populations increase, lactobacilli and bifidobacteria decrease. The intestinal barrier becomes more permeable, allowing toxins and other macromolecules to cross the GI tract barrier into the body.

Importantly, both lactobacilli (*Lactobacillus* spp.) and bifidobacteria (*Bifidobacterium* spp.) form biofilms in the intestines. This is a crucial element of the intestinal mucosal barrier. The biofilms formed by these symbiotic bacteria prevent adhesion of pathogenic bacteria to the bowel wall and limit the overgrowth of the normally present Gram-negative bacteria. A reduction in these bacteria, and the loss of the biofilms they create, results in structural and functional damage to the intestinal mucosal barrier, increasing its permeability. This, among other things, increases endotoxin loads in blood plasma, and makes many symptoms worse.

> *This is another reason why breaking up biofilms as an integral part of treating Lyme-group infections is a bad idea. It not only spreads more of the Lyme-group microbes throughout the body, it damages the mucosal integrity of the bowel, increases endotoxins in the blood, stimulates bowel permeability, and decreases the healthy bowel flora.*

Murine (mouse) research with *Salvia miltiorrhiza* found that the herb restores mucosal integrity, increases the population of healthy bacteria in the bowel (and their biofilms), improves intestinal microcirculation, and lessens portal hypertension. It restores the ecology of the bowel, reduces unhealthy bowel bacteria overgrowth, and increases the levels of healthy bacteria throughout the bowel.

A study of rats with endometriosis found that the herb reduced the cytokine markers associated with that disease, relieving symptoms.

The herb was used to treat chronic cerebral hypoperfusion in male Wistar rats. Levels of microglial activation, myelin basic protein (MBP), and the cytokines COX-2, IL-1β, and IL-6 were measured in the white matter of the brain and the hippocampus. Microglial activation was alleviated, MBP levels increased, and inflammation was reduced. The herb was found to attenuate white matter and hippocampal damage in the brain.

In mice, hypoxia/ischemia was induced, leading to neuronal damage in the brain. However, one day after hypoxia/ischemia, treatment with the herb reversed most of the damage. It showed strong neuroprotective and neurocorrective effects.

Other studies on diabetic rats found that the herb protects peripheral nerve function, alleviating diabetic neuropathy.

Inflammation after spinal cord damage causes apoptosis of affected cells. The use of the herb after injury (in rats) induced "significant" effects. It increased motor function, reduced tissue injury, reduced neutrophil infiltration, reduced myeloperoxidase activity, reduced expression of astrocytes, reduced apoptosis, and decreased expression of a range of inflammatory cytokines.

The herb stimulates osteogenesis (in rats) and bone marrow angiogenesis and inhibits bone resorption by osteoclasts, thus preventing bone loss in osteoporosis. Bone mineral density and mass both increase.

Numerous studies in both rats and mice found the herb to be highly protective of heart function and tissue. It prevents cardiac remodeling in hypertensive rats, reduces fibrosis in heart tissue, reduces fat buildup in arteries, reduces coagulation and thromboembolism tendencies in vascular functioning, reduces hypertension, and improves cardiac functioning.

Human Study

There have been several hundred human trials (at least) with the herb (or its constituents) on a variety of conditions. This includes pancreatitis, oral submucous fibrosis, fatty liver, polycystic ovary syndrome, hyperandrogenism, myocardial damage in people with severe burns, chronic artery disease in diabetics, coronary artery bypass, hypertension, elevated platelet thrombin levels in chronic hemodialysis, chronic heart disease, hypercholesteremia, hyperlipidemia, vascular endothelial dysfunction, chronic hepatitis B, liver cirrhosis, Henoch-Schönlein purpura nephritis, primary nephrotic syndrome, portal hypertension, infantile hypoxic-ischemic encephalopathy, hypertensive cerebral hemorrhage, chronic asthma, cervical erosion, chronic hepatitis, whooping cough, schistosomal hepatomegaly, shock, scleroderma, allergic rhinitis, glaucoma, enlarged spleen, insomnia, and angina pectoris.

Studies have been conducted on its use as prophylaxis for venous thromboembolism and for reducing skin flap ischemia and necrosis after mastectomy (with fewer side effects than pharmaceuticals), protecting the kidney from damage from extracorporeal shock wave lithotripsy during breakdown of kidney stones, ameliorating late-state COPD, preventing ischemic stroke recurrence, reducing damage from traumatic intracranial hematoma, ameliorating chronic fatigue, reducing hyphema, treating acute myocardial infarction, reducing severe inflammation due to infection, alleviating the effects of stroke, counteracting Alzheimer's disease, and aiding in cancer treatment.

Every study, irrespective of the condition, found the herb effective in helping alleviate or prevent the condition.

Many thousands of people have participated in the various clinical trials, many of them randomized and placebo-controlled. As only one example: An analysis of over 60 randomized clinical trials (with a total of 6,931 people) for the treatment of angina pectoris over a minimum of four weeks found the herb more effective than isosorbide dinitrate (ISDN).

The pharmacokinetics of the herb's constituents are very good, that is, they cross the GI tract membrane and circulate in high quantities in the blood and throughout the body. They also easily cross the blood-brain barrier. This is primarily due to the herb's inhibition of P-glycoprotein, one of the major mechanisms preventing compounds from crossing the various barriers that exist in the body.

Preparation and Dosage

There are a number of essential understandings necessary before using this herb. All concern the effects that different preparation methods have on the effectiveness of the herb. *These are crucial.*

1. As an initial step: please see "Collection and Root Preparation" above. The roots of this plant *must* be dried in the sun or under heat prior to preparation for the plant to be medicinally active to the degree necessary for use. In other words, the root should *never* be tinctured fresh. **The herb should *never* be tinctured fresh.** The salvianolic acids, such as SaB, are only present in minute quantities in the fresh root.

2. The concentrated powder or granules of this herb should *never* be used. Exhaustive studies on those compounds have found significant problems. Specifically, the hydrophobic (a.k.a. lipophilic) compounds, i.e., the tanshinones, are difficult to extract, and they are present only in very low quantities in many of the (Chinese-produced) concentrated forms of this herb, primarily because the manufacturers use water as their extractive medium. The hydrophobic compounds do not extract in water and without them the herb becomes significantly less effective for treating disease. Because it is impossible (at this point in time) to determine the extractive process being used in the production of any particular concentrated granules or powders, they should not be used.

3. Tanshinones are lipophilic, that is, "fat loving." They extract most efficiently in toxic substances such as methanol and hexane. (They do extract in ethanol, just not as efficiently.) Unfortunately, there has been very little work done on the most efficient ways to extract lipophilic compounds from herbs without utilizing sophisticated manufacturing processes. An analysis of the different medicinal components of herbs (which vary widely in their natures) and the most efficient extraction processes that can be used by community herbalists (whether in the United States or Africa or Asia or . . .) does need to be done.

Community practitioners do know a bit about this kind of difficulty already, but it is not widely recognized for its importance. For example, the extraction of herbs (such as *Artemisia annua*) containing both hydrophilic and lipophilic constituents in some regions (Asia) is accomplished using heated milk as the extracting medium.

4. Because the hydrophobic tanshinones do not extract well in water, infusions (teas) and decoctions are *not* recommended for this plant for use in treating the conditions discussed in this book. (The hydrophilic caffeic acid group does extract in water and is useful for a number of conditions, especially protecting endothelial integrity. However, that is not sufficient for counteracting the full range of physiological damage these Lyme coinfections cause. It is especially not sufficient for treating sepsis.)

5. The ethanol/water/herb tincture ratios that are commonly used with this herb vary considerably. In the U.K. the ratio is usually one part herb to three parts liquid (1:3), often with 25 percent alcohol (one part alcohol to three parts water), but I have seen formulations with 35 and 45 percent as well. In the United States 1:2 and 1:2.5 herb-to-liquid ratios are common, usually in 25 percent alcohol. There is also one 1:2 preparation, using cold percolation, with 50 percent alcohol/water, which is the only high-alcohol preparation I could find as this book was being written. (Hopefully this will change shortly.) **Note: There are significant problems with any tincture formulation of less than 50 percent alcohol.** Specifically . . .

The lipophilic tanshinones (a.k.a. the abietane diterpenoids) will *not* extract sufficiently in an ethanol concentration that low. (That amount of alcohol is barely enough to keep the tincture stabilized.) Studies of such formulations (in China) consistently find that there are little or no tanshinones present in them. Tinctures of this plant are highly useful as medicines (as is the dried root itself taken as powder or in capsules) but they need to be made with a much higher alcohol percentage than is common on the market. As researchers Song et al. (2009) comment:

> Chromatographic profiles from 12 manufacturers showed different patterns. HPLC profiles of granules from manufacturers A, C, G, H, and J were similar to those of aqueous extract of Danshen, which contained hydrophilic compounds but the contents of hydrophobic tanshinones were very low. The samples from B, D, E, F, I and K showed a similar pattern of 70% ethanol extract of Danshen, which contained both hydrophilic phenolic components and hydrophobic tanshinones.

Chinese researchers have found that a 70 percent ethanol extract produces the highest quantities of tanshinones. Other studies have found that a 50 to 60 percent ethanol extractive medium produced the most salvinolic acid B from the dried roots. (A 20 to 30 percent ethanol solvent extracted significantly less SaB than either a 50 or 60 percent solution.) I prefer a 60 percent alcohol to 40 percent water formulation for tincturing the root of this plant; it is what I suggest herein. That will efficiently extract both the hydrophilic and hydrophobic constituents in sufficient quantities for the herb to be useful in treating Lyme coinfections and sepsis.

Tincture

Preparation: 1:3, 60 percent alcohol.

Dosage: Varies considerably, anywhere from 1 to 2 milliliters (20 to 40 drops, a.k.a. a full dropper more or less) to 1 tablespoon, anywhere from 3x daily to every 15 minutes. Dosage specifics are:

- **For babesia:** ½ teaspoon 3x daily.
- **For ehrlichia/anaplasma:** 1 teaspoon 3–6x daily.
- **For severe pain:** up to 1 tablespoon every 15 minutes, reducing the dose as the pain subsides (thanks to Michael and Leslie Tierra for this one).

- **For sepsis:** 1 tablespoon every 15 minutes to 1 hour depending on severity.

Please note: There are one or two sources on the Internet insisting that this herb must never be taken in tincture form (they don't say why), however there is no support for this in the literature (in China or elsewhere).

Dried Herb

The dried herb is, in many respects, stronger than a tincture in that *all* the plant constituents are going into your body full strength. This allows your body to determine what it wants to pull from the herb and what it does not.

The Chinese, for the past two millennia, commonly used the dried herb. Dosage is high, as is normal in China, from 5 to 15 grams (about ⅕ to ½ ounce) up to several times a day. Up to 60 grams (2 ounces or so) is considered an acceptable single dose in severe, acute conditions.

- **For babesia:** ½ teaspoon powdered root, 3x daily.
- **For ehrlichia/anaplasma:** 1 teaspoon powdered root, 3–6x daily.
- **In acute conditions:** 1 tablespoon powdered root, 3x daily.

Infusions and Decoctions

Not recommended for this herb when treating Lyme coinfections or sepsis.

Side Effects and Contraindications

This herb is extremely safe, however since the herb is an anticoagulant, it is contraindicated for those with bleeding disorders (e.g., hemophilia, bleeding ulcers, and so on). Because it stimulates menstruation, it should not be used during pregnancy.

A few people are apparently allergic to this genus (as well as some of the constituents in danshen); rash, itching, and shortness of breath have been reported in a couple of instances. There are a few anecdotal reports of stomachache and/or decreased appetite when the tincture is used.

If side effects occur, stop using the herb.

Herb/Food Interactions

Soy and milk are reported to decrease the effectiveness of the herb; however, extensive searching in numerous databases and texts did not produce any support for this assertion. It seems to be one of those zombie ideas (herban legends) that show up for some reason and never go away no matter how many times you kill them.

Herb/Drug Interactions

The herb is an anticoagulant; it inhibits platelet aggregation and should not be used along with pharmaceutical anticoagulants such as warfarin, heparin, aspirin, and so on. (Excessive aspirin use is also contraindicated.)

Concurrent use of digoxin and danshen may result in falsely elevated serum digoxin concentrations when measured by fluorescence polarization immunoassay. A falsely lowered level may occur when measured by microparticle enzyme microassay.

The herb is a competitive inhibitor of liver CYP3A4, CYP2C9, CYP2E1, CYP2D6, and CYP1A2 activity. CYPs are major enzymes involved in drug metabolism and bioactivation in the liver. Inhibition of CYP3A, for example, has been found to decrease midazolam clearance and may affect the metabolism of other drugs. (There are numerous inhibitors of CYP3A that people commonly ingest, including clarithromycin, erythromycin, grapefruit juice, and quercetin, just so you know.)

Midazolam is used for acute seizures, for moderate to severe insomnia, and for sedation and amnesia prior to medical procedures. It is the most commonly used benzodiazepine as a premedication for sedation. Inhibition of CYP3A slows clearance of the drug from the body by 16 percent and increases the duration of sedation. The amount of losartan, an antihypertensive drug, in circulation is also affected by the herb. The effects on medications seems individual; theophylline, for example, is not affected by the CYP inhibition of the plant.

The root of this plant contains carboxylesterase inhibitors. Carboxylesterase is an enzyme in the human body that acts to metabolize many ingested substances, including drugs, thus increasing their solubility and activity in the body. The inhibition of carboxylesterase can reduce serum levels of the drugs in the body, thus lowering their effectiveness. This particularly affects esterified drug agents such as those in hormone replacement therapies and the anticancer prodrug irinotecan.

A number of constituents of danshen are competitive binders with salicylates (think aspirin) for albumin. Prior use of danshen displaces salicylates from albumin binding. This increases the amount of free salicylates in circulation. Prior use of aspirin displaces danshen binding with albumin; this increases the amount of danshen constituents in circulation.

The herb should be discontinued prior to surgery, not only because of its anticlotting properties but also because of its impacts on common anesthesia interventions.

Finding It
The dried root and tincture of the root are both fairly easy to find. Most of my recommended suppliers (see "Sources of Supply" at the end of the book) carry it. Horizon Herbs carries very high-quality seeds.

Angelica sinensis

This herb is most commonly known as *dong quai,* or Chinese angelica, which is, in the West, primarily known as a tonic herb for the female reproductive system (the "female ginseng"). The root is what is used.

As with most herbs, it is its general, widely known use that has dominated Western herbal thinking about it over the years. Until now, I haven't ever thought more deeply about the herb either. Its recurring presence in my research as a specific counteractant for HMGB1-initiated sepsis revealed that there was a lot more to the herb than I had realized. (A frequent occurrence with every plant medicine I have had only a superficial relationship with.)

The herb has been used in Chinese medicine for millennia and is considered specific for tonifying the blood, promoting blood circulation, relieving pain, as a specific for uterine/menstrual problems, and for helping normalize liver, spleen, and heart channels. Its major clinical uses are for dysregulation in menstruation and uterine function, for pain, and for early-stage infections of one sort or another. Nearly all herbalists in the West simply use it for female reproductive dysregulations of one sort or another.

Despite this traditional use, the Chinese have been extending its range considerably the past few decades. It has a profound impact on heart and circulatory functioning, and it acts as a vasodilator, lowering blood pressure and slowing both heartbeat and pulse rate. It functions well as a moderate heart tonic, protecting the heart from damage. The herb is also a moderate anticoagulant (with antifibrotic actions), decreases platelet activity, and stimulates hematopoiesis in the bone marrow (making it good for anemia for instance). Its use increases the numbers and activity of macrophages, fibroblasts, erythrocytes, granulocytes, and lymphocytes in the blood. The herb delays the aging of hematopoietic stem cells by inhibiting oxidative damage to them. It increases both thymus and spleen indices (increasing thymus weight and cellular production), and the numbers of red and white blood cells in peripheral blood, especially during myelosuppression. It increases the percentage of CD4+ cells and modulates the CD4+/CD8+ ratio.

The herb has reliable analgesic actions, helping with general aches and pains but also arthritic, abdominal, and postoperative pain. It has been successfully used in the treatment of chronic hepatitis and cirrhosis of the liver and acts as a hepatoprotector from both chemical and microbial insults. In fact it is pretty reliable for reducing fibrosis in organs, including the lungs, spleen, liver, and kidneys. It has some pretty good actions as a neuroprotector and relaxant. It stimulates the formation of new neural cells in the brain (promoting adult neurogenesis), thus helping to reverse cognitive impairments. It is pretty good at reversing any inflammatory-initiated cognitive impairments in the brain.

It is considered specific for chronic constipation in the elderly. In essence, the herb, as the Chinese have insisted for a while, is good for the heart, spleen, and liver channels.

Angelica has a number of cytokine impacts including rather strong inhibitions on TNF-α, reducing its apoptosis-stimulating actions, reducing the inflammatory pain it causes. It is an MIP-2 inhibitor and an IL-2 upregulator. It reduces NETs formation by inhibiting neutrophil elastase (NE). And it dose-dependently inhibits HMGB1 release and stops the progression of lethal sepsis. Circulating levels of HMGB1 are reduced, as are levels of IL-6. Angelica also inhibits the endothelial cell permeability HMGB1 causes. This is one of the specific herbs for use in treating sepsis and for counteracting myelosuppression and anemia.

Preparation and Dosage

The Chinese often prepare the herb as a decoction, 5–15 grams in water, divided into several doses daily. The powdered root is useful, 1–2 grams 3x daily. Dosage of the tincture of the dried root (1:5, 70 percent alcohol) runs ½ teaspoon–1 tablespoon 3x daily, depending on the severity of the condition.

Note: The herb is useful for pain, especially when combined with *Salvia miltiorrhiza;* take 1 tablespoon more every 15 minutes for pain, reducing the dosage and frequency as the pain lessens.

Side Effects and Contraindications

No real side effects to the herb; it is contraindicated in pregnancy, especially the first trimester, as it can stimulate menstruation. The herb does soften the bowel contents—not a good idea to use it during bouts of diarrhea.

Herb/Drug Interactions
Shouldn't really be used with anticoagulants.

Astragalus spp.

This is a huge genus of some 3,000 species that are prevalent through-out the world. The primary species used is *Astragalus membranaceus,* a.k.a. *A. membranaceus* var. *mongholicus,* a.k.a. *A. mongholicus* and so on, depending on the degree of taxonomitis that is occurring. The root is what is used for medicine.

Astragalus is an immune enhancer, modulator, stimulant, and restorative; antiviral; antibacterial; adaptogen; tonic; antihepatotoxic; hypotensive; diuretic; and organ tonic that enhances function in the lungs, spleen, and GI tract. It protects the heart from numerous insults as well (well, not verbal ones).

As an immune potentiator and modulator astragalus strongly reg-ulates IFN-γ and IL-2 levels. If IFN-γ levels are high, for example, it actively lowers them. The herb enhances CD4+ counts and balances the CD4/CD8 ratio, making it a very useful herb for these types of Lyme coinfections.

It is specific for immune atrophy and enhances function in the spleen and thymus, again making it a nicely functional herb for these conditions. The herb is specific as a preventive for infection from Lyme bacteria and for reducing severity of the disease. It is a very nice immu-nomodulator for the Lyme group of infections.

Astragalus has been a major herb in Chinese medicine for between 2,000 and 4,000 years. Its traditional uses are for spleen deficiency with lack of appetite, fatigue, and diarrhea. It is specific for disease condi-tions accompanied by weakness and sweating, stabilizes and protects the vital energy (qi), and is used for wasting diseases, numbness of the limbs, and paralysis. Other uses are: tonifies the lungs, for shortness of breath, frequent colds and flu infections; as a diuretic and for reduction of edema; for tonifying the blood and for blood loss, especially post-partum; for diabetes; for promoting the discharge of pus; for chronic ulcerations, including of the stomach, and sores that have not drained or healed well.

A considerable amount of scientific testing has occurred with astragalus, including clinical trials and both in vivo and in vitro studies. PubMed now lists over 5,700 citations for studies with astragalus and this does not include the many Chinese studies that have never been indexed for it. The Chinese database CNKI now has over 16,000 entries on the herb.

Most of the clinical studies and trials regarding immunostimulation have been focused on the use of astragalus in the treatment of cancer and/or as an adjunct to chemotherapy to help stimulate chemodepressed immune function. A number of other studies have examined its immune effects with a range of different conditions.

The herb has been used with children suffering tetralogy of Fallot after radical operation to correct the condition. Tetralogy of Fallot is a complex of four heart abnormalities that occur together, generally at birth. Surgery is used to correct it. Astragalus was found to decrease abnormal levels of IgG, IgM, C3, C4, CD8+, and CD19+ while increasing levels of CD4+ and CD56+. The ratios of CD4/CD8, CD3/HLA-DR, and CD3/CD16 normalized between the second and third week of use. IL-6 and TNF-α both began decreasing in the first week and by week four were in the normal range.

When used in the treatment of herpes simplex keratitis, levels of Th1, including IL-2 and IFN-γ, increased and Th2 levels, including IL-4 and IL-10, decreased, showing that the herb modulated Th1 and Th2 levels. This same kind of effect has been found in the treatment of numerous cancers. For example, in a study of 37 lung cancer patients astragalus was found to reverse the Th2 status normally present in that condition. Th1 cytokines (IFN-γ and IL-2) and its transcript factor (T-bet) were enhanced and Th2 cytokines were decreased.

In clinical trials with a number of different cancers and congestive heart conditions, astragalus has been found to increase CD4+ levels, reduce CD8+ levels, and significantly increase the CD4/CD8 ratio.

The plant has been found to have a broad immunostimulatory effect. Use of the herb with cancer patients undergoing chemotherapy found that white blood cell counts improved significantly (normalizing). The herb has been found to be specifically useful in preventing or reversing immunosuppression from any source: age, bacterial, viral, or chemical. Phagocytosis is enhanced and superoxide dismutase production from macrophages is increased.

Astragalus has been found to possess anti-inflammatory activity by inhibiting the NF-κB pathway and blocking the effect of IL-1β in leukotriene C production in human amnions. The constituent astragaloside IV inhibits increases in microvascular permeability induced by histamine. The whole herb decoction has been found to reduce capillary hyperpermeability. It is strongly inhibitive of TGF-β as well. It upregulates both IL-12 and MHC-II, inhibits TLR-4 (thus reducing HMGB1 levels), counteracts the suppression of Tregs by HMGB1, and counteracts endothelial cell permeability caused by HMGB1. Numerous studies have found that astragalus counteracts myelosuppression. It stimulates hematopoiesis, increasing blood cell progenitors in the bone marrow, and stimulates the production of both red and white blood cells.

Astragalus has been found to improve anisodine-induced impairment of memory acquisition and alcohol-elicited deficit of memory retrieval. After use of the herb the number of errors were reduced. The plant has been found to exert potent antioxidant effects on the brain, helping to prevent senility.

In one study, 106 newborns with neonatal hypoxic ishemic encephalopathy were separated into two groups. One received oral astragalus granules for seven months, the other nimodipine for three months, then pyritinol for an additional four. There was better recovery in the astragalus group, with less long-term negative effects from the initial condition. The incidence of cerebral palsy was markedly reduced. (Another study used injection, the outcomes were similar.) Studies on the use of astragalus injection in the treatment of cerebral palsy in children found that it significantly reduced symptoms.

Astragalus has been found effective in alleviating fatigue in heart patients and in athletes. In athletes given astragalus, the herb was found to positively influence their anaerobic threshold, enhance their recovery from fatigue, and increase their fatigue threshold.

A double-blind, randomized, controlled trial with 36 adults with chronic fatigue found that a mixture of astragalus and salviae radix (salvia root) significantly decreased fatigue scores.

Preparation and Dosage

Many astragalus formulations are standardized though I'm not sure that the literature really supports standardization with this herb. I think it is more a case of standarditis than anything else. The whole root contains constituents that are essential for carditis and enhanced immune function. And, indeed, the majority of the Chinese studies—clinical and laboratory—were with the whole herb. The herb may be taken as tea, powder, capsules, tincture, or in food.

Tincture

Tincture preparations vary considerably, from 1:2 and 1:3 up to 1:5 and with alcohol concentrations ranging from 25 to 60 percent. There doesn't seem to be a lot of data on why nor what is the best tincture preparation procedures. However, there is some good data suggesting it be done this way . . .

In general, many of the most potent actions of the plant come from its polysaccharides and polysaccharides are most efficiently released from the root cells by hot water. This is, in part, why many traditional uses of astragalus involve cooking it or using it as a tea.

So, if you are making an extract of, let's say, 5 ounces of astragalus powder, you would then use anywhere from two to five times the amount of water. Many of the manufacturers whose products I think are good use from 40 to 50 percent alcohol for their astragalus tinctures in either a 1:3 or 1:5 tincture ratio. For this example, let's do it this way . . .

Preparation: Take 5 ounces of astragalus root powder and 25 ounces of liquid (this makes it a 1:5 ratio). The liquid should be composed of half water and half pure grain alcohol, which will give you a 50 percent alcohol extraction medium. You would be using 12.5 ounces of water. Take the water *only* (starting with cold water), add the root to it—in a pot—and bring it to a boil. As soon as it comes to a boil, turn off the heat, and cover. Let it steep overnight. In the morning, put the whole mess in a jar, add the alcohol (12.5 ounces), and tighten the lid. Leave for two weeks, shaking when you remember to do so. Then decant.

Dosage: As a tonic, 30–60 drops up to 4x daily. In chronic illness conditions, 1 teaspoon 4x daily. As preventive (from viral infection), 1 teaspoon 4–6x daily. In acute conditions, 1 teaspoon 4–6x daily, generally every 3 hours.

Tea

Put 2 to 3 ounces of herb in a quart of hot water, let steep for 2 to 3 hours, strain, then drink throughout the day.

Powder

In chronic conditions, take 1 tablespoon 3x per day. In acute conditions, 2 tablespoons 3x per day. Your body's own bile and stomach acids will extract the constituents. You can go higher on these doses if you wish. The Chinese use very large doses of the powdered root, from 15 to 60 grams per day, essentially ½ to 2 ounces per day.

Side Effects and Contraindications

No toxicity has ever been shown from the regular, daily use of the herb nor from the use of large doses. The Chinese report consistent use for millennia in the treatment of colds and flu and suppressed immune function without side effects.

It is contraindicated, however, *for some people,* in certain kinds of late-stage Lyme disease because it can exacerbate autoimmune responses in that particular disease. For others it can alter the Th1/Th2 balance and reduce the autoimmune dynamics. Whether or not it acts as a modulator seems to depend on individual reactions to the herb; I haven't been able to find a reason why, for some people, it exacerbates their condition and for others it does not.

Herb/Drug Interactions

Synergistic actions: Use of the herb with interferon and acyclovir may increase their effects. The herb has been used in clinical trials with interferon in the treatment of hepatitis B; outcomes were better than with interferon alone. It has also shown synergistic effects when used with interferon in the treatment of cervical erosion; antiviral activity is enhanced.

Drug inhibitor: Use of the herb with cyclophosphamide may decrease the effectiveness of the drug. Not for use in people with transplanted organs.

Herb/Herb Interactions

Synergistic with echinacea and licorice in the stimulation of immune function.

Finding It

Herb stores everywhere and the Internet.

Bidens pilosa

There are a lot of different species of bidens. *Bidens pilosa* is the main species used medicinally (or at least on which most of the studies have been done) but there do seem to be a number of others in the genus that historical use and early research indicate can almost certainly be used similarly: *Bidens frondosa, B. tripartitus, B. ferulaefolia, B. alba* are all fairly potent, *frondosa* and *tripartitus* more so than *pilosa* in their antimalarial effects; *B. maximowicziana, B. pinnata,* and *B. campylotheca* are all fairly strong as well. (I use *B. pinnata* because it grows in my yard as a wild invasive. And, yes, the thousands of seeds that get stuck in my socks and pants every year are irritating.)

The aerial parts of the plant are usually used but the roots will often work as well. (Note: The plant is a great deal more active as an antibacterial and mucous membrane protectant if it is prepared fresh. The dried stuff is just not nearly as good.) The plant was originally native to South America but has escaped and is a potent invasive throughout much of the world. As it does mine, it probably grows around your house someplace.

The bidens are systemic herbal antibacterials with a fairly wide range of action against both Gram-positive and Gram-negative bacteria; they are also active against a fairly wide range of protozoa. They are antimalarial, antibacterial, antimicrobial, antidysenteric, diuretic, hepatoprotective, hypotensive, anti-inflammatory, hypoglycemic, antidiabetic, styptic, vulnerary, immunomodulant, antiseptic, neuroprotectant, blood tonic, astringent, carminative, galactogogue, mucous membrane tonic, and a prostaglandin synthesis inhibitor. In fact, bidens is one of the most potent PGE2 plant inhibitors known. Inhibiting PGE2 counteracts many tick salival proteins as well as stimulating dendritic cell maturation, helping fight the infection.

Bidens is exceptionally good for (in order of potency): 1) *any* systemic infections that are accompanied by problems in the mucous membranes anywhere in the body, especially chronic diarrhea, dysentery, UTI, vaginitis, and inflamed respiratory passages; 2) systemic staph; 3) malaria, babesia, leishmania.

The plant, in traditional use, has been used as a specific for a number of conditions: headaches, kidney problems, arthritis, ulcers, swollen spleen, coughs, lung and other infections, rheumatism, UTIs, rashes, and inflammation, and it's seen use as a neuroprotector. It has a long history of this kind of use in both Ayurveda and traditional Chinese medicine.

In China it is used for treating cardiac spasm, itching, gastroenteritis, appendicitis, colitis, irritable bowel syndrome, hemorrhoids, diarrhea, dysentery, difficulty swallowing, sore throat, tonsillitis, esoph-ageal enlargement, jaundice, acute or chronic hepatitis, malaria, boils, abscesses, infections, fever, chills, joint pain, traumatic injury, sprains, swelling, contusions, rheumatoid arthritis, gastric and esophageal can-cer, epilepsy in children, infantile fever with convulsions, malnutri-tion in infants, colds and flu, bronchitis, chest congestion, hemoptysis, allergies, lung irritation, pneumonia, insect bites, scorpion sting, and snakebite.

The Eclectic botanical physicians used it, primarily as an emmena-gogue and expectorant, for amenorrhea, dysmenorrhea, uterine prob-lems, severe cough, and asthma, as an infusion. An infusion of the seeds sweetened with honey was used for whooping cough. The plant was thought useful for heart conditions including palpitation, for colds, and for acute bronchial and laryngeal attacks.

The plant is a mucous membrane tonic and will not only stop the inflammation and act as a potent antibacterial in UTI infections but also heal the mucous membranes themselves. It has an affinity for mucous membranes and appears to act as a mucous membrane tonic. It is especially good for UTIs that are treated, return, are treated, return, *ad inuretherum*, especially if antibiotics have been used. The pain will usually go away in a day or two if you use bidens and within a couple of more days the problem should clear up.

It is specific for reducing elevated levels of uric acid in the blood, i.e., for treating gout or urate-based kidney stones. It is a decent diuretic and stimulates uric acid elimination from the body.

Because it is a mucous membrane tonic and is astringent, power-fully anti-inflammatory, and strongly antibacterial, bidens is specific for a number of troublesome diseases caused by resistant organisms: UTI, chronic diarrhea and dysentery, gastritis and ulcers (anywhere in the GI tract, from mouth to anus), inflamed mucous membranes in colds and flu and respiratory infections of any sort, sore throats from coughs or infection or even overuse of the throat, and vaginal infections. It's a good plant, too often overlooked.

Several of the plant's isolated polyacetylenes have been found to be more active than ampicillin, tetracycline, norfloxacin, and amphotericin B during in vitro studies. Ciprofloxacin and ofloxacin were more potent than the plant extracts. In one study, water extracts of the plant were found to be more effective against *E. coli* and *Bacillus cereus* than gentamicin. Bidens has been found to potentiate the activity of tetracycline if taken along with that pharmaceutical.

Bidens pilosa was found to be as effective as atropine, promethazine, neostigmine, and hydrocortisone in protecting mice from the venom of *Dendroaspis jamesoni*, a snake in Cameroon whose venom contains a potent neurotoxin. The plant extract also potentiated the normal antivenom normally used to treat those snakebites (as did atropine and promethazine). It is a very potent neuroprotector against neurotoxins.

A number of in vivo studies revealed the herbal tincture to be highly antiulcerogenic, inhibiting gastric lesions induced by alcohol, and to be more effective than sucralfate. The herb significantly protected gastric mucosa and initiated mucosal healing through a number of mechanisms.

Bidens has been found to be a strong antioxidant and anti-inflammatory. A double-blind, randomized crossover trial with 20 participants found the herb effective in the treatment of allergic rhinitis. In vitro and in vivo studies have found it highly effective in protecting erythrocytes from oxidative damage. The water-soluble fractions are more antioxidative than ethanol. The plant inhibits COX-2 expression (similarly to ibuprofen) and prostaglandin production. It is a prostaglandin synthesis inhibitor and a significant free-radical scavenger, comparable to alpha-tocopherol. It inhibits histamine release. Bidens also suppresses IL-1β, MAPK, and iNOS and inhibits lipid peroxidation by bacteria as well as NF-κB.

Bidens pilosa is a strong and reliable immune modulator. It has been found to modulate the differentiation of helper T cells and prevent Th1-mediated autoimmune diabetes in non-obese diabetic mice. This has been attributed to a number of polyacetylenic compounds and a butanol fraction. The butanol fraction also reduces Th2-mediated airway inflammation in mice. Hot water extracts of the plant stimulate IFN-γ expression. The plant will increase immune action if it is low, and decrease it if high.

Preparation and Dosage

The plant should be prepared in specific ways to be most effective. The problem appears to be threefold: 1) some of the plant's most potent constituents begin to degrade as soon as the plant is dried—the plant constituents oxidize easily; 2) heat destroys them as well; and 3) the most potent constituents are considerably more soluble in alcohol than in water. Water infusions still do have a decent range of potency (as can be seen from the plant's traditional uses as a tea in Africa) but are not nearly what they could be if they are prepared as a cold alcohol/water maceration. Water extractions of the plant (teas, infusions, decoctions) even if it is dried will possess about half the antibacterial activity of an alcohol tincture (depending on how old they are) but they *will* possess most or all of the other actions described in this material (anti-inflammatory, antiallergenic, immune-modulating, and so on), especially the anti-inflammatory and antipyretic actions. The fresher the dried plant material the better.

Water infusions lose potency fairly rapidly; they should be made and used daily. They won't keep. Additionally, the older the dried plant is, the less potent it will be—in either water or alcohol. The rapidity of degradation of the plant chemicals is, in part, why so many cultures that don't normally make alcohol tinctures resort to using the juice of the leaves of this plant, internally and externally, for disease.

So, for this herb, you'll want to use the tincture of the fresh plant, as follows:

Preparation: Tincture, 1:2, 95 percent alcohol, using the fresh plant leaves and stems.

Dosage: 45–90 drops in water up to 4x daily. In acute conditions (malaria, systemic staph), ¼–1 teaspoon and up to 1 tablespoon in water up to 6x daily for up to 28 days, depending on the severity.

Side Effects and Contraindications
None noted in the literature.

Herb/Drug and Herb/Herb Interactions
None noted, however . . . one study does show bidens potentiating tetracycline. Caution should be exercised in using the plant if you are on diabetes medications as it will alter your blood glucose and insulin levels.

Camellia sinensis (Green Tea and EGCG)

Green tea contains a number of catechins (which are polyphenols), the primary ones being epigallocatechin gallate (EGCG), epicatechin (EC), and epicatechin gallate (ECG). It also contains some important flavonoids: kaempferol, quercetin, and myricetin. Its myricetin content is higher than that in nearly all other plants. And of course, caffeine. Most of the research has occurred with EGCG but the other constituents are important and should not be neglected. If possible the best approach is to use a product that contains both the polyphenols *and* the flavonoids. (No, I don't know of one to recommend.)

Although not commonly thought of as an antibacterial, the catechins in both green and black tea have antimicrobial activity against a number of bacteria, including various mycoplasmas—especially *M. pneumoniae* and *M. orale*. They are also strongly reductive of the cytokine cascades various coinfections generate.

EGCG inhibits a wide range of cytokines, including TNF-α, NF-κB, IL-1β, IL-6, IL-8, ERK, CCL2, MMP-2, MMP-9, EGF, VEGF, PI3K, and p38 MAPK. EGCG also reduces peroxynitrite levels, reduces excess uric acid, reduces proteinuria, and protects rats, in vivo, from ischemia-reperfusion caused by bacterial lipopolysaccharides.

EGCG has been found to, in vivo, suppress induced autoimmune encephalomyelitis. It reduces clinical severity by limiting (and preventing) inflammation and reducing neuronal damage. It stops ROS production throughout the central nervous system. It reduces cerebral amyloidosis and modulates cleavage of the amyloid precursor protein. Studies have shown that it reduces age-related memory impairment in mice. EGCG apparently modulates the intracellular levels of free calcium in brain neurons (one of the causes of neuronal problems) and the hippocampus caused in such diseases as Alzheimer's and a number of coinfections.

EGCG also has some good protection for mitochondria. Besides the anti-inflammatory actions it also increases the accumulation of zinc in the mitochondria and cytosol.

EGCG helps with arthritic inflammation, attenuates the overexpression of pro-inflammatory cartilage cytokines, and modulates the antioxidant status in arthritic rats. It reduces edema in arthritis, suppresses lipid peroxidation, and increases the levels and activity of superoxide dismutase, glutathione, and catalase in cells. It is strongly inhibitive of acetylcholinesterase.

EGCG reduces lesions generated by inflammatory cytokines in peridontitis and colitis. It inhibits angiogenesis and has been found to have a strong impact on cancer cells, inhibiting inflammation and metastasis.

Green tea and EGCG are both synergistic with some herbs and supplements. EGCG, resveratrol, and gamma-tocotrienol (a form of vitamin E) are more effective against breast cancer cells when combined than when separated. The same is true for prostate cancer cells when EGCG is combined with quercetin and genistein. Effectiveness is enhanced against osteosarcoma cells when it is combined with lysine, proline, arginine, and ascorbic acid.

EGCG is synergistic with tetracycline against staph bacteria; it inhibits the efflux pump the bacteria use against the antibiotic. It potentiates beta-lactam antibiotics against resistant bacterial species. And does the same with carbapenems and ampicillins against MRSA (methicillin-resistant *Staphylococcus aureus*). It is synergistic with doxycycline.

EGCG and green tea in general have a number of actions that are directly useful during coinfections but there are a number of problems in the use of EGCG as a supplement, essentially its bioavailability. (It also can increase nitric oxide production, a potential problem in some cases, but excellent for treating babesiosis.)

Unfortunately only about 40 percent of the EGCG taken will get through the GI tract membranes. Most of the EGCG absorption takes place in the small intestine but fairly substantial amounts remain in the GI tract. Once it reaches the colon it is metabolized by the microflora in the gut. (Epicatechin gallate levels, if all the catechins are ingested, are much higher in the blood than EGCG levels.) The EGCG that does get into the blood undergoes extensive methylation, glucuronidation, and sulfation in the liver, where it is broken down into much less effective metabolites.

How to Take It

Plasma levels of EGCG are highest if it is taken on an empty stomach just after rising in the morning. Peak plasma concentrations are reached in one to two hours; they remain high for about three hours and then begin to decline, reaching zero by the next morning. (So, you have to take EGCG every three to four hours.)

The amount of EGCG, and the other tea catechins, that gets into the blood and does remain active depends on a number of factors, few of which are usually taken into consideration when using it as a supplement.

1. Serum albumin levels need to be highish. Human serum albumin contributes to transport and stabilization of EGCG and the other catechins. If it is low, bioavailable levels of EGCG are low.
2. EGCG and the catechins degrade in humidity and hot air temperatures. They have to be stored in a cool, dry location to remain active (think "refrigerator").
3. Since EGCG is a potent antioxidant, exposing it to the air over any length of time will activate its oxidative actions, caus-

ing auto-oxidation and rendering it relatively useless once you ingest it.

4. Taking EGCG with hard water affects its absorption into the body. The harder the water, the less that can be absorbed into the body. Soft water is essential.

5. Ingesting it with milk will inactivate it.

The bioavailability of green tea and EGCG can be significantly enhanced, however, if you take them with certain other substances. Quercetin (1,200 mg daily) or ascorbic acid (200 mg) or omega-3 fatty acids (1,000 mg), for instance, will all increase their availability. Quercetin increases the bioavailability of green tea catechins and decreases their methylation, in vitro and in vivo. Quercetin is itself a very good supplement for treating cytokine cascade problems. It inhibits NF-κB, TNF-α, IL-1β, EGF, iNOS, NO, and JNK. I would highly suggest, at minimum, a quercetin/EGCG combination (and no, nobody sells one, so buy them separately). EGCG is also much more effective if combined with resveratrol (knotweed), vitamin E, and/or N-acetylcysteine.

And . . . there is evidence, as usual, that the whole herb—the green tea itself—is and remains much more bioavailable than the isolated constituents.

If you do wish to use EGCG, it is really good, but bear all the necessary restrictions on its use in mind *and* combine it with other things, most especially quercetin.

Dosage

Try to get a supplement with at least 80 percent total catechins, at least that amount of polyphenols, and 50 percent or so of EGCG. A supplement with the natural green tea flavonoids would be even better. Dosage range is 400 to 800 mg daily. For greater effectiveness in treating *Babesia*-generated endothelial cell damage, for instance, take it with 1,200 mg quercetin daily—both at the same time, in the morning.

Note: There is about 100 mg EGCG in a cup of green tea. I would imagine that drinking green tea itself throughout the day would be a good approach and it produces better bioavailability.

Comment

EGCG is a very good supplement to use to normalize endothelial cells that are being targeted for inflammation, especially during *Babesia* and *Bartonella* infections.

Ceanothus spp. (Red Root)

There are 50 or 60 or a million species of *Ceanothus* in the Americas, from Canada to Guatemala, no one seems to know exactly how many there are. The genus isn't native anyplace else but it has been planted as an ornamental throughout the world, especially in Europe. Most species can be used medicinally; the most common are *C. velutinus*, *C. cuneatus*, *C. integerrimus*, *C. greggii*, and *C. americanus*. All species are apparently identical in their medicinal actions. My personal favorite is *Ceanothus fendleri*, a.k.a. Fendler's ceanothus, which grows in my region and which I have been using for over 25 years.

Red root is an important herb in many disease conditions in that it helps facilitate clearing of dead cellular tissue from the lymph system. When the immune system is responding to acute conditions or the onset of disease, as white blood cells kill bacterial and viral pathogens they are taken to the lymph system for disposal. If the lymph system clears out dead cellular material rapidly the healing process is increased, sometimes dramatically. The herb shows especially strong action whenever any portion of the lymph system is swollen, infected, or inflamed. This includes the lymph nodes, tonsils (entire back of throat), spleen, appendix, and liver. (Yes, it will help reduce an inflamed liver, though milk thistle is better.)

Essentially, if the spleen is swollen, that is, inflamed due to excess cytokine activity and immune cell production, the lymph system clogged, the nodes enlarged, the immune system depressed, and a chronic condition in place, red root is specifically indicated. The herb helps tone and modulate function in the nodes and spleen and is highly protective of the spleen from microbial damage.

Red root has a very long history of use in the Americas. The indigenous cultures used the plant for a wide range of complaints from arthritis to influenza, though it was primarily used as an astringent. The early American herbalists loved it and the Eclectic botanical physicians developed the use of the plant considerably, using it as an astringent, expectorant, sedative, antispasmodic, and antisyphilitic. It was used specifically for gonorrhea, dysentery, asthma, chronic bronchitis, whooping cough, general pulmonary problems, and oral ulcerations due to fever and infection. Its primary use, however, was for enlarged spleen and, to some extent, enlarged liver.

In recent years there has been a minor amount of exploration on the antimicrobial actions of red root. Several of the root compounds have been found active against various oral pathogens including *Streptococcus mutans, Actinomyces viscosus, Porphyromonas gingivalis,* and *Prevotella intermedia.* The flowers are active against *Staphylococcus aureus* and a couple of candida species; the roots probably are, too.

Betulin and betulinic acid, which are fairly prominent in the root, have a broad range of actions, both in vivo and in vitro: antiplasmodial, anti-HIV, anti-inflammatory, anthelmintic, antioxidant, antitumor, and immunomodulatory. Ceanothane, another constituent, is fairly strongly antistaphylococcal, antiplasmodial, and antimycobacterial. It does have some antimicrobial action against protozoa.

There is some evidence that red root's activity in the lymph nodes also enhances the lymph nodes' production of lymphocytes, specifically T cells. Clinicians working with AIDS patients, who have historically low levels of T cells, have noted increases after the use of red root. It is especially effective in reducing inflammations in the spleen and liver from such things as excessive bacterial garbage, white blood cell detritus in the lymph, and red blood cell fragments in the blood in diseases like babesiosis. There is clinical evidence that it has broad action throughout the lymph system and helps reduce not only the spleen but also the appendix when inflamed and that it stimulates lymph drainage as well in the intestinal walls.

Preparation and Dosage

Preparation: Tincture of the dried root, 1:5, 50 percent alcohol.

Dosage: 30–90 drops up to 4x daily. In acute conditions, 1 teaspoon up to 6x daily.

Side Effects and Contraindications

No side effects have been noted; however it is contraindicated in pregnancy. It should not be used if there is excessive chance of intravascular coagulation—*Salvia miltiorrhiza* should be used instead.

Herb/Drug Interactions

Red root should not be used with pharmaceutical coagulants or anticoagulants.

Chelidonium majus (Greater Celandine)

Greater celandine is native to Europe and western Asia; it's pretty widely established throughout the world now, including North America (some people even say it is native here). And, dear to my heart, it is an invasive, quite common in areas where coinfections are endemic. Specifically, chelidonium is invasive in most of the central and northeastern United States, from Georgia north throughout Canada and west to the Mississippi River. It is also invasive in Montana, Utah, Washington State, and Nebraska.

Greater celandine has a long history of use both in the West and in China. In Chinese medicine the herb has been used to treat blood stasis, as a pain reliever, to promote diuresis in edema, for ascites, for jaundice, and for cough. Its primary functional use in the West has been as a pain reliever, cough suppressant, antitoxin, and anti-inflammatory. It has been used for a very long time as a specific for jaundice, gout, toothache, ulcers, bronchitis, pulmonary infections, eye problems, infected wounds, wasting, GI tract problems, as a topical for abnormal growths, and as a blood tonic.

Its primary use now is as a mild sedative, antispasmodic, detoxifying herb, and for relaxing the muscles of the bronchial tubes, GI tract, and reproductive tract.

The plant has a nice cytokine-cascade suppressive effect. It inhibits NF-κB, TNF-α, IL-6, NO, Rho kinase, ERK, 5-LOX, 12-LOX, IFN-γ, B-cell proliferation, and gamma delta T cells in the spleen. Importantly, it is strongly inhibitive of the overactivation of the P2X(7) receptors in the brain, perhaps more than any other plant, making it specific for the kind of neurological problems that coinfections can cause.

The plant is strongly anti-inflammatory due to its cytokine cascade inhibition, which is part of its pain-relieving actions. It is used in Korea as an anti-inflammatory (among other things) especially in the treatment of rheumatoid arthritis. Studies with mice (in Korea) found that the herb significantly reduced the levels of IL-6 and TNF-α in the spleen and lymph nodes and strongly suppressed the progression of arthritis in the knee joint of mice, as well as "dramatically" reducing the erosion of cartilage in the joint.

It has a decent range of antimicrobial activity. It was found strongly active against *Bacillus, Staphylococcus, Streptococcus, Enterococcus* (including resistant strains), and 98 percent of human dental plaque pathogens. It has some antiviral actions against HIV, herpes virus, poxvirus, and grippe virus. It is potently active against the tick-borne encephalitis virus in vitro and reduces the impacts of the disease in mice given aqueous extracts, thus making it useful for that particular coinfection of Lyme. And it is antifungal against various candidas, resistant strains as well. It is strongly anthelmintic against *Dactylogyrus intermedius* parasites in fish. It is a biofilm inhibitor as well—a number of the compounds in the plant are active against the biofilm formation of various *Staphylococcus* species. It also is inhibitive of bacterial adhesion to human cells, probably from the herb's content of chelerythrine (see below). This range of actions bears out the plant's traditional uses for infected wounds and gums.

The plant has shown immunomodulatory activity in the spleen and bone marrow and has been found to strongly stimulate the production and release of bile, to be hepatoprotective and antiulcerogenic, to be antitumor, antispasmodic, radioprotective, and antiosteoporotic—primarily during in vivo and human trials.

One human trial found it to improve cellular and humoral immunity and nonspecific resistance to disease, significantly reducing the number of recurrences in children of chronic tonsillitis. Another clinical trial found that it was effective in reducing severe abdominal pain when compared with placebo.

The traditional uses of the plant and the range of actions that have been verified in scientific studies show it has a broad range of activity in many of the areas where Lyme coinfections have impacts. However, the most interesting are those that occur from one of its major constitutents: chelerythrine.

Greater celandine has over 30 different alkaloids, the main ones being coptisine (as in *Coptis chinensis*), sanguinarine (as in bloodroot and Mexican and opium poppy), chelidonine, and chelerythrine. The root has the most chelerythrine, running 2 to 3 percent by weight.

Chelerythrine is a very potent, and selective, protein kinase C (PKC) inhibitor (at tiny doses of 0.66 micromolar), ATPase inhibitor, and alanine aminotransferase (ALT) inhibitor. It also very strongly blocks the P2X(7) receptors in the brain that ATP stimulates.

Chelerythrine is also a potent ATPase inhibitor. *Babesia, Ehrlichia,* and *Anaplasma,* when acute (and most mycoplasmas), release ATP into the system. ATPase inhibitors can reduce many of the symptoms of more acute coinfections as well as mycoplasmas' ability to adhere to host cells by 50 percent. Inhibiting ATPase reduces the degree of impact that these coinfections can have on host cells and keeps energy levels higher in the host.

High ATP levels in the brain lead to tremendous damage to the

brain and central nervous system (CNS). ATP is also particularly stimu-
latory of the brain's P2X(7) receptors. Over time this produces neuronal
excitotoxicity. In other words, excessive stimulation of P2X(7) receptors
in oligodendrocytes is toxic to those cells. This causes oligodendrocyte
death, myelin damage, and axon dysfunction.

Excess ATP production also leads to white-matter ischemia. Loss of
motor and sensory function, neurobehavioral problems, and cognitive
impairments can all result. Cell damage causes significant ATP release
from the damaged cell cytoplasm into the extracellular environment,
where it quickly activates P2X(7) receptors on all cells in the brain,
including astrocytes. This causes a dramatic increase in intracellular
calcium levels, mediated by the P2X receptors, which begins to cause
significant damage in the CNS/brain. Levels of ATP (a neuroexcitant)
continue to increase and levels of adenosine (a neuroprotectant) to
decrease. P2X(7) receptors are highly expressed in microglial cells in
the white matter, on all myelin sheaths, and on oligodendrocytes. High
levels of ATP immediately cause myelin destruction, oligodendrocyte
cell death, and death of the microglia in the white matter, leading to
small foci of necrosis throughout the white matter.

Preventing P2X(7) receptor activation has been shown to reduce
or even eliminate this. Activation of P2X(7) receptors is a root cause
of neural pain as well. Deactivation will help alleviate peripheral nerve
pain during many coinfections. Reducing P2X(7) activation will significantly reduce damage to the brain and CNS.

Preparation and Dosage

Preparation: The plant should be tinctured fresh, 1:2, 95 percent
alcohol.

Dosage: The typical American dosage is 10–30 drops 3x daily for
30 days. The English dosage is higher, generally 40–80 drops 3x
daily. Chinese dosages are usually higher than that. I would begin
with the American dosage and see how you respond. Then consider the English dosage if all goes well. In general, use for 30 days,

wait a week, reinitiate use as necessary depending on physiological response to the herb.

Chelidonium is an important herb in the treatment of many coinfections, including mycoplasma, especially if there is severe brain and CNS inflammation. There are, however, some side effects to be concerned about.

Side Effects

Chelidonium is used by millions of people worldwide every day. In general, it is *very* safe. However, in recent years concern has been raised because it *occasionally* causes severe impacts on the liver. There are some 40 instances in the literature of chelidonium causing liver disease, specifically cholestatic hepatitis. This is jaundice with bile stasis due to severely inflamed intrahepatic bile ducts. More women than men are affected by it, usually older (56 years average), and the herb was taken for about a month before the first symptoms appeared. All recovered upon discontinuance of the herb. Because of this the herb needs to be used with awareness. In general what the herb does, in those it affects this way, is to inflame the bile duct openings, causing them to swell and close. This creates the condition. This action of the herb is, in essence, an overstimulation. Many people use the herb to increase bile flow; for some people it just stimulates things too much. There has been a lot of overreaction to this, especially by herb-hostile physicians. So . . .

To put this in context, many antibiotic drugs will cause this condition; it is not uncommon—though with antibiotic drugs, the condition is not always reversible. Liver damage, often severe, is common as well with acetaminophen (i.e., Tylenol). Death and liver transplants are sometimes necessary. In contrast, this herb is extremely safe. Still . . .

The symptoms of cholestatic hepatitis are jaundice, itching, abnormal stools, and, sometimes, pain in the region of the gallbladder. In general, again, you have to take the herb for at least a month to develop symptoms. If you stop the herb, the condition will improve almost immediately, with no long-term effects. So . . .

Pay attention to the impact the herb has on you and take action accordingly. In spite of this problem greater celandine is a very good herb for some of the Lyme coinfections; its use is warranted.

Contraindications
Obstructed bile duct, pregnancy.

Cordyceps spp.

Cordyceps really is a very potent and very good medicinal with a wide range of actions. And, as you will see, it is very specific for many of the problems that Lyme coinfections cause.

It is a strong immunomodulator and immunoadaptogen, mitochondrial adaptogen (increases oxygen utilization in the mitochondria, stimulates ATP production by the mitochondria, protects mitochondria from adverse events), anti-inflammatory, antioxidant, neuroprotective, antitumor, antimetastatic, hepatoprotective (autoimmune protection, reduces fibrosis, reduces and inhibits cirrhosis, anti-hepatitis B), renoprotective (protects from toxicity, inhibits renal failure, reverses glomerulonephritis), cardiotonic (hypotensive, strengthens heartbeat, antiarrhythmic, improves myocardial ischemia), nerve sedative, sleep regulator, anticonvulsant, antitussive, antiasthmatic, expectorant, bronchial regulator, antipyretic, adrenogenic, steroidogenic, hypolipidemic, hypoglycemic, antibacterial, animicrobial, insecticidal. It is highly protective of the bone marrow, reversing myelosuppression from a variety of causes (microbial to radiation).

Cordyceps is a rather potent immunoadaptogen. If immune activity is high, it reduces it, if low, it enhances it. When taken regularly, if the immune system is stressed by, say, a bacterial organism, the herb will stimulate the immune system in just the right way to respond to the stressor while lowering the levels of or inhibiting entirely the bacterial-induced cytokines that are generated. It affects nearly all the crucial cytokines at play during coinfections.

Specific Uses

The herb is specific for fatigue and weakness, especially after long illness or in chronic infections, poor mitochondrial function, chronic wasting, unproductive cough from no known cause, general inflammation in the brain or joints, mental fog and confusion, low libido, lung infections, kidney infections, thick mucous in the lungs that will not move, immune dysregulation, dizziness, tinnitus, nocturia, cancer. It is especially effective for mycoplasma infections.

In traditional Chinese medicine, cordyceps is described variously as having a neutral property and sweet taste or as being sweet/acrid with a "warm" property. It acts on the lung and kidney channels, is lung-nourishing, kidney-vital-essence- and vital-energy-tonifying, hemostatic, and phlegm resolvent, that is, a mucolytic. It is generally prescribed for overall debility after sickness and for the aged. It is considered to be one of the three primary invigorating medicinals in Chinese medicine along with Asian ginseng and deer antler.

It is specific for tonifying the lungs, arresting bronchial bleeding, dispelling phlegm, chronic cough, asthma, wasting, and tonifying the kidneys. It is also used for impotence, low libido, poor seminal emissions, aching of loins and knees, and as a tonic for spontaneous sweating, aversion to cold, tinnitus, chronic nephritis, general weakness, and sexual hypofunction.

Important

To be effective for anything, cordyceps *must* be dosed appropriately. That means a minimum dose of 3 grams daily but the best results occur with 6 grams daily as the baseline, especially in acute conditions. The renal studies usually used from 3 to 4.5 grams. This dose range can also work for lung problems, except in truly acute conditions when it should be 6 to 9 grams.

Note: There is a ridiculous herban (or is it urban) legend that if a person has a candida infection (or any kind of yeast or fungal infection or overgrowth, e.g., thrush) they can't take any kind of mushroom (IT'S A FUNGUS!) as it will cause the yeast/fungal infection to grow out of control. This is totally and completely untrue. It is akin to saying that I have an allergy to eggplant, so I can't eat any other plants. Some people do have allergic reactions to fungi, and if you do, don't use this one. But it will NOT, absolutely NOT, cause candida or any other kind of intestinal or systemic yeast or fungal infection to "bloom."

Preparation and Dosage

Cordyceps needs to be viewed as a medicinal *food*, not a raw drug to be taken in minute doses. Again, the Chinese tonic dosages are normally rather large, 3 to 9 grams per day, and during acute disease conditions they can go as high as 50 grams, nearly 2 ounces, per day.

The tepid U.S. dosages, 500 to 1,000 milligrams daily, are useless for any active disease condition. I repeat: *useless.*

If you think of the herb as a food, then eating 2 ounces, say, as you do of asparagus or potatoes, doesn't seem like all that much. In China, cordyceps is often added to soups and stews (just as astragalus is) as a food ingredient for chronic illness. Sometimes the Chinese decoct it in water and drink it as a tea, however traditional healers for millennia in Tibet and India (and in parts of China) used the herb only after soaking it in an alcohol/water combination, usually the local alcoholic drink. And in fact a number of the constituents are only extractable in alcohol.

The best way to use the herb is either as a powder preparation, taken directly by mouth (allowing the stomach acids and bile, etc., to extract for you), or as a tincture.

Bulk Powder

For Lyme coinfections I would recommend you buy the powder in bulk from someone such as 1stChineseHerbs.com. Dosage: 3–4 tablespoons blended in water or juice 3x daily.

Capsules

The Chinese brands, if you buy capsules, run around 900 to 1,000 mg per capsule and the suggested dose is 6,000 milligrams (6 grams) per day—just for a tonic dose. If you want to use the capsules for an active coinfection I would double that.

Tincture

Preparation: 1:5, 50 percent alcohol.

Dosage: As a tonic, ¼–½ teaspoon 3x daily; for an active infection, ½–1 teaspoon 3–6x daily.

Some sources recommend taking cordyceps with vitamin C to help assimilation. There isn't anything in the scientific literature on this and the Asians used the herb (and noted its beneficial effects) for thousands of years before vitamin C was discovered, so . . . not sure where that herban legend came from.

Side Effects and Contraindications

There are no side effects noted in the literature. Up to 5 grams per kilogram of body weight per day have been used in rats long term with no side effects. That would be 350 grams—i.e., about 12 ounces or ¾ pound—in a person weighing 150 pounds. Double that dose was used with rabbits for three months with no side effects.

The only reported side effects I can find are occasional reports of dry mouth, nausea, diarrhea. One case of an allergic reaction (a general allergy to fungi) that subsided when the herb was discontinued.

Herb/Drug and Herb/Herb Interactions

Cordyceps sinensis is synergistic with cyclosporin A and the amount of the drug needed is lessened if cordyceps is taken. The hypoglycemic actions of the herb also reduce the dosage needs for those on antidiabetic medications. There is some concern as well that cordyceps might be synergistic or additive with anitretroviral drugs, thus affecting dosage requirements, but nothing has yet been reported in the literature.

Vitamin C is reputed to help assimilation and may, if this is true, increase the impact of the herb in the body.

Finding It

You can get bulk powder and capsules from 1stChineseHerbs.com as well as many other online purveyors. If you want to spend enormous amounts of money, you can also buy the wild-crafted mushroom itself. Or . . . you can join the local mycological society (find a fun one, usually it *won't* include guys with mathematically shaven beards) and learn to find it in the wild. In the United States this will almost always be *Cordyceps militaris,* but this is interchangeable with more traditional Chinese cordyceps (*Cordyceps sinensis*).

Crataegus oxyacantha (Hawthorn)

The berries of the hawthorn bush (and sometimes the leaves and flowers) have been used as a heart tonic for at least 2,000 years in Western medicine and for a bit less than 700 years in China. They are specific for nearly every manifestation of heart disease: atherosclerosis, cardiac arrhythmia, congestive heart failure, hypertension, and peripheral vascular disease. In vivo studies have found that the herb lowers blood pressure, increases blood vessel dilation throughout the body, lowers cholesterol levels in the blood, and is powerfully antiarrhythmic, slowing and normalizing heartbeat.

In vivo and in vitro studies have shown that hawthorn increases both the amplitude of heart contractions and the heart's stroke volume. Studies also show that if blood pressure is too low, hawthorn raises it; if it is too high, hawthorn lowers it. It is in fact a normalizer of blood pressure and a regulator of blood flow within the body. Dozens of clinical trials have been conducted with hawthorn extracts on thousands of people with heart disease. All have confirmed the herb's remarkable effectiveness. In general, hawthorn is a pretty good heart protectant and tonic.

Hawthorn has a direct effect on the diameter of blood vessels and arteries, causing them to dilate, generally through increasing the endothelial cells' production of NO. (This makes it especially useful during Lyme coinfections.) This increases the oxygen being received by the heart. Hawthorn also changes the rhythm and pattern of the heartbeat. The heart beats more slowly, the beats last longer, and the power is increased. The longer the herb is used, the more healing occurs in vessel walls and the more toned the muscle of the heart becomes.

Hawthorn does have some cytokine inhibitory actions. It inhibits TNF-α, IL-6, NO, and protein tyrosine phosphatase.

Preparation and Dosage

Take 120–900 mg of the herb daily, or ¼–½ teaspoon 3x daily of the tincture (1:5, 60 percent alcohol).

The dosage range in most clinical studies has been from 120 to 900 mg daily. Most of these have used nonstandardized (i.e., raw herb) extracts, either in capsules or as an alcoholic tincture. Some practitioners are suggesting that the extracts be standardized for 1.8 percent vitexin-4'-rhamnoside or 10 percent procyanidin content. I think that a bit of overkill; the herb seems fine all on its own.

Side Effects and Contraindications

Hawthorn is a food-grade herb; it is tremendously safe. It is about as dangerous as its close relative apples. An incredibly tiny number of people have experienced headache, nausea, and palpitations from the herb.

Herb/Drug and Herb/Herb Interactions

The main problem is that hawthorn can lower blood pressure, so if you are taking blood pressure medications, caution is indicated. It may enhance the actions of digoxin. The herb is additive in its effects with knotweed and motherwort. Just take care if you are mixing the herb. Don't stand up suddenly as you might experience light-headedness.

Stand s l o w l y.

Cryptolepis sanguinolenta

There are a number of species in this genus, most of them in the Asian regions. The primary systemic antibacterial among the genus is *Cryptolepis sanguinolenta*. This is the species I have used for the past 15 years; it is very reliable as a broad-spectrum antibiotic, especially for protozoal infections and MRSA. Some people think the Ayurvedic species *C. buchanani* works similarly, I have not seen enough study on it to be sure, nor have I used it. The root is usually the part used medicinally.

Cryptolepis is antiparasitic, antimalarial, antibacterial, antipyretic, hypothermic, antimicrobial, antimuscarinic, renal vasodilator, noradrenergic, hypoglycemic, antithrombotic, anti-inflammatory, antiprotozoal, mildly antiviral.

It is active against a wide range of Gram-positive and Gram-negative organisms, protozoa, and yeasts. Tests have found the plant to be a stronger antibacterial than the pharmaceutical antibiotic chloramphenicol. Generally, it is more broadly active against Gram-positive bacteria (which are usually easier to treat due to their cellular structure) but does have potent activity against a number of Gram-negative bacteria. I have found it specifically effective for systemic infections, especially malaria, MRSA, streptococcus, babesia, campylobacter, urinary tract infections, and sepsis.

Cryptolepis has been successfully used for centuries by traditional African healers in the treatment of malaria, fevers, and diarrhea, which is essentially how it came to the attention of Western practitioners.

Among the traditional healers of Guinea-Bissau it's used to treat fever, hepatitis, and jaundice. Healers in Zaire and Senegal use it for stomach and intestinal disease. In Ghana it's used for malaria and fevers; in Nigeria for urinary tract infections, upper respiratory tract infections, colic, and stomach troubles; in Senegal, Democratic Republic of Congo, and Uganda for colic and stomach complaints; for wounds, snakebite, and hernia in Uganda; and in Senegal and Nigeria for venereal disease, rheumatism, and as a general tonic. In the DR Congo it's used for amoebic infections, including dysentery. Some

African practitioners have used it for the treatment of insomnia, and others for hypertension.

Cryptolepis buchanani has been used in traditional Ayurvedic practice for millennia. It is widely distributed throughout Pakistan, India, Nepal, Bhutan, Myanmar, China, Thailand, and Sri Lanka. It is considered an invasive weed in many areas. (A useful sign of medicinal importance.) It's been used as an antidiarrheal, antibacterial, antiulcerative, anti-inflammatory, blood purifier, demulcent, diaphoretic, and diuretic, and for treating paralysis and rickets and as a general tonic for overall health. It is commonly used for urinary tract infections, for coughs as an expectorant, as a febrifuge (antipyretic), and for abdominal disorders such as dysentery and stomach complaints. In Thailand alcohol extracts of the plant have been used as a primary anti-inflammatory in the treatment of arthritis, muscle and joint pain, and rheumatism.

Cryptolepis was discovered by the West because of the resurgence of pharmaceutically resistant plasmodial parasites. In an attempt to find new treatments for malaria, researchers began looking at traditional treatments for the disease. Initial studies revealed both *Cryptolepis sanguinolenta* and *Artemisia annua* as powerfully active against resistant strains. Artemisia was the first to be developed into a drug (with the same predictable problems as most antibacterial pharmaceuticals cause, including resistance); cryptolepis lagged but in the past 15 years a tremendous amount of research has been conducted on the plant. Initially, most of it was concerned with malaria. Cryptolepis is potently active against the malarial parasite, *Plasmodium falciparum*. (It is also active against other members of the genus: *P. berghei berghei, P. berghei yoelii,* and *P. vinckei petteri*.) Scores of studies have found it to be effective against the malarial parasite *no matter the degree of its resistance to pharmaceuticals.*

The herb has been remarkably potent against malaria in human clinical trials. One such trial compared the effectiveness of cryptolepis (a hot water infusion of the powdered root) with chloroquine, the usual synthetic drug for malaria treatment, in comparative patient populations at the outpatient clinic of the Centre for Scientific Research into Plant Medicine at Mampong-Akuapem in Ghana, West Africa. Clinical symptoms were relieved in 36 hours with cryptolepis, and 48 hours with chloroquine. Parasitic clearance time was 3.3 days in the cryptolepis group, and 2.3 days in the chloroquine group—a remarkably comparable time period. Forty percent of the patients using chloroquine reported unpleasant side effects necessitating other medications, whereas those using cryptolepis reported *no* side effects.

Because many of the antimalarial compounds in cryptolepis are water soluble and water-soluble extracts had previously worked well in clinical trials, a local company in Ghana hoped that a pre-made tea of cryptolepis would work well against malaria. With 2.5 grams of the dried, powdered root of *C. sanguinolenta* per bag of tea, the preparation is called Phyto-Laria and can be purchased over the counter in Ghana. (Similar products called Malaherb and Herbaquine are available in Ghana, and another called Malarial is available in Mali.) A clinical trial was carried out. Forty-four people with uncomplicated malaria participated in the trial, which was performed on an outpatient basis. Each participant prepared a strong tea (they steeped the tea bag in hot water for 5 to 10 minutes for each cup of tea) and drank it three times daily for five days. There was a post-treatment followup for the next 28 days. More than half cleared the malarial parasite from their blood within 72 hours; mean clearance time was 82.3 hours. Fever clearance time was 25.2 hours compared with the drug chloroquine's clearance time of 48 hours. Chills, vomiting, and nausea were cleared in all patients in 72 hours. There were two instances of late recrudescence (return of the disease) but the researchers are unsure whether this resulted from reinfection or relapse; no genetic testing was done on the initial infection. Overall the cure rate was 93.5 percent. Nii-Ayi Ankrah, of the Department of Clinical Pathology at the University of Ghana, remarked, "The present result is indeed welcome news since it advances the vision to incorporate plant medicine into the health care delivery system in Ghana" (Ankrah 2010). How different than in the United States.

Other studies, in mice, have found that the intake of a cryptolepis tea prior to inoculation with the malarial parasite does confer some degree of protection against infection. Taking it daily as a preventive as so many in Africa do seems to work well.

I have found the herb specific for babesial infections, though not quite as effective as it is for malaria. In most people it will clear the infection when used by itself, even those with a wide range of genetic variants. However about 30 percent of people need to utilize the other herbs in the *Babesia* protocol (see page 94) in order to successfully clear the infection.

Preparation and Dosage

You can take cryptolepis as powder, capsules, tea, or tincture.

Tincture

Preparation: 1:5, 60% alcohol.

Dosage: 20–40 drops up to 4x daily.

- **For resistant staph:** In the treatment of severe systemic staph infection (whether resistant or not) the usual dose is ½ teaspoon–1 teaspoon 3x daily. In very severe cases up to 1 tablespoon 3x daily can be used.
- **For babesiosis and malaria:** 1 teaspoon–1 tablespoon 3x daily for 5 to 30 days; repeat if necessary.

Tea

Preparation: Use 1 teaspoon in 6 ounces water to make a strong infusion. While the herb will work if infused in cold water, studies have found that the hot water extraction is more effective. It is nearly as strong as the alcohol tincture.

Dosage: As a preventive, drink 6 ounces once or twice daily. In acute conditions, drink up to 6 cups a day.

Note: The alkaloids in cryptolepis are water soluble, but if the pH of the water is alkaline the alkaloids will not dissolve well. The pH scale ranges from 1 to 14, where 1 is the most acidic, 14 the most alkaline, and 7 neutral. The word *alkaloid* means "alkaline-like." The more alkaline water is, the less the alkaloids will dissolve in it. You have to have a pH of at least 6 for the alkaloids to dissolve in the water. Hard water is alkaline. (A water softener makes hard water soft—that is, acidic rather than alkaline.) If you have hard water (you can call your city's water department to find out the average pH) or if you don't know, add a teaspoon of vinegar or lemon juice to the boiling water you are using to make your cryptolepis tea.

Capsules
As a preventive, take 3 "00" capsules 2x daily; in acute conditions take up to 20 capsules a day.

Note: Cryptolepis is taken as a regular tonic for years at a time in some parts of Africa and India. One or two cups a day of the tea or two to three droppers of the tincture (60 to 90 drops) a day is fine for extended, long-term use.

Side Effects and Contraindications
None noted. Considerable research has taken place to determine the potential adverse reactions from using the plant, and none have been found, either in human clinical use or with in vivo testing on mice, rats, and rabbits. The plant is taken, often for years, as a general tonic by many people in Africa with no sign of adverse effects. However . . .

Researchers in some instances have noted that people taking cryptolepis have elevated levels of ALP (alkaline phosphatase) and uric acid, which return to normal after the herb is discontinued. There have been no reported side effects from this.

There is one report in the literature of adverse effects of cryptolepis in mouse pregnancy. I can find nothing in traditional use that substantiates an extrapolation to humans nor any studies in the literature that show negative effects for pregnancy in people.

One of the herb's constituents, cryptolepine, has been found to be cytotoxic, which raises concerns in some people. A few points:

- Cryptolepine is an isolated constituent, and like most isolated constituents that are made into pharmaceuticals, it produces side effects that don't appear when the whole herb is used. *Cryptolepis itself has not been found to be cytotoxic to people.*
- The word *cytotoxic,* when used in reports, generally means it kills cancer cells and indeed cryptolepine does.
- Cryptolepine is cytotoxic because it intercalates DNA. DNA is a double helix, two joined twisted ladders. Cryptolepine inserts itself between the two ladders—that is, intercalates—and as a result interferes with cellular division, which is why it is useful in cancer treatment. Cryptolepine is a potent inhibitor of topoisomerase II, which it inhibits once it intercalates. The function of topoisomerase II is to allow DNA replication by unwinding the DNA helix, using it as a template, and then winding it again after replication. If topoisomerase is inhibited, DNA replication and cellular division can't occur.

Herb/Drug Interactions

None noted. However . . . cryptolepis has been used in traditional medicine to help rectify insomnia. One mouse study has supported that effect of the plant. There is some potential for the plant to synergize with hypnosedatives or central nervous system depressants. Caution should be exercised. However, there have been no reported adverse effects in these situations to date.

Finding It

The herb has been somewhat difficult to obtain in the United States but more companies are selling it every year. The main supplier I have used over the years is Woodland Essence. *Cryptolepis buchanani* may (I repeat, *may*) be a decent substitute for *C. sanguinolenta*, and it is somewhat easier to find.

Eupatorium perfoliatum (Boneset)

Boneset is antiviral, immunostimulant (increases phagocytosis), diaphoretic, febrifuge, mucous membrane tonic, smooth muscle relaxant, anti-inflammatory, cytotoxic, mild emetic, peripheral circulatory stimulant, gastric bitter, analgesic, and mildly antibacterial. It does have some decent actions against protozoa, especially the malarial parasite; it is something of a midlevel antimalarial herb in its actions. This makes it a fairly nice adjunct for babesiosis, especially when its other actions are taken into consideration.

The plant, indigenous to North America, has been used by Native American peoples for millennia, specifically for intermittent fevers and chills, with pain in the bones, weakness, and debility. The American Eclectics used it for intermittent (i.e., malarial), typhoid, and remittent fevers, and for general debility, pneumonia, cough, epidemic influenza, colds, catarrh, and pains accompanying those conditions. It was one of their primary remedies.

The sesquiterpene lactones in boneset have a large range of actions including some nice immunostimulatory effects. The specific lactone active against the malarial (and babesial) parasite is considered to be a dimeric guaianolide. It has a range of antiplasmodial actions but is strongest against *Plasmodium falciparum*. The action is mild (compared to herbs such as cryptolepis) but if boneset is added to a traditional antiprotozoal that is strong, such as cryptolepis, the effects are mutually supportive.

I consider the plant a useful adjunct botanical for any intermittent or relapsing infections such as flu, malaria, babesia, and dengue, and not a primary treatment botanical. It will really help lower fevers. It will help with the aches and pains of these kinds of infections. It *will* make you sweat (if taken hot as a tea, as it should be). And it does help eliminate these kinds of relapsing infections if they just keep coming back no matter what you do. (It is especially good for this purpose if combined with bidens.)

Note: Because of the common name *boneset* some people think this eupatorium good for setting bones. Others, however, insist that the name came from a common, ancient name for dengue, breakbone fever, and that the herb has never been used for setting bones and, more, indigenous peoples never used it for that either. (Feelings run high.) I have taken various sides in this over the years but did think it highly amusing a number of years ago when a well-respected indigenous herbalist (from the United States) who had used the herb for over 50 years (and who had learned its use from *her* teacher when she was very small) informed a rather self-satisfied group of herbalists that she used the herb primarily for setting broken bones (as a compress/poultice) and had done so all of her life. (So, now I read fiction novels and don't think about why it is called what it is called.)

Preparation and Dosage

The herb is bitter, and a tea made from it is about as much fun to drink as a tea made from earwax. Honey helps considerably . . . and if you have the kind of flu where you can't taste anything. Generally, the herb is taken as tea or tincture but few take the tincture directly on the tongue. Too bitter.

Tea

Cold infusion: 1 ounce of herb in 1 quart boiling water, let steep overnight, strain, and drink throughout day. The cold infusion is better for the mucous membrane system and as a liver tonic. If you want to help fevers, you need to take the tea hot.

Hot infusion: 1 teaspoon herb in 8 ounces hot water, steep 15 minutes. Drink 4–6 ounces up to 4x per day. Boneset is only diaphoretic when hot and should be consumed hot for active infections or for recurring chills and fevers.

Tincture

Fresh herb: Fresh herb in flower, 1:2, 95% alcohol; take 20–40 drops up to 3x daily in hot water.

Dry herb: 1:5, 60% alcohol; take 30–50 drops in hot water up to 3x daily.

- **In acute viral or bacterial upper respiratory infections:** Take 10 drops of tincture in hot water every 30 minutes up to 6x daily.
- **In chronic conditions:** If the acute stage has passed but there is continued chronic fatigue and relapse, take 10 drops of tincture in hot water 4x daily.

Side Effects and Contraindications

Boneset is an emetic when taken in large doses, so an early sign that you may be taking too much is *nausea*. Generally, the cooler the tea the less nausea. The herb *may* be contraindicated in pregnancy but no one really seems to know why. *Sometimes* some people have an allergic reaction to plants in this family—chamomile, feverfew, ragwort, tansy—so if you are allergic to those, careful with this one.

Herb/Herb and Herb/Drug Interactions

None noted.

Finding It

Fields and streams in the eastern United States, the Internet, herb stores here and there. Horizon Herbs sells the seeds.

Forsythia suspensa

This is one of the 50 fundamental herbs in Chinese medicine. It is a weeping forsythia, a large shrub, and quite pretty. It has escaped cultivation and is moderately invasive throughout the United States. (Again, an important sign that we are going to be needing its help fairly soon.)

It is called either *qing qiao* or *huang qiao* in Chinese medicine, depending on whether the green or fully ripe yellow fruit is used as medicine. The unripe fruit is considered to be the strongest. (Rarely, the stem bark and leaves are used.) The dried fruit, whatever its ripeness, is used for fever, headache, restlessness, delirium, lymph gland enlargement, general inflammations, erysipelas, boils, epidemic febrile diseases, acute liver and kidney infections, swelling in the small bronchioli, tonsillitis, sore throat, retina hemorrhage, and pus formations (foci or necrosis) in organs, especially the lungs.

The herb is a pretty good antiviral as well as being anti-inflammatory, antioxidant, vasorelaxive, antibacterial, antiparasitic, antiemetic, cytoprotective, and diuretic (antiedema). It is primarily used for clearing heat and toxins in Chinese medicine, essentially colds and flus, especially with lung, spleen, liver, kidney, and lymph involvement.

The herb has some good cytokine suppressive effects, especially for those activated by microorganisms. It tends to act most strongly in organs affected by cytokine cascades and to protect them from developing focal necrosis. This makes it a useful plant for Lyme coinfections that affect the organs. But the strongest reason for its presence herein is its impacts on some rather strongly impactive cytokines, especially MPO and HMGB1. This makes it especially useful for sepsis or acute inflammation during coinfections.

Dosage

The Chinese primarily use the dried herb either as tablets (or dried herb) or in a decoction, often in combination with *Lonicera* spp. The normal dosage is 9 to 15 grams per day, usually in divided doses. It is rarely used by itself.

Side Effects

A rather benign herb; no side effects are noted that I can find. It is recommended to avoid it in pregnancy but I can't seem to find a reason for that.

Genistein

Genistein, while first found in dyer's broom (*Genista tinctoria*, hence its name) is, these days, almost always derived from soy. It is common in lupins, fava beans, soybeans, kudzu, and coffee of all things. Genistein is a rather potent antioxidant and anthelmintic (removing intestinal parasites), but it is primarily known for its estrogenic effects. It is considered a rather potent phytoestrogen. The compound also has a number of other actions including protecting against endothelial barrier dysfunctions caused by cytokines, inhibiting leukocyte-endothelium interactions (making it specific for these Lyme coinfections), and inhibiting cancer formation and angiogenesis (though it can exacerbate breast cancers and inhibit their treatment due to its estrogenic actions). It helps prevent and correct both cardiovascular disease and osteoporosis.

The supplement's primary use is for treating *Ehrlichia* coinfections. Genistein inhibits protein histidine and tyrosine kinases. Studies have found that it significantly decreases the numbers of intracellular ehrlichial bacteria during infections. In other words, it specifically inhibits the ability of the bacteria to gain access to their preferred cellular habitat. The bacteria require the rapid activation of protein kinases to gain access to monocytes and macrophages. Genestein prevented the entry, internalization, and proliferation of both *Ehrlichia chaffeensis* and *Neorickettsia risticii,* a close relative, into target cells. The higher the concentration of genistein and the earlier it is ingested, the greater the inhibitory actions. The supplement is not directly biocidal against the organisms but rather specifically inhibits their ability to enter and proliferate in target cells, thus stopping the infection.

The supplement is also a fairly strong neutrophil elastase (NE) inhibitor, reducing NETs formation in the body. This makes it highly useful for sepsis.

The supplement is extremely bioavailable. Within one hour plasma levels increase substantially, reaching a maximum concentration around four hours later.

Dosage

Normal dosage is 20 to 80 mg of genistein daily. However for ehrlichial infections a much higher dose is recommended, 250 mg twice daily for 30 to 60 days. (There are some high-dosage formulations on the market; they are much more expensive.) High-dose usage should be limited to 60 days due to potential side effects, especially in men (who are twice as likely to be infected by *Ehrlichia* anyway).

Side Effects and Contraindications

Overall, this supplement is extremely safe. However, it is a phytoestrogen. It can aggravate breast cancer and interfere with breast cancer treatment. It will raise estrogenic levels in men. It should not be used at this kind of high dosage if you are pregnant or nursing, have breast cancer, or wish to remain manly.

Note: There has been quite a bit of phytohysteria about this supplement and soy in general. However, Asian women and men generally have high levels of genistein in their systems from their regular soy intake (tofu, soy sauce, and so on) without apparently suffering the kinds of impacts phytohysterians routinely regurgitate as imminent. In this instance we are looking at high-dose usage over a limited time frame as an antibacterial interventive.

Glycyrrhiza spp. (Licorice)

Licorice is an unusual medicinal. It is potently antiviral, moderately antibacterial (but fairly strong against a few bacterial species such as *Staphylococcus* and *Bacillus* spp.), immune modulating and potentiating, and a very potent synergist. It is one of the best, most widely acting, and useful of all herbal medicines. However, *it should rarely be used alone or in large doses for extended periods.* There are a lot of unpleasant side effects if it is used alone, at high doses, for too long.

The root is usually what is used medicinally. Licorice has been used as a food plant and medicinal for between four and five millennia. All licorice species have been used as medicine wherever they have grown and by every culture that has had access to them.

Actions

Major broad-spectrum antiviral, potent synergist (enhancing the actions of other herbs and pharmaceuticals), antibacterial, prevents biofilm formation, antistressor, adrenal tonic, thymus stimulant, immuno-modulant (will reduce immune levels if they are high, increase them if too low), expectorant, antitussive, antiulcerative, mucoprotective, hepatoprotective, neuroprotective, anti-inflammatory, antioxidative, cardioprotective, anticancer/tumor inhibitor, smooth muscle relax-ant, antispasmodic, protects from the effects of radiation exposure, gentle laxative, demulcent, analgesic, antihyperglycemic, reduces gas-tric secretions, stimulates pancreatic secretions, estrogenic, adrenal cor-tex stimulant, inhibits the enzymes tyrosinase and xanthine oxidase, antihemolytic.

Licorice is a fairly potent synergist. It has been found to poten-tiate the action of antituberculosis drugs, increasing positive out-comes in treatment. It potentiates the action of oseltamivir against resistant influenza strains. It reduces toxicity and potentiates other medications in the treatment of rheumatoid arthritis. It potentiates the effect of the neuromuscular blocking agent paeoniflorin. During tincturing it enhances the solubility of compounds from other plants (e.g., the sapogenin isoliquiritigenin from astragalus, the saikosa-ponins from ginseng) by a factor of up to 570, and it increases the immune-stimulating action of other herbs such as *Echinacea purpurea* significantly.

It takes four to eight hours (depending on what and how it is taken) for licorice's glycyrrhizin to reach maximum serum concentration after oral ingestion, then it is slowly excreted, and eventually eliminated entirely about 72 hours after ingestion. (Most of it is gone after 24 hours.) It stays in the body a long time.

Ayurveda

Variously known as *mulathi, yasti-madhu, jasti-madhu, madhuka, mithiladki,* and so on. The plant is considered cooling, tonic, demulcent, expectorant, diuretic, and a gentle laxative. It's used for treating poisoning, ulcers, diseases of the liver, bladder, and lungs. It is specific for any inflammation in the mucous membranes anywhere in the body. It is used for cough, sore throat, hoarseness, fever, and as a general tonic in debility from long-term disease conditions, especially pulmonary and GI tract conditions. It is considered a synergist, a specific additive to other herbal formulations.

Traditional Chinese Medicine

Known as *gan cao* in Chinese medicine, licorice has been used in China for 3,000 years or so. The herb is considered sweet and mild. It regulates the function of the stomach and is a qi tonic, lung demulcent, expectorant, latent-heat cleanser, antipyretic, detoxicant, anti-inflammatory, spleen invigorative, and a synergist in many herbal formulations. The herb is used in pharyngolaryngitis, cough, palpitations, stomachache due to asthenia, peptic ulcer, pyogenic infection, ulceration of the skin, hepatitis, encephalitis B, measles, and all types of respiratory infections.

Western Botanic Practice

The ancient Egyptians used the plant as a major medicinal; the plant has often been found in their tombs. The Greek Theophrastus, in the third century BCE, noted the plant's use for asthma, dry coughs, and respiratory problems. The Romans called the plant *liquiritia,* eventually corrupted to the word *licorice.* It was a primary medicine in ancient Rome for coughs. It was used throughout Europe as a primary medicinal and although harvested in the wild originally, it has been a main agricultural crop for over a thousand years.

The American Eclectics used it intensively, as did most medicinal practitioners in the Americas. The Eclectics used it for coughs, catarrhs, irritation of the urinary passages, diarrhea, and bronchial diseases. It was an early agricultural medicinal, grown by most people in their medicinal gardens. The indigenous tribes of the Americas used the indigenous species similarly, that is, for sore throat, chest pains, swellings, coughs, diarrhea, stomachache, fevers, toothache, skin sores, spitting blood, and as a general tonic.

Actions

The medicinal species have been intensely studied for years; there are over 2,000 citations on PubMed alone and thousands more on the Chinese database CNKI.

Licorice and its constituent glycyrrhizin are very reliable immune modulators, raising immune action if needed, lowering it if it is too high. In other words, if an infectious organism begins a cytokine cascade by initiating NF-κB activity (common), the herb will begin to normalize cytokine levels in spite of what the bacteria or viruses are doing. Another component of licorice root, isoliquiritigenin, also has potent effects on cytokines, especially NF-κB. Specifically it blocks the induction of VCAM-1 (vascular cell adhesion molecule 1), E-selectin, and PECAM-1 (platelet endothelial cell adhesion molecule 1). It interferes with THP-1 monocyte adhesion to TNF-α–activated endothelial cells, and abolishes many of the cytokine effects of TNF-α. It does this by blocking the nuclear translocation of NF-κB, essentially acting as an upstream cytokine cascade blocker in bacteria- or virus-initiated inflammatory processes.

In vivo studies have found licorice to be potently antioxidant, to stimulate immune activity, to be anticonvulsant, to be potently anti-inflammatory on skin eruptions, to be liver protective, to be cerebro-protective, to heal aspirin-induced ulcers, to be antispasmodic to the lower intestine, to be strongly antitussive, and to protect the mitochondria from damage.

As discussed in chapter 8, licorice and its constituent glycyrrhizin are important adjuncts in treating HMGB1-related sepsis.

Preparation and Dosage

Licorice is used as tincture, as a tea, and in capsules. **Again:** This herb is best used with other herbs in a combination formula.

One of the primary things to keep in mind when using licorice is that the higher the glycyrrhizin content, the more antimicrobial the herb will be. If you're using the herb as an antimicrobial you *should not* use deglycyrrhized licorice.

Tincture

Preparation: Dried root, 1:5, 50% alcohol.

Dosage: 30–60 drops up to 3x daily.

In acute conditions: ½ teaspoon (2.5 ml) 3–6x daily—blended with other herbs—generally for a maximum of 6 weeks at this dose, and only if you take the additional supplements described with the contraindications below.

Infusion

Preparation: ½–1 teaspoon of powdered root in 8 ounces water, simmer 15 minutes, strain.

Dosage: Drink up to 3 cups a day.

In acute conditions: Drink a cup every 2 hours.

Decoction

The traditional preparation in Japan (standard now in the Japanese pharmacopoeia) is as follows: 6 grams powdered root in 500 ml (about 16 ounces) water, bring to a boil, uncovered, and let boil moderately until the liquid is reduced to 250 ml. (This will be fairly mucilaginous.) Then add enough water to bring the volume up to 1,000 ml. Drink throughout the day. Tests in Japan found that this preparation will have about 50 mg/g of glycyrrhizin. (I assume here that the powdered root they used conformed to the Japanese standard of 2.5 percent glycyrrhizin.)

Capsules or Powder

Take 4,000 mg (i.e., 4 grams) daily in three divided doses. Note: ¼ tea-spoon of the powder is about 2,000 mg. *However* . . . Chinese doses run high, as they tend to do, up to 9 grams daily. Oddly, the WHO mono-graph lists the dosage range as 5 to 15 grams daily, somewhat higher. Assuming that you are getting a 4 percent glycyrrhizin content in the root, that will give you 200 to 600 mg of glycyrrhizin daily, which is the WHO suggested limit. The European Union standards suggest people not consume any more than 100 mg of glycyrrhizic acid per day. In Japan glycyrrhizin intake is suggested to be kept to 200 mg per day. So, as usual, you have a range to choose from. *If* you are struggling with a severe infection, for which this herb is specific, especially if it is severe encephalitis, there is no reason, keeping the contraindications in mind, not to use the higher WHO dose during limited treatment of 4 to 6 weeks' duration. Again, please keep in mind the side effects and contraindications.

Side Effects and Contraindications

Generally, licorice is nontoxic, even in high doses. However, long-term use, especially if you use the herb as a single (rather than in combina-tion), and most especially if you use large doses, can cause a number of rather serious side effects. Even the use of a tea over several years will do it, and every now and then, due to the rather good range of effects the herb has, someone does. (This makes anti-herb proponents *very* excited.)

Note: *This herb should rarely be used in isolation or in large doses or for long time periods*—that is, longer than 4 to 6 weeks. (However, see the comments in the next paragraph.) The side effects can be severe: edema, weak limbs (or loss of limb control entirely), spastic numb-ness, dizziness, headache, hypertension, hypokalemia (severe potassium depletion)—especially in the elderly. Additional problems are decreases in plasma renin and aldosterone levels, and at very large doses decreased body and thymus weight and blood cell counts. Essentially, this com-plex of symptoms is a condition called pseudoaldosteronism, which licorice can and indeed does cause if you take too much of it for too long. However . . .

If you take licorice along with some other supplements, it *can* reduce or even eliminate the tendency of the herb to produce pseudoaldosteronism. There is an intravenous form of glycyrrhizin commonly used in China that contains 40 mg aminoacetic acid (glycine), 2 mg L-cysteine, 1.6 mg sodium sulfite, and 4 mg monoammonium glycyrrhizinate (glycyrrhizin) per 2 ml vial. Normal dosing is 40 to 60 ml IV and up to 100 ml. The oral therapeutic dose is as high as 200 mg daily. This combination eliminates pseudoaldosteronism as a side effect. You can add both glycine and L-cysteine to your protocol to limit the potential for pseudoaldosteronism if you are taking large doses of licorice for extended periods. (Glycine, minimum 2,000 mg daily; L-cysteine, minimum 500 mg daily.) The addition of potassium (5,000 mg daily) will also help prevent the hypokalemia. *Again:* Licorice should be taken in combination with other herbs—this reduces the tendency for side effects by itself. And, if you do need to take largish doses of licorice, even with other herbs, for severe infections, please add these supplements to your regimen and carefully monitor for side effects.

Because of licorice's strong estrogenic activity it will also cause breast growth in men, especially when combined with other estrogenic herbs. Luckily all these conditions tend to abate within 2 to 4 weeks after licorice intake ceases. Caution should be used, however, in length and strength of dosages.

A number of studies have found that large doses of licorice taken long-term during pregnancy have detrimental effects on the unborn children. Low doses are apparently safe. Again, this plant should not be used in large doses or for lengthy periods of time *especially if you are pregnant.*

The herb is contraindicated in hypertension, hypokalemia, pregnancy, hypernatremia, and low testosterone levels. However, for short-term use in those conditions (10 days or less), in low doses combined with other herbs, it is very safe.

Herb/Drug Interactions

The plant is highly synergistic. It is also additive. It should not be used along with estrogenic pharmaceuticals, hypertensive drugs, cardiac glycosides, corticosteroids, hydrocortisone, or diuretics such as thiazides, loop diuretics, spironolactone, or amiloride.

Finding It

You can buy very good-quality organic licorice root from Pacific Botanicals, my preferred source for high-quality grown herbs. Regrettably there is no way to determine the glycyrrhizin content of their product. (I still like it though; it *feels* good.) 1stChineseHerbs.com has the Chinese-grown *G. glabra,* which, while not organic, is definitely supposed to be at least 4 percent glycyrrhizin by weight. Seeds can be had from Horizon Herbs in Oregon or Richters Herbs, an international seed merchant.

Note: Some of the licorice in commerce comes from eastern Europe (which possesses some of the highest levels of soil and air pollution in the world). It makes no sense to buy potentially contaminated herbs to use for their broad-spectrum immune and liver actions.

Houttuynia spp.

Houttuynia cordata is the primary species used. Some people think there is only one in the genus, others two. (Pistols at dawn.) There is a lot of speculation that there are significant *sub*species (or chemotypes) of *H. cordata,* mostly determined by their taste. Whatever it is, there is definitely something going on that the tongue is noticing even if the brain is not. This does have an impact as the herb is reportedly hard to ingest for a number of people—all because of the taste.

The Chinese/Vietnamese chemotype is reported to possess a taste/smell similar to coriander; the Japanese chemotype, according to one anonymous reporter, has "a strange lemon or orange odour that is often compared with ginger." To others, however, the taste of the plant, irrespective of chemotype, is apparently very close to rotten fish. This plant may be the herbal equivalent of cilantro. Some people love it but for those who do not, hate is the closest word to describe their reaction.

I have tasted it, and just to be biologically contrary, I experience it in none of those ways. It's not a lot of fun, but then, I've had worse. (Saw palmetto tincture—fetid soap.)

There are a lot of cultivars of this plant; it is common in gardens everywhere, so you get a lot of names for the thing: heart-leaved houttuynia, lizard tail, Chinese lizard tail, chameleon plant (as opposed to the specific variety called 'Chameleon'), heartleaf, fishwort, fishmint, bishop's weed, *doku-dami* (Japan), and *yu xing cao* (China). The Chinese name literally means "fishy-smell herb" because, well, it smells like fish—to someone, someplace, I guess. (My favorite synonym is *Houttuynia foetida*.) Generally, the aerial parts are used for medicine, rarely the roots. The Chinese consider the fresh plant the strongest form of the herb. If you are making tinctures use the fresh plant picked just at flowering.

The herb has a wide range of actions. It is antiviral, antibacterial, antifungal, antimicrobial, anthelmintic, larvicidal, anti-inflammatory, antioxidant, anticancer, immunomodulatory, astringent, diuretic, emmenagogue, febrifuge, hypoglycemic, laxative, depuritive, analgesic, hemostatic, antitussive, antileukemic, and opthalmic.

The herb is specific for respiratory and intestinal infections, mycoplasma infections, any serious infections in the lungs especially with abscesses, infections in the urinary passages and kidneys, genital infections, dysentery and any bacterial diarrheal conditions, various diseases of the eye (fresh juice or tea applied topically), skin infections with pus or boils. It is especially indicated if any of these conditions are accompanied by foul-smelling discharge.

There is a lot of indigenous and local use of the plant throughout its native ranges, for both food and medicine, but the most extensive use of the plant, historically, has been by, no surprise, the Chinese.

In traditional Chinese medicine the herb is considered to be slightly cold, pungent, and specific for the lung channel. It has traditionally been used for removing toxic heat, eliminating toxins, reducing swelling, discharging pus, and relieving stagnation. It is specific for promoting drainage of pus, lung abscess with purulent expectoration, heat in the lung with cough, dyspnea, carbuncles and sores, dysuria, acute dysentery, and acute urinary infections. It is considered latent-heat clearing, antipyretic, detoxicant, anti-inflammatory, and diuretic. It has been traditionally used for virulent carbuncle, lung abscesses, cough with thick sputum, leukorrhea, and edema. The fresh juice for snakebite and skin infections. Common medicinal use in China is for chronic nephritis, inflamed pelvis or cervix (pelvic inflammatory disease), gonorrhea, rheumatism, anal prolapse, hemorrhoids, inflamed respiratory tract (including pneumonia and bronchitis with or without edema), prevention of postoperative infections, inflammation and pus in the middle ear, measles, tonsillitis, chronic sinusitis, nasal polyps, inhibiting anaphylactic reactions, and various cancers.

Most of the scientific studies have occurred in China, often with injectable forms of the herb. Numerous others have been conducted in India and Thailand. Few have occurred in the United States. (The herb tastes funny.) In general, the studies found that the effects were dose dependent—in other words, the more they gave, the better the outcome. Since the herb has shown no toxicity from oral ingestion (up to 16 grams per kilogram in mice, a huge dose), that would indicate that largish doses can be used very effectively.

In vitro studies found that the herb (water extract) significantly increases IL-2 and IL-10 cytokines. IL-10 is also known as cytokine synthesis inhibitory factor; it is an anti-inflammatory cytokine. It essentially downregulates other cytokines and blocks NF-κB activity. It is specific for counteracting the effects of mast cell–initiated allergic reactions, which is why the herb is good for stings and bites and anaphylactic reactions. The herb also stimulates the production of CD4+ lymphocytes. It is especially active in the spleen. The herb reduces Th2 cytokines, specifically IL-4 and IL-5. It inhibits HMC-1 cell migration. It also inhibits topoisomerase 1 activity.

Houttuynia liquid extract protected and restored white blood cell counts in mice X-rayed and administered cyclophosphamide. It normalized connective tissue growth factor and increased levels of adiponectin in streptozotocin-induced diabetes in rats.

The herb (water extract) was used to treat bleomycin-induced pulmonary fibrosis in rats. The herb significantly decreased SOD, malondialdehyde, hydroxyproline, IFN-γ, and TNF-α. The morphological appearance of the lung was markedly improved.

A number of studies found that the herb strongly inhibited induced-oxidation events in rats. It specifically inhibited NF-κB, TNF-α, NO, COX-2, and PGE2. Houttuynia inhibited IgE-mediated systemic passive cutaneous anaphylaxis (PCA) in mice, reduced antigen-induced release of IL-4 and TNF-α, reduced NF-κB, and inhibited degradation of IκB-α. It specifically inhibited antigen-induced phosphorylation of Syk, Lyn, LAT, Gab2, and PLCG2. Further downstream it also inhibited Akt (a.k.a. protein kinase B or PKB) and MAP kinases ERK-1 and ERK-2 and JNK-1 and JNK-2 but not p38.

Extracts of the herb protected rat kidneys when rats were injected with streptozotocin. TGF-β1 and collagen levels in renal tissues decreased; BMP-7 (bone morphogenetic protein 7) increased. A modified form of houttuynin both protected mice from and corrected induced membranous glomerulonephritis in mice. It inhibited the expression of NF-κB and MCP-1.

A water extract of the herb protected rat primary cortical cells from beta-amyloid–induced neurotoxicity, specifically through modulating calcium influx and protecting mitochondria. In another study, the mortality of chicks challenged by *Salmonella* was significantly reduced when the herb was included in their feed. PGE2 synthesis decreased, CD4+ lymphocytes increased, the CD4+/CD8+ ratio balanced, immune function in all chicks was enhanced.

The herb's constituents move fairly rapidly into the bloodstream and maintain a high presence. The absorption half-life after oral ingestion is 3.5 hours. The herb's constituents are present in the highest amounts in the lungs, heart, liver, kidneys, and serum in that order. Elimination of constituents, metabolized or not, in the urine and feces is very low; the main route of excretion is the lungs (breath). Radioactively labeled houttuynin was found to persist in rat tissues for up to 48 hours. The highest levels were in the bronchi (especially at one and four hours postinjection) and in descending order in the gallbladder, liver, ovary, intestine, spleen, kidneys, and lungs. Oral dosing found the highest levels in the bronchi after 24 hours.

Preparation and Dosage

The fresh plant is much more antibacterial/antiviral (as is the tincture made from it) than the dried plant, and it is traditionally pounded to make juice for oral administration internally, or for use externally on wounds or as eye drops. The remaining mashed plant can be used as a paste applied topically to wounds and bites; the decoction (allowed to cool) can be used for an external wash. The Japanese use a tea, taken regularly, as a tonic medicine.

Tincture

Preparation: The tincture of the fresh leaves (1:2, 95 percent alcohol) is the most potent form of the plant as medicine. I would not use a dried plant tincture unless that is all you can find.

Dosage: ¼–½ teaspoon up to 6x daily for viral infections, or ½ teaspoon 3x daily for Lyme coinfections.

There are a few companies selling the tincture for absurd prices, which, given that the plant is an invasive and very easy to grow, I find obscene.

Decoction

Traditionally the herb (sometimes the root) is used, either dried or fresh, to make a decoction. For dried, 15 to 30 grams (about ½ to 1 ounce) of the dried plant is decocted (that is, briefly boiled), allowed to cool, then consumed. For fresh, 30 to 50 grams of the fresh herb is decocted similarly. Examination of the decocted herb has, however, revealed that it loses much of its antibacterial/antiviral actions upon boiling (which is why the Chinese tend to boil it really, really briefly). If decocted intensively, the plant works well to stop diarrhea but is relatively inactive antimicrobially. Apparently the Chinese boil it at all simply to alter the taste; the fishy taste is significantly reduced if even boiled briefly.

Again: It can taste nasty, very fishy, to some, so put it in something with a strong taste to cover it (fish soup?). Otherwise it can be hard to get it down.

Powder

You can also find the powder, sometimes concentrated at 5:1, sometimes just the regular old powdered herb, from some Chinese herb companies. You can encapsulate the powder if you cannot take the taste of the tincture or decoction. I have been unable to locate any pre-encapsulated forms on the market. The herb really isn't that popular at this point.

If you do encapsulate it yourself, use "00" capsules. I would begin with two capsules 3x daily and see how it goes, adjusting the dose depending on how it works for you. I have never been sure of how to dose the 5:1 concentrated powders that the Chinese often make; presumably you would take one-fifth the dose of the nonconcentrated form.

Side Effects and Contraindications

Fishy-smelling breath (maybe). The taste can be terrible to the point of gagging (some say). Other than the nausea from the taste there are no reported side effects in the literature from oral ingestion of the plant.

It does have emmenagogue actions (though oddly enough the herb is not traditionally used for starting menstruation) so it should not be used in pregnancy. However, a few individual reports from China say it can, very rarely, cause congestion in the vagina (but I can't really tell what that means).

The Chinese sometimes use it as an injectible and there have been some severe anaphylactic reactions to that. So . . . don't inject it.

Herb/Drug and Herb/Herb Interactions
None have been noted in the literature or in any anecdotal reports that I can find.

Finding It
If you want a very good fresh tincture at a decent price try Woodland Essence. The dried herb (in both powder and cut form) is available from 1stChineseHerbs.com.

L-Arginine
L-arginine is an amino acid normally present in the body. Its levels can drop during many microbial infections, including those from *Babesia, Bartonella,* and *Mycoplasma.* L-arginine is a rather crucial amino acid. It is needed for the replication and division of cells, the protection of endothelial integrity, the healing of wounds, healthy immune function, and proper hormone activity. It is strongly protective of bones and helps repair microbial damage to them. It significantly *decreases* the amount of time needed for wounds to heal.

L-arginine is important to use during *Babesia* infections in that it strongly protects the endothelial cells from the kinds of damage the *Babesia* cause. It reduces the cytokine cascade the protozoa initiate and stops them from creating more habitat.

L-arginine is also potently effective in improving endothelial dysfunction during any type of circulatory system disorder. It normalizes endothelial function, inhibits adhesion to endothelial cells (of all blood cell types), inhibits hyperplasia, reduces endothelial activation, stimulates the production of NO from endothelial cells (which will kill the protozoa), corrects induced NO deficiency in the body, and generally restores healthy vascular functioning.

L-arginine is the primary supplement to use to protect and restore endothelial function during *Babesia* infection. It will, by itself, counteract the majority of detrimental effects that occur during babesiosis. Studies have found that simply supplementing the body with L-arginine will reduce or even eliminate babesial infection from the body.

Dosage
Take 1 or 2 500 mg capsules up to 3x daily.

Side Effects and Contraindications
L-arginine should be avoided in cases of active shingles or herpes as it can exacerbate the outbreak. L-arginine will not usually initiate an outbreak but once an outbreak occurs, existing viruses can use arginine to enhance their replication.

Supplement/Drug Interactions
L-arginine can affect blood sugar levels and should be used with caution if you are diabetic. It can also lower blood pressure so should be used with caution if you are taking blood pressure medications.

Leonurus cardiaca (Motherwort)
Motherwort is an important supportive herb in that it provides protection for mitochondrial integrity and function and is very good at reducing anxiety and sleeplessness.

Motherwort has been found to be strongly neuroprotective, especially in ischemia-reperfusion–induced mitochondrial dysfunctions in the brain, including the cerebral cortex. It significantly improves neurological outcomes and reduces ischemia-reperfusion impacts in the brain. It decreases ROS levels in the brain mitochondria and, importantly, reduces mitochondrial swelling and restores mitochondrial membrane potential. Motherwort decreases the expression of the Bcl-2 protein in the brain. Increased Bcl-2 levels in the body have been implicated in the generation of various cancers, including prostate, as well as various psychiatric disorders of the central nervous system and autoimmunity problems. Part of the function of the protein is interfering with apoptosis, that is, cell death. Motherwort decreases its expression and increases the levels of Bax. Bax is a protein, closely related to Bcl-2, that acts to increase apoptosis in cells. Bcl-2 and Bax normally exist in a modulated balance and their expression is controlled by a protein, p53. This protein is intimately involved in controlling the emergence of cancers in the body as well as protecting the genome from damage. It is sometimes referred to as "the guardian of the genome."

Many coinfections decrease Bax and increase Bcl-2. This not only leads to cancer formation by mycoplasmas over long infection periods but also keeps cells that are infected by mycoplasmas from dying. This allows the bacteria to invade cells and scavenge their genome. Physiologically, in this instance, the mitochondria swell as they are infected, but cannot die, and are kept artificially alive while they are scavenged for nutrients. A major outcome of this is loss of energy due to mitochondrial malfunction. More crucially, it leads to damage in the brain that contributes to the psychiatric problems associated with mycoplasma infection.

Motherwort stops this process and protects the mitochondria in the brain, and presumably other cells in that location as well since it also decreases the production, and impact, of ROS in the brain. The herb exerts anti-inflammatory actions throughout the central nervous system and also exerts a moderate pain-relieving action as well. Motherwort contains a number of chemical compounds, among which is ursolic acid, which has been found to be a potent inhibitor of intracellular ROS induced by bacteria. Some studies have found that motherwort is higher in its antioxidative actions than both hawthorn and ginkgo.

Water extracts of motherwort completely inhibit tick-borne encephalitis (TBE) and induce resistance to the TBE virus in mice infected with it.

Motherwort slows and strengthens the heartbeat and has traditionally been used as a heart medicine. It is also a reliable and strong relaxant for anxiety. During anxiety episodes heart rate increases; motherwort calms it down through a variety of mechanisms. In combination with this, it also significantly decreases anxiety by its actions in the central nervous system. Double-blind studies have found it to significantly help in the treatment of anxiety. It also has been found to significantly decrease sensitivity to light—a problem that often occurs during Lyme and a number of coinfections.

Its actions are dose dependent.

Preparation and Dosage
Use the tincture.

Preparation: 1:2, 95 percent alcohol, of the freshly harvested, not dried, plant.

Dosage: ¼ teaspoon up to 6x a day. *Fresh plant tincture only.*

Side Effects and Contraindications
The herb is contraindicated in pregnancy, stomach irritation has been so rarely reported as to make me question the source, and I don't know what to make of the one report of diarrhea. Tremendously high levels have been reported to cause uterine bleeding but I can only find one source for this and nothing in the journal papers that are so often hysterical about herbs. The herb has traditionally been used as an emmenagogue, that is, a substance to start a delayed menstrual cycle, so perhaps this is why it is reported to cause uterine bleeding.

The plant does lower blood pressure, so if you already have low blood pressure, be careful with it. But just to make things more difficult the herb is also reported to raise blood pressure. I haven't seen this in practice in 25 years of use so I am not sure what to make of that assertion.

Herb/Drug and Herb/Herb Interactions
Will produce additive effects if taken along with blood pressure–lowering pharmaceuticals.

N-acetylcysteine (NAC)

NAC is specific for a number of Lyme coinfections. For example, researchers, studying the cytokine impact of *M. pneumoniae,* found that significant elements of that cascade, specifically intracellular levels of ROS (reactive oxygen species) in epithelial cells, phosphorylation of JAK-2 and STAT-3, STAT-2 DNA-binding activity, and IL-8 expression caused by the bacterial lipid membrane proteins, were inhibited by NAC *in a dose-dependent manner.* In other words, the higher the dose, the greater the reduction. NAC is a precursor of the potent antioxidant glutathione. During mycoplasma infection of the lungs the ROS it stimulates within the cells also causes DNA double-strand breaks. Researchers found that by stopping the ROS increases the DNA strands remained whole.

NAC also strongly inhibits hydrogen peroxide, a common problem in some Lyme coinfections. Other studies have noted that NAC inhibits the production of TNF-α, PI3K (phosphatidylinositol 3-kinase), p38 MAPK, JNK, IL-6, IL-1β, and MMP-9.

NAC is also strongly mucolytic, meaning it thins, loosens, and clears mucus from the lungs and airways. It is strongly protective of the cilia. NAC is also helpful in septic shock—an overwhelming infection that causes a resultant severe drop in blood pressure. Studies of the supplement in treating septic shock—and endotoxin shock—have found it can reverse those conditions, even if taken post-shock.

More interestingly, the levels of glutathione in red blood cells are significantly increased by NAC, thus protecting them from bacterial oxidation and lysis. TNF-α levels are decreased. (NAC is synergistic with pharmaceuticals and herbs in the protection of red blood cells from oxidative death.) NAC has a strongly protective effect on red blood cells, protecting them from oxidative events. This type of protection also occurs in synovial tissues, where it reduces inflammatory cytokines and inhibits collagenase, which breaks down collagen. And it is also protective throughout the reproductive systems, male and female.

NAC has strong protective effects against neurotoxicity throughout the central nervous system and can correct neurotoxic effects in the brain, especially in the hippocampus. It protects brain mitochondria from oxidative effects, eliminating membrane depolarization, keeping the mitochondria from swelling, bursting, and releasing ATP. It inhibits brain edema and as well acts throughout the entire peripheral nervous system to inhibit inflammation. It has also been found to protect the fetus during development from the impacts of inflammation induced by bacterial membrane lipids. NAC also inhibits biofilm formation by bacteria, reducing that particular form of protection that many bacteria use.

NAC is a very good systemic; it is widely dispersed in the body within one hour and reaches peak at four hours. Levels remain high for 12 hours. It is predominantly concentrated in the liver, kidneys, skin, thymus, spleen, eyes, brain, and serum.

These actions of NAC are consistent whether in vitro, in vivo, or in human studies.

Dosage

The usual dose in most studies on rats has been 20 mg/kg per day. That would translate to 1,400 mg daily for a 150-pound person. However, a University of Florida study with people found that a better dose for adults is 4 to 6 grams per day—for children 60 mg/kg. The best dose for Lyme coinfections, based on this, would be 2,000 mg in the morning and 2,000 mg in the evening just before bed.

Paeonia lactiflora

The root of this peony, and of several others, has been used in Chinese medicine for over 2,000 years. It is variously referred to as white and red peony root, depending (on the colors of the flowers according to some, not so! say others). The root is generally boiled and then dried in the sun and ultimately sliced and stored for use. It is used for nourishing the blood, acting on the liver and spleen channels, reinforcing yin, nourishing the liver to reduce liver pain, and reducing liver yang.

It is used for irregular menstruation, liver pain, abdominal spasm and pain, pain in the extremities, and headache due to liver stagnation. It is tonic, anodyne, alterative, diuretic, carminative, lowers fevers, relieves colds, and alleviates neurological problems. It helps protect the brain from the deleterious effects of microbial inflammation. It helps reduce ataxia and is antidepressant. It is an anticoagulant and inhibits platelet aggregation.

The herb is a pretty good cytokine modulator, especially for inflammatory conditions. It downregulates MPO and TLR-4 and HMGB1, making it highly useful in treating sepsis. It also inhibits RAGE, TGF-β, MCP-1, NF-κB, TNF-α, IL-1β, IL-6, p38 MAPK, E-selectin, ICAM-1, PGE2, and IL-17. It upregulates caspase-3, stimulating apoptosis in damaged and infected cells. It reduces microbe-induced permeability of endothelial cells. Like a number of other herbs that possess actions along these lines, the herb helps prevent fibrosis in infected organs such as the liver, lungs, and kidneys. It is particularly good for this. The herb is usually combined with other medicinals.

Preparation and Dosage
Chinese doses are, as usual, high: from 5–10 grams for tonic doses, or 15–30 grams for acute conditions, decocted in water. The tincture (1:5, 60 percent alcohol) dosage is ½–1 teaspoon up to 3x daily. It is usually best combined with other herbs (e.g., angelica for anemia, licorice for dysmenorrhea).

Side Effects and Contraindications
Mild GI tract disturbances, including occasionally diarrhea. Not for use during pregnancy or while on blood-thinning medications.

Panax ginseng
This herb has, perhaps, the longest history of use of any plant in Asian medicine, perhaps as long as 4,000 years in China. The Asian root, this species, is stronger than the American (*Panax quinquefolium*) . . . more

yang as they say. I consider it to be an adaptogenic stimulant, whereas the American root is more tonic in its actions. The herb is primarily considered to be an immunomodulator with a wide range of effects, including increasing androgens for men in middle and old age, and helping alleviate type 2 diabetes. The dried root is usually used for medicine or making tinctures.

Within the Chinese system it is considered to act on the spleen, lung, and heart channels, to powerfully replenish chi, and to tonify the spleen and lungs, calm the nerves, tranquilize the mind, and improve mental power. It is used for shortness of breath, listlessness, weak pulse, deficiency after prolonged illness, and excessive loss of fluids. It is specific for yang depletion (loss of vital energy) with profuse sweating and/or cold limbs.

In general, the herb improves resistance to stress, increases stamina and endurance, improves overall health and vitality, and increases mental performance.

It is important in the treatment of these Lyme coinfections because of its numerous cytokine and immune effects. It upregulates caspase-3, MHC-II, and IL-12. It inhibits TNF-α, TLR-4, CXCL10, CXCL11, CXCL1, and CCL3 and 4. And it has tremendous impacts on bone marrow progenitor stem cells, strongly counteracting myelosuppression in the marrow. The numbers of all hematopoietic cells are increased by the herb, helping counteract their suppression in the bone marrow. It is markedly good for anemia caused by such suppression.

Preparation and Dosage

In China, the dosage is 5 to 10 grams (as a powder) daily, in 1- to 2-gram doses taken two or three times daily. For deep and prolonged chronic conditions, up to 15 to 30 grams per day are used. Tincture (1:5, 70 percent alcohol) dosages tend to be smallish, from 10 drops up.

Side Effects and Contraindications

Should not really be used with stimulants (caffeine, amphetamines, and so on) and should be avoided if you have high blood pressure or are consumed by anxiety. Not really for use during pregnancy.

Polygala tenuifolia (Chinese Senega Root)

This is one of the 50 fundamental herbs of Chinese medicine and is known as *yuan zhi*. It is used in China primarily as an expectorant and to help lung inflammations. But it also has strong impacts on cognitive function, enhancing memory, alleviating neurotoxicity, and producing positive impacts in the treatment of Alzheimer's, dementia, depression, and degenerative diseases. It is a very good anti-inflammatory and inhibits NF-κB, NO, iNOS, COX-2, PGE2, TNF-α, and IL-1β in microglial cells. One of the more important activities of the herb is that it enhances the secretion of nerve growth factor (NGF) in the brain, spinal cord, and peripheral nervous systems. NGF is a small protein that is crucial for the growth, maintenance, and survival of neurons. When neuronal damage occurs, higher levels of NGF are essential in stimulating axonal regeneration. This is perhaps the best plant for stimulation of NGF.

Preparation and Dosage

The dosage is 30 drops of the tincture of the dried root (1:5, 50 percent alcohol) 3x daily for 30 days. It is contraindicated in those with ulcers or gastritis.

Polygonum cuspidatum (Japanese Knotweed)

Japanese knotweed is a world-class invasive originally native to Japan, north China, Taiwan, and Korea. It is another significant invasive that is specific for emerging bacterial infections. The root is the part of the plant used for medicine.

The herb has a wide range of actions: antibacterial, antiviral, antischistosomal, antispirochetal, antifungal, immunostimulant, immunomodulant, anti-inflammatory, angiogenesis modulator, central nervous system relaxant, central nervous system (brain and spinal cord) protectant and anti-inflammatory, antioxidant, antiathersclerotic, antihyperlipidemic, antimutagenic, anticarcinogenic, antineoplastic, vasodilator, inhibits platelet aggregation, inhibits eicosanoid synthesis, antithrombotic, tyrosine kinase inhibitor, oncogene inhibitor, antipyretic, cardioprotective, analgesic, antiulcer (slightly reduces stomach acid and protects against stress ulcers), hemostatic, and astringent.

A broadly systemic plant, Japanese knotweed modulates and enhances immune function, is anti-inflammatory for both arthritic and bacterial inflammations, protects the body against endotoxin damage, and is a potently strong angiogenesis modulator, highly protective of the endothelia of the body. It crosses the blood-brain barrier and is potently anti-inflammatory in the brain and central nervous system. It is highly specific for *Bartonella* and Lyme disease infections and is a very useful adjunct for a number of the other coinfections, especially when endothelial dysfunction is present.

Knotweed is a very strong inhibitor of cytokine cascades initiated by bacteria. During Lyme infection, for instance, there is a spirochete-stimulated release of a number of matrix metalloproteinases (MMPs). The most common are MMP-1, MMP-3, and MMP-9. Production of MMP-1 and MMP-3 in Lyme arthritis occurs through a particular grouping of pathways—those of the mitogen-activated protein kinases (MAPKs), specifically JNK, p38, and ERK-1 and ERK-2. MMP-9 production occurs through the JNK pathway and another, the PKC-delta pathway.

While there are a number of herbs that can reduce autoinflammatory conditions stimulated by MMP-1 and MMP-3 (e.g., curcumin), the only herb that specifically blocks MMP-1 and MMP-3 induction through these three particular pathways is *Polygonum cuspidatum*. Resveratrol (one of the plant's constituents) is also directly active in reducing MMP-9 levels through both the JNK and PKC-delta pathways; it has been found to specifically inhibit MMP-9 gene transcription. Another component of the plant, rhein, inhibits the JNK pathway for MMP-1, MMP-3, and MMP-9 expression. Knotweed is also a formidable inhibitor of NF-κB, IL-8, PI3K, E-selectin, and VEGF.

Polygonum cuspidatum's constituents cross the blood-brain barrier, where they exert actions on the central nervous system: antimicrobial, anti-inflammatory, as protectants against oxidative and microbial damage, and as calming agents. The herb specifically protects the brain from inflammatory damage, microbial endotoxins, and bacterial infections.

Knotweed enhances blood flow especially to the eyes, heart, skin, and joints. This makes it especially useful in Lyme and its coinfections as it facilitates blood flow to the areas that are difficult to reach to kill the organisms. It is a drug and herb synergist, facilitating the movement of other herbs and drugs into these hard-to-reach places when taken with them.

It is also extremely effective for treating coinfection-initiated inflammatory arthritis. Its most potent constituents are the resveratrols, emodin, and polydatin. The plant root is so high in resveratrols that it is the main source of the supplement throughout the world.

While there is a long historical use of the plant in Asia, especially China and Japan, stretching back 2,000 years, there has been little knowledge of the plant in the West until recently. Research on and subsequent use of the plant as a phytomedicinal has been primarily because of its high content of resveratrol, a potent vasodilator and inhibitor of platelet aggregation (among other things).

The plant's compounds easily move across the gastrointestinal mucosa and circulate in the bloodstream.

In traditional Chinese medicine the herb is used for invigorating and clearing the blood, and for its antipyretic, detoxicant, anti-inflammatory, antirheumatic, diuretic, expectorant, antitussive, and stasis-eliminating and channel-deobstructant actions. Primarily, it is used in the treatment of jaundice, rheumatic pain, strangury with turbid urine and leukorrhea, dysmenorrhea, retained lochia, bleeding hemorrhoids and anal fissure, wounds and injuries.

Other uses include respiratory infections and damage to the skin: scalds and burns, carbuncles, skin infections, snakebite (usually as a poultice). It's also used for bacterial dysentery, acute infectious hepatitis with jaundice, hepatitis B (surface antigen positive), chronic active hepatitis, neonatal jaundice, cholelithiasis, cholecystitis (with damp heat or severe heat syndrome), trichomonas, bacterial vaginitis, hyperlipidemia, and psoriasis. (Basically, it is used to treat pathogenic heat in the blood, cough from lung heat, constipation from accumulated heat in the GI tract, jaundice and liver inflammation due to damp heat, and accumulated heat in the skin.)

There are literally hundreds of studies on the plant and its constituents. In the West these studies have primarily focused on the actions of resveratrol, followed (in descending order) by the whole plant and the constituents trans-resveratrol, emodin, and polydatin. The scores of clinical and laboratory studies in China have been primarily on the whole plant and the single constituent polydatin.

The plant and its constituent resveratrol interfere with the actions of NF-κB. This transcription factor is strongly linked to inflammatory and immune responses. It is active in the regulation of cell proliferation and apoptosis, cell transformation, and tumor development. It controls the gene expression of cytokines, chemokines, growth factors, cell adhesion molecules, and some acute-phase proteins, including the inflammatory mediators iNOS and COX-2. Bacteria such as *Borrellia* and its coinfections can activate NF-κB, causing a cascade of immune-mediated cellular reactions. The herb apparently modulates the actions of NF-κB rather than acting simply as its suppressor. Resveratrol also modulates IFN-γ-induced neopterin production and tryptophan degradation. Resveratrol also inhibits IL-6, IL-8, TNF-α, ERK-1, and ERK-2.

Another component of knotweed, emodin, is highly protective of brain neurons and reduces pain by inhibiting the activation of the P2X(7) receptors in the brain. It reduces impacts on the P2X(2/3) receptors as well.

The herb, in fact, is a potent immunomodulator. It normalizes immune response, especially in diseases where autoimmune reactions are stimulated (such as Lyme disease and lupus). It seems able to bring up immune function when necessary and reduce its local manifestations when overstimulated, e.g., in rheumatoid arthritis. This is a very strong aspect of the plant's actions.

Clinical studies have found the herb to be effective in acute icteric viral hepatitis, inflammation of the bone and bone marrow, psoriasis, herpes, and cervix erosion. The herb and its constituents have also been found to enhance and potentiate the action of other drugs and herbs when taken with them. Japanese knotweed and its constituents also possess strong actions in the central nervous system and brain, and this range of activity is where a great deal of interest in the plant is being generated.

Knotweed and the constituents trans-resveratrol and resveratrol have been found to be strongly neuroprotective through a variety of actions in numerous studies. One of the herb's mechanisms of action in this regard is as an antioxidant. One study found that resveratrol and trans-resveratrol protected rat embryonic mesencephalic cells from a powerful pro-oxidant, tert-butyl hydroperoxide. Another study found that regular use of trans-resveratrol prevented streptozotocin-induced cognitive impairment and oxidative stress in rats (an Alzheimer's-like condition). And yet another found that trans-resveratrol protected and reversed many of the impacts of induced stroke in rats.

While the herb's antioxidant actions are important, trans-resveratrol, for example, has been found in a number of studies to strongly protect neuronal structures from damage through mechanisms other than antioxidant activity alone. Resveratrol has been found specific for protecting the brain from neurotoxic substances such as the beta-amyloid peptides, which are associated with Alzheimer's disease.

Resveratrol and trans-resveratrol are specific for reducing inflammation in the brain and central nervous system. In spinal cord injuries resveratrol "remarkably" reduced secondary spinal cord edema, significantly suppressed the activity of lactate dehydrogenase, reduced malondialdehyde content in the injured spinal cord tissue, and markedly improved NA+/K+-ATPase activities. It immediately stimulated microcirculation to the injured tissues.

Low-level, chronic inflammation in the brain and central nervous system plays a major role in many neurodegenerative conditions. Both the herb and its constituents are specific for such inflammations. They have been found active for such things as amyotrophic lateral sclerosis and other motor neuron diseases, Parkinson's disease, Alzheimer's disease, bulbar atrophy, dementia, Huntington's disease, myasthenia gravis, stroke, multiple sclerosis, frontotemporal dementia, encephalomyelitis, traumatic brain injury, cerebral ischemia, and so on. The resveratrols specifically protect brain cells from assault, whether chemical or microbial in origin. The herb and its constituents, as well, stimulate microcirculation in the brain.

Preparation and Dosage
Capsules, powder, or tincture.

Capsules: Capsules of pure knotweed root can be had (try Green Dragon Botanicals at www.greendragonbotanicals.com) or you can buy "resveratrol," which is in fact only a standardized knotweed root formulation. That is, it is knotweed root standardized for the presence of a certain percentage of resveratrols. Most of the brands on the market are usable. Just make sure they are made from knotweed root (it will say on the package someplace in tiny print) and not grapes. Dosage for Lyme and its coinfections is 3 capsules 3x daily.

Powder: I actually prefer, these days, to use the powdered root in a liquid of my choice, usually 1 teaspoon–1 tablespoon 3x daily. (I am tired of swallowing capsules.)

Tincture: ¼–½ teaspoon of the tincture of the dried root (1:5, 50 percent alcohol) 3x daily.

Contraindications and Side Effects

While a very safe herb, Japanese knotweed is contraindicated in pregnancy. Side effects of high dosages are primarily gastrointestinal in nature—dry mouth, bitter taste in mouth, nausea, vomiting, abdominal pain, diarrhea. If gastrointestinal side effects occur, reduce the dose. A couple of notes . . .

Note: A very few people have reported a loss of their ability to taste from using the herb. This definitely is a potential side effect, even though it occurs in less than 1 percent of the people using the plant. It can take a while to return (months).

Note: Some people have reported rather strong negative physical responses to the Source Naturals resveratrol. I am not sure why this is; however, those that do, having switched to another product by Paradise Herbs, report a better outcome. Just an FYI on that one.

Herb/Drug and Herb/Herb Interactions

Should not be used with blood-thinning agents. Discontinue use of the herb 10 days prior to any surgery. The plant is a synergist and may potentiate the effects of pharmaceuticals and other herbs.

Pueraria lobata (Kudzu)

Though originally native to Japan, kudzu is an invasive vine in the southern United States. It is particularly impressive, being able to grow 12 inches per day and up to 100 feet per year. It can't be stopped, it can't be reasoned with, nothing will kill it, and it knows where you live. It is the root that is used for medicine.

Kudzu has long been used in both China and Japan as medicine and food. It increases blood circulation, relieves tension in the face and neck, is somewhat antiviral, lowers blood pressure, and is anti-inflammatory. It can help the headaches that occur from encephalitis, will reduce Bell's palsy, and reduces inflammatory cytokine cascades. Kudzu root has very strong antifever actions as well and will reduce severe fevers fairly quickly; the effects last about eight hours.

Kudzu root and its major constituents (puerarin and kakkalide and irisolidone—a metabolite of kakkalide produced by intestinal microflora that is more potent than kakkalide) inhibit TNF-α, IL-1β, NF-κB, ERK, iNOS, PGE2, COX-2, AP-1 (activator protein 1), ICAM-1, VCAM-1, E-selectin, CRP (C-reactive protein), and the phosphorylation of IκB-α. They have targeted and potent effects on cytokine-activated microglial cells and will reduce damage by cytokines in the central nervous system.

Kudzu and puerarin are strongly protective of the brain and central nervous system, especially in ischemia-reperfusion injury. They have a strong protective effect against beta-amyloid–induced neurotoxicity in hippocampal neurons, protect mitochondria from ROS, and stimulate peripheral nerve regeneration. Neuron pain receptors P2X(3) and P2X(2/3), similar to P2X(7), in the brain are inhibited by puerarin, making this a very good companion herb to use with greater celandine (see page 242). The root is, in fact, strongly anti-inflammatory in the brain and central nervous system. It significantly inhibits neutrophil respiratory bursts, reducing autoimmune dynamics in the brain. Similarly to motherwort (page 278), it modulates Bax/Bcl-2 actions in the mitochondria in the brain and inhibits caspase-3 and iNOS expressions. It is strongly neuroprotective during inflammation disturbances in the brain and central nervous system.

It is a good herb for these types of cytokine cascades, especially so since it is invasive and there is no dearth of supply. *Anywhere* encephalitis occurs and kudzu grows, use kudzu.

Dosage

In traditional Chinese medicine the usual dose is 6–12 grams per day of the powdered root. Normally dosing in the West is 1 gram per day. Tincture (1:5, 50 percent alcohol) dosage for Lyme coinfections is ½ teaspoon 3–4x daily.

Quercetin

Quercetin is abundant in plants, including most medicinal and food plants. We get a lot of it in our diet. It has a wide range of actions, including antioxidant, anti-inflamatory, antiplatelet activity, antineo-plastic, antiviral, antihistaminic, and so on. It is of import for use in these types of Lyme coinfections due to its effects in three areas: 1) sepsis; 2) cytokine inflammation; and 3) *Ehrlichia/Anaplasma* infections.

The supplement inhibits MPO and NE, meaning that it suppresses NETs formation and presence in the body; it also inhibits HMGB1. This makes the supplement, in high doses, very good for treating sepsis. The herb also reduces TNF-α and MIP-2 cytokines. And it is a fairly good inhibitor of histidine kinase, which means it will interfere with or even eliminate the ability of both *Ehrlichia* and *Anaplasma* bacteria to infect white blood cells. It is an excellent supplement for all stages of infection by those bacteria, including acute conditions and sepsis.

Dosage
Take 1,000 milligrams 2x daily during treatment of Lyme coinfections.

Side Effects and Contraindications
This supplement is well tolerated—high dosages taken daily for months produced no adverse side effects. It should not be taken along with digoxin; there is a possibility of negative side effects (speculative).

Rhodiola spp.

No one knows just how many rhodiola species there are, but they do guess a lot: 36, or maybe 60, or probably 90. The primary medicinal that most people use is *Rhodiola rosea* but many of the related species are used medicinally in the regions in which they grow. Because of the interest in *R. rosea,* the genus is being intensively studied for activity: I have found medicinal studies of one sort or another on *R. crenulata, R. quadrifida, R. heterodonta, R. semenovii, R. sachalinensis, R. sacra, R. fastigiata, R. kirilowii, R. bupleuroides, R. dumulosa, R. imbricata,*

R. rhodantha, and *R. integrifolia.* The roots are what are used as medicine. *All* the *Rhodiola rosea* plants, irrespective of where they grow or in what country, have nearly identical chemistry. They are all perfectly usable as medicine.

Rhodiola is an adaptogen, immune tonic, nervous system tonic, neural protectant, hippocampal protectant and tonic, mitochondrial tonic and protectant, endocrine tonic, adrenal protectant, ergogenic, antidepressant, antifatigue, antistressor, strong antioxidant, potent cardiotonic, potent hypoxia antagonist, anticancer. A mental and muscular stimulant. Possibly a synergist; the plant is a strong inhibitor of CYP3A4 and P-glycoprotein.

It is specific for chronic, long-term fatigue, recurrent infections, recovery from long-term illness and infections, nervous exhaustion, chronic fatigue syndrome, chronic disease conditions with depression, low immune function, brain fog, acceleration of recovery from debilitating conditions.

Rhodiola, as far as I can tell, and in spite of assertions that it is a long-standing traditional Chinese medicinal, was a contribution to the medicinal plant world by the Russians due to their interest in adaptogens. This is pretty much a Russian-introduced category of medicinal herb—a plant that enhances general overall functioning, somewhat like a tonic but one that increases the ability of the organism to respond to outside stressors of whatever sort, diseases included. It enhances an organism's general resistance to multiple adverse influences or conditions. Rhodiola, like the stronger preparations of eleutherococcus, is considered to be not just adaptogenic but an adaptogenic stimulant—part of the reason it can cause jitteriness and wakefulness in some.

Numerous rhodiola species have been found to be highly neuroprotective and neuroregenerative.

In vitro studies have found that compounds in both *Rhodiola sacra* and *R. sachalinensis* protect neurons against beta-amyloid–induced, staurosporine-induced, and hydrogen peroxide–induced death. Salidroside, a common compound in many rhodiolas, protects cultured neurons from injury from hypoxia and hypoglycemia; protects neuro-nal PC12 cells and SH-SY5Y neuroblastoma cells against cytotoxicity from beta-amyloid and against hypoglycemia and serum limitation; and protects neurons against hydrogen peroxide–induced death. It does so by inducing the antioxidant enzymes thioredoxin, heme oxygenase 1, and peroxiredoxin 1, downregulating the proapoptotic gene Bax, and upregulating the antiapoptotic genes Bcl-2 and Bcl-xL. It also restores mitochondrial membrane potential and intracellular calcium levels fol-lowing hydrogen peroxide–induced loss.

Studies have shown that *Rhodiola rosea* enhances the level of 5-hydroxytryptamine in the hippocampus, promotes the prolifera-tion and differentiation of neural stem cells in the hippocampus, and protects hippocampal neurons from injury. *R. rosea* protects against cognitive deficits, neuronal injury, and oxidative stress induced by intra-cerebroventricular injection of streptozotocin. Salidroside protects rat hippocampal neurons against hydrogen peroxide–induced apoptosis. A combination of rhodiola and astragalus protects rats against simulated plateau hypoxia (8000 m/24,000 feet). It inhibits the accumulation of lactic acid in brain tissue and serum.

The herb also has a number of antifatigue/antistress actions. In vitro studies found that salidroside stimulates glucose uptake by rat muscle cells, but more importantly, *Rhodiola rosea* extracts stimulate the synthesis or resynthesis of ATP and stimulate reparative processes in mitochondria.

In vivo trials found that *Rhodiola rosea* extracts increased the life span of *Drosophila melanogaster,* lowered mitochondrial superoxide lev-els, and increased protection against the superoxide generator paraquat; salidroside protected the hypothalamic/pituitary/gonad axis of male rats under intense stress—testosterone levels remained normal rather than dropping, secretory granules of the pituitary gland increased, and mitochondrial cells were strongly protected; *R. rosea* extract completely reversed the effects of chronic mild stress in female rats; rhodiola sup-pressed increased enzyme activity in rats subjected to noise stress—

alanine aminotransferase (ALT), alkaline phosphatase, and creatine kinase levels all returned to normal, while glycogen, lactic acid, and cholesterol levels in the liver also returned to normal; *R. rosea* reduced stress and CRF-induced anorexia in rats; and so on.

In one clinical trial 24 men who took rhodiola while living at high altitude for a year were tested to see its effects on blood oxygen saturation and sleep disorders—rhodiola increased blood oxygen saturation significantly and increased both sleeping time and quality; in a double-blind, placebo-controlled study of the effects of *R. rosea* on fatigue in students caused by stress, physical fitness, mental fatigue, and neuro-motoric indices all increased (other studies found similar outcomes); *R. rosea* intake in a group of healthy volunteers reduced inflammatory C-reactive protein and creatinine kinase in the blood and protected muscle tissue during exercise; *Rhodiola rosea* in a placebo-controlled, double-blind, randomized study increased physical capacity, muscle strength, speed of limb movement, reaction time, and attention—in other words it improved exercise endurance performance; a phase three clinical trial found that rhodiola exerts an antifatigue effect that increases mental performance and concentration and decreases cortisol response in burnout patients with fatigue syndrome; other studies have found similar outcomes including the amelioration of depression and anxiety.

The plant has also been found to be highly antioxidant in numerous studies, to be liver protective, and to be highly protective of the cardiovascular system.

The plant is adaptogenic, that is, it increases the function of the organism to meet whatever adverse influences are affecting it, whether stress or illness. Most of the attention has been paid to its ability to increase endurance and mental acuity but its effects on the immune system, though less studied than those of eleuthero, are similar.

Dosage

Tincture (dried root, 1:5, 50 percent alcohol) . . .

As a tonic, 30–40 drops 3–4x daily, usually in water.

In acute conditions, ½–1 teaspoon 3x daily for 20–30 days, then back to the tonic dose.

Side Effects and Contraindications
Some people experience jitteriness from the herb; you should not take it at night until you know if you are one of them.

Herb/Drug and Drug/Drug Interactions
None that I can find.

Scutellaria baicalensis (Chinese Skullcap)

S. baicalensis is the primary species used in China and the one meant when Chinese skullcap is talked about. It most definitely ***does not*** mean the American skullcap, *Scutellaria lateriflora*—or any of the other American species. It is the root that is used. (The leaves of the American species, which are the part commonly used, are not suitable for these Lyme coinfections.)

Chinese skullcap has a wide range of actions. It is antiviral, anti-inflammatory, antioxidant, nervine, neuroprotective, anodyne, mildly sedative, anticonvulsant, hepatoprotective, antihypertensive, anticholesterolemic, cholagogue, antianaphylactic, antispasmodic, astringent, expectorant, hemostatic, antioxidant, antiangiogenic, antitumor, antimetastic, antibacterial, antifungal, antidiarrheal, antidysenteric, febrifuge, diuretic, and synergist.

Chinese skullcap root is a truly remarkable herb for use during Lyme coinfections. It is a synergist, a cytokine normalizer, and a tonic for much of the body. It is a top-notch herb for respiratory infections, pneumonia, infections that affect the central nervous system (meningitis, encephalitis, mycoplasma, Lyme, and so forth), impaired brain function, fevers, intermittent fevers, GI tract disorders with accompanying inflammation, diarrhea and dysentery, liver and kidney inflammation, urinary tract infections, nervous irritability, epileptic seizures, convulsions, sleep disruptions, and as supportive therapy in cancer. It is also a fairly potent synergist with pharmaceuticals, herbs, and supplements, helping increase the presence of those compounds in the body by getting them past the GI tract and brain barriers.

This species of scutellaria is one of the 50 fundamental herbs of Chinese medicine and has been used in traditional Chinese medicine for over 2,000 years. It is one of the most widely used herbs in Chinese medicine.

It is considered to be bitter and cold, to dispel heat (fever reducer, anti-inflammatory), and to expel damp heat (e.g., lung infections). It is used as a detoxicant, to stop bleeding, and to prevent abnormal fetal movements. It is specific for fever, cough, pneumonia, hemoptysis, jaundice, hepatitis, dysentery, diarrhea, bloody stool, vexation, insomnia, headache, enteritis, acute conjunctivitis, uterine bleeding, abnormal fetal movements, hypertension, carbuncle, and furuncle.

Most of the scientific studies on this plant have been conducted in China and there are a lot of them. The compounds in the root are, not surprisingly, synergistic with each other. All of them that have been studied are potently antiviral, anti-inflammatory, antioxidative, and free-radical scavenging. Wogonin is the most potent NO inhibitor, while oroxylin is the most potent in inhibiting lipid peroxidation. Together they produce effects beyond the individual constituents.

The herb has strong cytokine impacts, reducing NO, iNOS, IL-3, IL-6, IL-17, COX-2, PGE2, NF-κB, IκB-α, IL-1β, IL-2, IL-12, TNF-α, VEGF, and tends to upregulate IL-10. It inhibits the production of IgE, thus suppressing the expression of histamine. It has especially strong impacts in the spleen. It attenuates the activity of c-Raf-1/MEK-1/2, ERK-1 and ERK-2, p38, and JNK MAPKs.

In Vitro Studies

Flavones from the root are strongly neuroprotective. Baicalein strongly inhibits the aggregation of neuronal amyloidogenic proteins and induces the dissolution of amyloid deposits. Wogonin stimulates brain tissue regeneration, incuding differentiation of neuronal precursor cells.

Baicalin promotes neuronal differentiation of neural stem/progenitor cells by modulating p-STAT3 and bHLH (basic helix-loop-helix) protein expression. Wagonin is neuroprotective against cerebral ischemic insult, and at tiny micromolar concentrations completely suppresses the activity of NF-κB and inhibits the migration of microglial cells to ischemic lesions, thus reducing inflammation at the site of injury. It inhibits the movement of the cells in response to the chemokine MCP-1. Baicalein attenuates the induced cell death of brain microglia in mouse microglial cells and rat primary microglia cultures by strongly inhibiting NO through the suppression of iNOS. The compound inhibits NF-κB activity in the cells as well.

Baicalin suppresses IL-1β–induced RANKL (receptor activator of NFκ-B ligand) and COX-2 production at a concentration of 0.01 mcg/ml. The longer the constituent is applied the stronger the effect. Used on human peridontal ligament cells it shows highly protective effects. Baicalein inhibits IL-1β and TNF-α–induced inflammatory cytokine production from human mast cells via regulation of the NF-κB pathway. It inhibits NF-κB and IκB-α phosphorylation. Baicalin promotes repair of DNA single-strand breakage caused by hydrogen peroxide in cultured fibroblasts.

There are scores of other in vitro studies such as these, all showing potent anti-inflammatory and cytokine-modulating actions of the herb and its constituents.

In Vivo Studies

In rats, oroxylin A markedly enhanced cognitive and mnestic function in animal models of aging brains and neurodegeneration. Baicalein has been shown to be anticonvulsive, anxiolytic, and sedative in rats.

Flavonoids from the stems and leaves of *Scutellaria baicalensis* improved memory dysfunction and reduced neuronal damage and levels of abnormal free radicals induced by permanent cerebral ischemia in rats. Other studies found that the compounds could enhance and improve learning and memory abilities and reduce neuronal pathological alterations induced by a variety of chemicals in mice.

The plant reduced symptoms associated with chronic cerebral hypo-perfusion (and chronic lipopolysaccharide infusion), including spatial memory impairments, hippocampal MAPK signaling, and microglial activation.

Baicalein protected mice hippocampal neuronal cells against damage caused by thapsigargin (TG) and brefeldin A (BFA). The constituent reduced TG- and BFA–induced apoptosis of hippocampal cells, reduced the induced expression of endoplasmic reticulum stress-associated proteins, and strongly reduced the levels of MAP kinases such as p38, JNK, and ERK. It reduced ROS accumulation and levels of MMPs. It strongly protected the mitochondria from oxidative damage.

S. baicalensis (in combination with bupleurum) was strongly neuro-protective against iron-induced neurodegeneration in the nigrostriatal dopaminergic system in rat brains, showing it to be useful for treating central nervous system neurodegeneration.

Mice, subjected to transient global brain ischemia for 20 minutes, were treated with baicalein (200 mg/kg once daily). Neuronal damage was minimal compared to controls, and MMP-9 activity in the hippocampus was inhibited. Pretreatment with baicalein was, in addition, found to be preventive.

Wogonin is also strongly protective in the brain. Rats were damaged by either four-vessel occlusion or excitotoxic injury (systemic kainate injection). Wogonin conferred protection by attenuating the death of hippocampal neurons. It inhibited the inflammatory activation of the microglia by inhibiting iNOS, TNF-α, NO, IL-1β, and NF-κB. In vitro studies at the same time found that lipopolysaccharide-activated macrophages were protected similarly.

An ethanol extract of *S. baicalensis* prevented oxidative damage and neuroinflammation and memory impairments in artificial senescense mice. The hippocampus and the mitochondria were strongly protected and neuroinflammation sharply reduced. Expressions of COX-2, iNOS,

NO, PGE2, Bax, cleaved caspase-3 protein were all reduced. Bcl-2 was increased. The effects were dose dependent and were most effective at 100 mg/kg (that would be 7 grams for a 150-pound person, just in the dosage range usually used in China).

Baicalin reduced the severity of relapsing-remitting experimental autoimmune encephalomyelitis induced by proteolipid protein in a mouse model of multiple sclerosis. All the histopathological findings decreased in the mice given the extract.

Baicalein has been found to be antidepressant in animal models of depression. It reversed the reduction of extracellular ERK phosphorylation and the level of BDNF (brain-derived neurotrophic factor) expression in the hippocampus of CMS (chronic mild stress) rat models.

Oral administration of baicalein in mice infected with Sendai virus resulted in a significant reduction of viral titers in the lungs and reduced death rates.

Oral administration of baicalein in mice infected with influenza A virus showed significant effects in preventing death, increasing life span, inhibiting lung consolidation, and reducing lung virus titer in a dose-dependent manner. Amounts as low as 1.2 mcg/ml of baicalin (the metabolite of baicalein) resulted in significant inhibition of the virus. (Note: Plasma levels of baicalin from the ingestion of skullcap root are significantly higher than this after dosing with 3 to 9 grams per day.)

Baicalein and wogonin inhibit irradiation-induced skin damage by suppressing increases in MMP-9 and VEGF through the suppression of COX-2 and NF-κB. *S. baicalensis* was effective in reducing IL-6 and TNF-α in mouse models of pelvic inflammatory disease; the herb was both anti-inflammatory and antinociceptive. *S. baicalensis* extract stimulated the formation of red blood cells and their precursors under conditions of cyclostatic myelosuppression and sleep deprivation.

The root decoction has been used in a number of clinical treatment situations in China to effectively treat scarlet fever, chronic bronchitis, and epidemic cerebrospinal meningitis.

Preparation and Dosage

Again, use the root of Chinese skullcap *and please do not attempt to substitute the American skullcap for this one.* The herb reaches peak levels in the plasma and body organs in about one hour and only lasts in the body for about four hours, so you really do need to dose about every three to four hours.

Tincture

Preparation: 1:5, 50 percent alcohol.

Dosage: ¼–½ teaspoon 3x daily. In acute conditions, double that.

Dried Herb

The Chinese dosages are large, as usual, generally 3–9 grams at a time. Most of the clinical studies and trials used similar dosing. If you are using capsules this is the dosage range you should be exploring, divided into three equal doses every four hours or so.

Side Effects and Contraindications

Side effects from scutellaria are rare, mostly gastric discomfort and diarrhea. It should not be used during pregnancy. Caution should be exercised if you are taking pharmaceuticals as it can increase the bioavailability of the drugs, thus increasing their impacts. It may interact additively with blood pressure–lowering drugs. Type 1 diabetics should exercise strong caution with the herb as it can affect insulin and blood sugar levels.

Herb/Drug and Herb/Herb Interactions

Lots. Chinese skullcap is a synergist, perhaps as efficacious as licorice, ginger, and piperine, and should probably be added to that category of herbs. Among other things it inhibits the NorA efflux pump, which inactivates some forms of antibiotic resistance. Like the other synergists I know of, it is also a strong antiviral, which is beginning to stimulate speculation. Nevertheless, the herb strongly effects pharmaceuticals and herbs taken along with it.

Baicalein, one of the major compounds in *S. baicalensis*, is synergistic with ribavirin, albendazole, ciprofloxacin, amphotericin B.

S. baicalensis is strongly inhibitive of CYP3A4, a member of the cytochrome oxidase system. It is a type of enzyme, strongly present in the liver, and is responsible for catalyzing reactions involved in drug metabolism. Many of the pharmaceuticals that are ingested are metabolized by the CYP3A4 system, meaning that some portion of the drug is inactivated. In some instances it is the metabolites created by CYP3A4 that are active as medicinals. Since the herb inhibits the CYP3A4 system, dose dependently, it can enhance the presence of a number of drugs in the system, specifically acetaminophen, codeine, cyclosporine, diazepam, erythromycin, and so on. It does affect the degree of antibiotics that enter the system.

One of the herb's constituents, oroxylin A, is a strong P-glycoprotein inhibitor. P-glycoprotein is strongly present in the blood-brain barrier, the lining of the GI tract, renal tubular cells, capillary endothelial cells, and the blood-testes barrier. It stops substances from crossing over those barriers. Additionally, cancer cells use P-glycoprotein as a form of efflux pump in order to eject from themselves drugs designed to kill them. P-glycoprotein inhibitors allow more of a substance to cross over barriers high in P-glycoprotein. That means that oral ingestion of a substance will produce more of it in the bloodstream if it is also taken with a P-glycoprotein inhibitor. This means that Chinese skullcap will act through two mechanisms to increase drug and herb uptake in the body.

It will also increase the effectiveness of anticancer drugs by inhibiting P-glycoprotein–mediated cellular efflux. Paclitaxel uptake, for example, was increased over twofold when administered with oroxylin A.

The herb ameliorates irinotecan-induced gastrointestinal toxicity in cancer patients.

The herb will increase the uptake of herbal medicines similarly, again by inhibiting the CYP3A4 system and P-glycoprotein.

Finding It

Try any of the suppliers listed in "Sources of Supply" at the end of the book.

Sida acuta

There are a lot of different sidas around the world. They live primarily in the tropics and subtropics but some species extend into temperate regions. The main medicinal species studied has been *Sida acuta*; however as research has deepened on this species other sidas are coming to light as similarly potent, particularly *S. rhombifolia* and *S. cordifolia*. Two other species, *S. tiagii* and *S. spinosa,* have not been studied as extensively but their traditional uses, and some research, indicate they may possess the same medicinal actions. The sidas are invasives—in general, potent medicines that are making themselves known through insistence. I like them immensely. In the United States they tend to grow along the Gulf Coast and here and there in New Jersey and Pennsylvania.

The sidas are potent broad-spectrum systemic antibacterial plants with a wide range of actions and contain one of the most potent systemic plant antibacterials, cryptolepine (as does *Cryptolepis* spp.). They are antimalarial, antiprotozoal, antimicrobial, antibacterial, hematotonic, hematoregenerator, hematoprotectant, antioxidant (mild), anticancer (antineoplastic, antiproliferative), adaptogenic, analgesic, antipyretic, anthelmintic (fresh leaf juice), antiamoebic, antifertility activity (inhibit egg implantation in mice; however, see the discussion of contraindications and side effects, below), insecticidal, anti-inflammatory, hepatoprotective, antivenin, antiulcerogenic, hypoglycemic. They are strongly protective of red blood cells, especially from microbial invasion. They are pretty good adaptogens.

Sida acuta is widely used in traditional medicinal practice around the world to treat malaria, fevers, headache, skin diseases, infected wounds, diarrhea, dysentery, snakebites, asthma, GI tract problems, systemic infections, renal inflammation, toothache, sore gums, hysteria, bruises, eye infections (as eye drops), breast cancer, abscesses, neuralgia, and arthritis. James Duke's database lists 12 species of sida that have been used in traditional medicine, all for a similar range of complaints. The heaviest hits occur with *acuta, cordifolia, rhombifolia,* and *veronicaefolia.*

Various sida species have been used in India for over 5,000 years; it has a long history of use in Ayurvedic medicine. It has a wide range of use, including for nervous and urinary diseases and disorders of the blood and liver, strangury, hematuria, gonorrhea, cystitis, leukorrhea, chronic dysentery, epilepsy, facial paralysis, asthma, spermatorrhea, rheumatism, lingering debility from previous illnesses, intermittent diseases, rheumatic conditions, and cardiac complaints.

In traditional Chinese medicine the plants are used, just not as much. They are considered to be antibiotic, anti-inflammatory, analgesic, diuretic, and tonic. Sidas are commonly used for depression, bronchitis with cough and wheezing, and urinary tract inflammations. Less common uses are for dermatosis, itching, eczema of the scrotum, sores and boils, stomach pain, dysentery, gastritis, enteritis, tonsillitis, liver problems, jaundice, cervical tuberculous lymphadenitis, malaria, colds and flu, kidney stones.

Importantly, sida is an extremely potent protector of red blood cells, strongly active in protecting them from infestation by such organisms as *Plasmodium* and *Babesia.* It has been found in vivo to neutralize venom from the snake *Bothrops atrox,* a common and very poisonous pit viper in South America. The snake's venom is a hemotoxin that destroys red blood cells (rather than the neurotoxin more common to cobras and rattlesnakes). With snake venom, rather than its antimicrobial actions killing an infective organism, compounds in the plant neutralize a hemotoxic compound. In this sense sida represents a unique category of herbal medicines: hematotonic, hematoregenerator, hematoprotectant. It is especially useful for anemia and I believe there are strong indications that the herb will be significantly useful for the treatment of certain forms of myeloma—cancer of the red blood cells. It is the only herb I know of that is specific in this way for red blood cells.

Sida increases glutathione levels in the blood (important in Lyme coinfections), increases red blood cell numbers (making it good for anemia), and increases total white blood cell count, indicating an immune potentiation effect that may tie in with its reported adaptogenic actions in traditional practice. Numerous studies have found *Sida cordifolia* to possess very potent anti-inflammatory and analgesic activities, some of these coming from its ability to increase glutathione levels. The sidas are strong inhibitors of lipid peroxidation from bacterial membranes, inhibit quinolinic acid in the brain, and significantly reduce both LOX and COX. (A tincture of the plant has been found as active as the drug selegiline.) Unfortunately, in spite of consistent anti-inflammatory outcomes, few studies have been conducted on the sidas' effects on cytokine cascades. Use of the plant after myocardial injury showed significantly increased endogenous antioxidants in heart tissue.

In vivo studies have found *Sida acuta* to have a strong and reliable antiulcer effect—that is, it protects the stomach lining from the formation of induced ulcers. In vivo research has also found a strong analgesic action.

Several compounds from the plant have been found to inhibit induced preneoplastic lesions in mouse mammary tissue. *Sida tiagii* during in vivo research has been found to have antidepressant and antiseizure effects (mice).

Tincture and the hot water extract are the strongest medicinal forms of the herb for internal use.

Preparation and Dosage

Tincture

Preparation: Dried leaf, 1:5, 60 percent alcohol.

Dosage: 20–40 drops up to 4x daily. In the treatment of severe systemic staph infection the usual dose is from ½ teaspoon to 1 tablespoon, 3–6x daily. I prefer to not use this high a dosage for longer than 60 days. That is usually sufficient.

Hot Tea

As a preventive, 1–2 teaspoons of the powdered leaves in 6 ounces water, let steep 15 minutes, drink 1–2x daily. In acute conditions drink up to 10 cups a day.

Side Effects and Contraindications

The main side effect I have seen is that, for some people, sida can increase fatigue and symptoms of coinfection. If this occurs, reduce the dose. That will generally end the problem. This kind of side effect is not noted any-place in the literature. My speculation is that sida breaks down biofilms and, in diseases such as bartonellosis, once that happens, instead of the bacteria being limited to one location, they are then spread more widely throughout the body, increasing their negative impacts. In the literature, there are no side effects noted, known, or reported; however . . .

- The herb is used traditionally to prevent pregnancy. It does inter-fere with egg implantation in mice. The herb should not be used if you are trying to get pregnant or if you are newly pregnant.
- Even though the herb is traditionally used in pregnancy, caution should be exercised if you are pregnant. I would be uncomfortable using it if I were pregnant but then, I would be uncomfortable anyway if I were pregnant.
- The herb contains ephedrine, although not in large quanti-ties. There has been a lot of inaccurate, hysterical reporting on ephedra, even among researchers who should know better. Wikipedia is now among the worst offenders of overly conserva-tive fearmongering—a departure from its original mission.

Although the main reason cited for banning ephedra in the United States is adverse effects, including death, what *is* accurate is that:

1. Weight loss and "natural energy" companies were the ones who marketed the supplements containing the herb (usually along

with caffeine and other stimulants). Herbalists did not support this use of the herb.

2. People wanting to lose weight or increase their energy took the supplements—often in huge doses, far beyond sanity.

Basically the herb was a way to make money off an aspect of the United States' cultural insanity about how one should look to be beautiful or how much one should work to be useful, with, of course, predictable results.

In spite of this, the primary reason the ephedra was banned was that meth labs were using the herb to make meth. The adverse reactions from improper use of the herb were just the excuse. Ephedra is very safe when used properly; it really didn't need to be banned. The companies using it improperly just needed to be prohibited from doing so.

Nevertheless, just be aware that the herb contains *minute* (I repeat: *incredibly tiny*) amounts of ephedra and that a mild raciness or wakefulness may occur from using the herb—but it probably won't.

Herb/Drug and Herb/Herb Interactions
None known or reported; however . . .

- Since the herb is hypoglycemic, it *may* affect medications for diabetes. Just watch your blood sugar levels if you are diabetic.
- Since the herb contains ephedrine, it probably should not be used with pharmaceuticals that possess similar effects.

Silybum marianum (Milk Thistle Seed)
Milk thistle has a wide range of actions, much of it on the liver. It is a hepatoregenerator, hepatoprotective, hepatotonic, antihepatotoxic, choleretic, anticholestatic, an anti-inflammatory for both the liver and spleen, and an immunostimulant.

Milk thistle is strongly protective of the liver against the deleterious effects of microbial pathogens and chemical toxins. It stimulates the regeneration of damaged liver tissue and will tonify, restore, and normalize liver function. It will reduce liver and spleen inflammation and is particularly useful in combination with red root (*Ceanothus* spp.; see page 240). It stimulates bile production and flow. It will enhance supportive immune functions, especially the stimulation of IL-4, IL-10, and IFN-γ.

Milk thistle does reduce a number of cytokines as part of its actions. It inhibits TNF-α, NF-κB, E-selectin, hydrogen peroxide, and c-JNK. This herb, if standardized, will strongly protect the liver from inflammatory damage, reduce inflammatory infiltrates, protect the Kupffer cells, reduce ALT and AST levels, and help remodulate the JAK/STAT pathway.

It is specifically indicated in cirrhosis or severe liver impairment, acute or chronic hepatitis, elevated liver enzymes, bile insufficiency, liver or spleen inflammation, feelings of abdominal pressure, fatigue, poor appetite.

Milk thistle is one of the most potent herbs for protecting the liver against hepatotoxins and helping damaged liver tissue to regenerate. It is also the most extensively studied in clinical trial. The major active constituent is believed to be silymarin, which is found only in the seed and pericarp. Silymarin is actually a combination name for three separate constituents of the herb. Milk thistle is also high in a number of other constituents including betane, the primary constituent of beets.

Milk thistle and silymarin have been extensively tested in human trials for many years. Human trials have followed from as few as 6 patients to as many as 2,000 for up to four years. All have found the herb useful.

The trials have found that in cases of chronic alcoholic liver disease, toxic liver damage, type II hyperlipidemia, and "fatty liver," use of the herb enhanced immune function (T-cell and CD8+ counts were raised); symptoms of tiredness, abdominal pressure, poor appetite, nausea, itching were relieved; superoxide dismutase activity of white and red blood cells increased; significant improvement in liver function occurred; total cholesterol levels decreased; there was normalization of serum transaminases and BSP (sulfobromophthalein) retention; ALT and AST levels decreased; serum total and conjugated bilirubin levels decreased; gamma-Gt and LAP values normalized; a marked decrease in triglycerides occurred; there was improvement in inflammation and toxic/metabolic lesions verified through biopsy; and there was major improvement in liver enzyme activity.

There have been numerous clinical trials focusing on the use of milk thistle seed in treating hepatitis and cirrhosis. In hepatitis B trials there has been marked improvement of hepatic dysfunction and disappearance of HBsAG (the surface antigen of hepatitis B virus) after treatment. Three trials focusing on acute hepatitis found shortened treatment time as determined by ALT levels; improvement of serum levels of bilirubin, AST, and ALT; and much faster return of biochemical values to normal than with placebo. Nine studies focusing on chronic hepatitis found significant improvement in the patient population, normalization of liver function as determined by biopsy, and relief of bloating, abdominal pressure, weakness, nervousness, insomnia. In general, the average time necessary for improvements to be seen in treating hepatitis was 30 to 40 days.

Eleven studies focusing on cirrhosis observed longer mortality rates; significant improvement in liver function tests (especially AST, ALT, and serum bilirubin); regression of inflammatory changes and regression of toxic/metabolic lesions; significant improvement determined by liver cell permeability, metabolic efficiency, and excretory function; reduction of symptoms such as bloating, insomnia, abdominal pressure, and increased body weight.

Perhaps the most impressive studies of the actions of milk thistle have been in cases of poisoning with *Amanita phalloides* mushrooms. These mushrooms contain one of the most potent liver toxins known—phalloidin. A number of interventions in poisoning cases in Germany found that milk thistle protected the liver from the action of the toxin and reversed the damage to the liver. Optimum results occurred if the poisoning cases were treated within 48 hours. Deaths were reduced from 50 to 10 percent.

Preparation and Dosage

I strongly prefer the use of standardized milk thistle for any disease condition. I feel the seeds themselves are fine for general tonic use, but not so much so if you already are ill.

Standardized tincture: Standardized to somewhere around 80 mg silybum flavonoids (40 drops 3x daily) or 140 mg silybum flavonoids (25 drops 3x daily).

Standardized capsules: 1,200 mg daily just before bed.

Note: These dosages can go much higher during acute liver damage.

Side Effects and Contraindications

Milk thistle is a food-grade herb. It is about as dangerous as potatoes. An incredibly tiny number of people have experienced GI tract upsets of various sorts from it.

Herb/Drug and Herb/Herb Interactions

None that I know of.

Withania somnifera (Ashwagandha)

There are six species in this genus. *Withania somnifera* is the most commonly used, though two other *Withania* species, *Withania obtusifolia* and *W. coagulans,* are used in much the same manner. The root is pretty much all that is used in Western practice but the whole plant is used in the rest of the world.

The root does have a nice range of actions, especially for Lyme coinfections. It is an immune tonic and modulator, stress-protective, alterative, anxiolytic, nerve sedative, neuroprotector, chondroprotector, collagenase inhibitor, alterative, reliable tonic sedative for insomniac conditions (especially if from stress or disease), antifatigue, amphoteric, antioxidant, anti-inflammatory, hematopoietic, antibacterial, diuretic, antipyretic, antitumor, and astringent. The leaves and stems are a nerve sedative, antipyretic, febrifuge, bitter, diuretic, antibacterial, antimicrobial, astringent, antitumor. Seeds: hypnotic, diuretic, coagulant. Fruit: immune tonic, antibacterial, alterative, astringent.

Ashwagandha has been a major medicinal plant in India for at least 3,000 years. They consider it tonic, alterative, astringent, aphrodisiac, and a nervine sedative. It has been used for tuberculosis, emaciation of children, senile debility, general debility, rheumatism, nervous exhaustion, brain fog, loss of memory, loss of muscular energy, and spermatorrhea. Its primary use is to restore vigor and energy in a body worn out by long-term constitutional disease or old age.

Use of the herb (in several studies) found that it produces a marked increase in hemoglobin levels by the end of 30 days. Packed cell volume, mean corpuscular volume, serum iron, and hand grip all increase by 60 days. In a double-blind study with 101 healthy men aged 50 to 59, each took 3 grams per day of ashwagandha for one year. All showed significantly increased hemoglobin and red blood cell counts, improvement in melanin levels, and decreased erythrocyte sedimentation rate, and three-quarters reported increased sexual performance.

The plant (or its extracts) has been found to be analgesic and antipyretic, and the root extract highly chondroprotective of damaged human osteoarthritic cartilage matrix and inhibitive of the gelatinase activity of collagenase type 2 enzyme.

The plant has also shown to have anxiolytic and antidepressant actions, to have strong antioxidant activities, to be neuroprotective (correcting scopolamine-induced memory loss in mice), to stimulate neuritic regeneration and synaptic reconstruction in damaged cortical neurons, and to completely inhibit dendritic atrophy. Treatment of rats for 14 days significantly improved nitropropionic acid–induced cognitive dysfunction and oxidative damage; there have been at least 30 studies finding cognitive improvements in various animal species from the use of the root.

The plant has shown strong anti-inflammatory activity in various rheumatological conditions, it significantly reduces induced leukopenia in mice and significantly increases thyroid production of T3 and T4, and there have been at least 30 studies on the immune-potentiating and immune-modulating actions of the root in various animal species.

Preparation and Dosage
Tincture (dried root, 1:5, 70 percent alcohol), 30–40 drops up to 3x daily. Higher dosages can be used if desired.

Side Effects and Contraindications
Avoid high doses in pregnancy; may be abortifacient in large doses. May cause drowsiness. Take the herb after dinner to find out just how sleepy it makes you before using it during the day. In rare instances: diarrhea, GI tract upset, vomiting at large doses.

Herb/Drug and Herb/Herb Interactions
May potentiate barbiturates (anecdotal); don't use with sedatives and anxiolytics.

10

What the Future Holds

Until man duplicates a blade of grass, Nature can laugh at his so-called scientific knowledge . . . it is obvious that we don't understand one millionth of one percent about anything.

THOMAS EDISON

If you are not skeptical of your own skepticism you are not a skeptic but merely someone afraid to believe in anything other than your own sequestered, and very narrow, worldview.

THE AUTHOR

We live in interesting times. If you look with any depth at the incidence of emerging and resistant infections over the past 30 years, especially the types of infections many people are calling stealth pathogens, it is clear that our relation to the microbial world is changing very quickly—and not in ways we are likely to enjoy.

We have taken the word of experts about our capacity to control bacteria and their movements into our lives. We have been told that bacteria are not very intelligent, that with the use of science we can defeat bacterial disease completely; we have been told that if we only wait, all diseases will be cured. And so we stopped thinking for ourselves, stopped using our own abilities to perceive, to see what is right in front of us.

In some ways, the many people who have contracted Lyme or one or more of the many coinfections of Lyme, as well as the many people contracting resistant infections, are much like the canaries once used in coal mines. Canaries were taken down into the mines in earlier centuries because they would succumb to the effects of carbon monoxide and methane long before people did. They were in fact members of a group of what are called sentinel animals, animals that respond more sensitively to environmental dangers and so serve as warnings to people that something dangerous is occurring.

Like the subtle damage caused by environmental disruption, carbon dioxide and methane are invisible, odorless, and tasteless. We don't notice them until it's too late. Emerging and resistant infections are invisible, odorless, and tasteless. But the many people falling ill with them are sentinels to us, informing us that we need to pay attention at a deeper level to what is happening around us.

Our future will increasingly be filled with these kinds of diseases. There is little we can do to stop them from spreading. But we can begin to take charge of our own health, learn about our bacterial neighbors, understand how to approach them and how to treat the diseases they cause. And most importantly, we can learn how to keep our immune health high so that we can find some sort of balance with the pathogens we will encounter throughout our lives. We can begin to take charge of ourselves and our health. It isn't the easiest thing to do but it sure beats the alternative.

The more I study these diseases and the more I learn of their functions in the ecology of this planet, the more fascinating it becomes to me that so many of the herbs that are useful for these diseases are invasives: Japanese knotweed, kudzu, isatis, houttuynia, greater celandine, *Eleutherococcus spinosus*, bidens, phellodendron, sida, ailanthus. There is something deeply wonderful, and not graspable by the reductive mind, in the emergence of invasives that are specific for these conditions just as they are emerging so strongly in the human community.

Please understand, if you had to—*if you had to*—you could treat Lyme and all its coinfections, and most resistant bacteria, solely with these invasive plants. (And, perhaps not so surprisingly, many of them are very good edibles. I suspect we will all be getting a bit hungry by and by.) Instead of trying to eradicate them we should be asking why they are here and what they are doing.

The emergence of the Lyme group of pathogenic microbes is deeply related to ecosystem disruption. At the same time, plants specific for both these microbes and the underlying ecosystem disruption are emerging, of their own accord, into the world's ecosystems. These plants do have many functions in healing ecosystem damage; they also have tremendous potential for healing ecosystem damage in us. But, much like our bacterial cousins, they are overlooked, thought to be merely dangerous un-American illegal aliens that should be eradicated to make our country safe.

That picture of the world isn't going to work much longer. It is time to begin to see what is right in front of us, to begin to rearrange our perceptions of the world around us. Time to respond to what the ecosystems of this planet are telling us. Time to take charge of our own lives and health.

It is a challenge when these kinds of illnesses come into our lives. But we can learn to heal, learn to use the plants that are around us, learn to enhance our own health. And we don't need experts to do it for us.

Perhaps in many ways that is the deep lesson of our time: that the solutions to our troubles are all around us, if only we will look around ourselves and begin to act on what we perceive, if only we stop waiting for Santa Claus, or an expert, to do it for us.

One thing is for sure: stepping outside that expert paradigm opens up a world that is much more vital than the one the experts live in. There really is nothing quite like not being afraid anymore.

I invite you to join us.

APPENDIX

The Sophisticated Synergy of Plant Compounds

Standardization Rant (Wonkish)

Materialism contains a prodigious depth that materialists are a long way from fully grasping.

ERNST JUNGER,
IN *THE DETAILS OF TIME* (1986)

To understand Gaia, we must let go of the mechanistic compartmentalizing conditioning imposed on us since childhood by our society. From an early age nearly all Westerners (and especially young scientists) are exposed to the concept that life has come about due to the operation of blind, meaningless laws of physics and chemistry, and that selfishness underpins the behaviour and evolution of all plants and animals. A child's mind becomes totally ensnared by this style of intellectuality, so that the intuitive, inspirational qualities of the mind are totally ignored. The mind's intuitive ability to see each part of nature as a sub-whole within the greater wholes is destroyed by this sort of education. The result is a totally dry, merely intellectual ecology, not a genuine perception of the dynamic power, creativity, and integration of nature.

STEPHAN HARDING,
"GAIA THEORY AND DEEP ECOLOGY,"
IN *GREENSPIRIT*, ED. MARIAN VAN EYK MCCAIN (2010)

*We have been trained to think of patterns, with the exception of those of music, as fixed affairs. It is easier and lazier that way but, of course, all nonsense. In truth, the right way to think about the pattern which connects is to think of it as **primarily** a dance of interacting parts.*

GREGORY BATESON, *MIND AND NATURE* (1979)

Despite the multiple, synergistic actions of the scores of other constituents in *Salvia miltiorrhiza*, reductionists (such as the developers of the Herbal Medicines Compendium) are pushing for standardization of the herb, insisting that it contain a minimum of 0.1 percent tanshinone IIA, 0.2 percent total tanshinones (i.e., the sum of cryptotanshinone, tanshinone I, and tanshinone IIA), and 3.0 percent salvianolic acid B. As has been commonly known for more than 30 years, this approach fails to understand the complex reality of herbal medicines. In some instances (e.g., for milk thistle seed, or ginkgo) this approach is legitimate, but *only* when it is applied to the final product, especially when they are used to treat acute conditions. In the case of most plants however, including *Salvia miltiorrhiza*, the approach is flawed. First, there is an inaccurate understanding (which is not correctable) of the true numbers of constituents in the plants. Second, there is absolutely no knowledge nor recognition of the importance of the synergistic interactions between the constituents that *are* known.

While it is true that plants tend to create some constituents that produce marked results when used as isolated chemicals, when these same constituents are examined *in situ* more subtle elements of the reality in which we are embedded begin to emerge. To truly understand medicinal plants, it is fundamental to recognize that none of these constituents were developed by plants in isolation. They were generated in the midst of a spectrum of chemicals and behaviors while the plant was immersed in an ecological scenario to which it was responding. The constituent being viewed in isolation is *in reality* an expression of a complicated chemical communication in which *none* of the other parts are irrelevant to its actions. Even a simple look from a minimally broader perspective reveals errors in the "active constituent" approach. For instance . . .

Berberine, a strong antibacterial found in goldenseal and many other plants, is very active against a large number of resistant and non-resistant bacterial organisms. It is considerably more active, however, in the presence of another constituent in goldenseal (and other berberine-containing plants), 5'-methoxyhydnocarpin (5'-MHC). The constituent 5'-MHC is in fact a multidrug efflux pump inhibitor. It reduces or eliminates the ability of resistant staphylococcus bacteria to eject, from inside their cellular membrane, antibiotic substances that might harm them.

In response to plant bacteria generating resistance to berberine (millennia ago), the plants created a new chemical, 5'-MHC, which has no known function other than to act as an efflux inhibitor, enabling the berberine to remain effective.

> *Plants can't run, they can't hide, they can't call a doctor,*
> *or go to the hospital. They have to make their own*
> *medicines and they are incredibly good at it, much better*
> *than we will ever be. They have had, after all, between*

170 and 300 millions years of practice. We have
had less than a century.

Goldenseal's creation of 5'-MHC is one of the reasons the plant is such an effective antibacterial herb in the treatment of resistant infections of the GI tract. However, standardization acolytes never speak of standardizing the plant for this compound, indicating a serious lack of understanding on their part about the true nature of herbal medicines. And, at the same time, ultimately creating obvious downstream usage problems similar to those that have accompanied the unrestrained use of pharmaceutical antibiotics in the absence of any real understanding of bacteria.

Compounds such as 5'-MHC are why plants are often more effective than single constituents in treating disease conditions. If goldenseal were standardized for berberine content and if, for some reason, the standardized compound contained no 5'-MHC, its effectiveness as an antimicrobial would be significantly diminished. Yet 5'-MHC is not considered important enough as a standardization marker since it is not an "active" constituent. Numerous other compounds, rarely recognized by reductionists, are essential for the "active" constituents to actually be effective in practice.

And this is only a tiny glance at a very complex phenomenon. Some compounds in plants, for example, have no known function in the plants other than to reduce the side effects of more pharmacologically active constituents. Plants intentionally generate side effect–ameliorating compounds for themselves in order to allow them to utilize their potent antimicrobial compounds without suffering the side effects so often experienced by people who use pharmaceuticals. (They are actually a lot smarter than we are.) These compounds are not, and most likely never will be, considered active constituents. They aren't sexy enough. They just help. Nevertheless, without these other compounds, the "active" compounds would not work nearly so well. In some instances they would not work at all.

Such complexities are hardly limited to the berberine plants. For instance, the anticonvulsant actions of the kavalactones in *Piper methysticum* (i.e., yangonin and desmethoxyyangonin) are much stronger when used in combination with other kava constituents that are generally considered irrelevant in any standardization missives. As well, concentrations of yangonin and another lactone, kavain, are much higher in the brain when the *whole plant* extract is used instead of the purified lactones themselves. In other words, some of the other constituents in kava help move the bioactive lactones across the blood-brain barrier and into the brain where they will do the most good. Blood plasma concentrations of kavain are reduced by 50 percent if the purified compound is used rather than an extract of the plant itself.

Plant compounds in *Isatis tinctoria,* a potent antiviral and anti-inflammatory herb, are also highly synergistic. Tryptanthrin, a strong anti-inflammatory in the plant, possesses very poor skin penetration capacity; however, when the whole plant extract is applied to the skin, penetration of tryptanthrin is significantly enhanced. In other words, applying a salve of pure tryptanthrin to the skin, despite its anti-inflammatory nature, won't do you much good. But if you make the plant itself into a salve, the tryptanthrin moves rapidly into the skin and helps reduce skin inflammation. Tryptanthrin is, unfortunately, the compound that is considered important to standardize in the plant. No notice is taken of the other, rather crucially important, constituents that facilitate skin penetration.

Artemisinin is much more active against malarial parasites if administered with the artemisia flavonoids artemetin and casticin that are normally found in the whole plant extracts. The additional flavones chrysoplenetin and chrysospenol-D also act as potent synergists for the so-called "active" compounds. These latter two compounds are also P-glycoprotein inhibitors, thus facilitating the movement of artemisinin and the plant's other constituents through the intestinal membrane and into the blood, significantly enhancing the actions of artemisinin in the body. One of the real problems with the use of pure artemisinin is that it does not move easily across the intestinal membrane. In consequence, lower levels of the drug actually reach the areas that need it. As well, by removing the isolated constituent from the plant and marketing it as a malarial drug (to combat drug-resistant malarial organisms), we lose the other constituents in the plant that specifically act to inhibit resistance mechanisms in the malarial protozoa. This is why the protozoa worldwide are developing resistance to the drug now that it has been pharmaceuticalized for profit.

Regrettably, the medical reductionists involved in herbal medicine throughout the Western world, and most especially in the United States, have little cognizance of these kinds of complexities. Their view is just too linear. And that linear view does not allow them to understand that plant medicines are in fact so complex that a linear approach will never produce reliable control over the medicinal activity in herbal medicines.

A simple look at some of the other constituents in *Salvia miltiorrhiza* shows just how inept the reliance of the Herbal Medicines Compendium on such standardization criteria is when it comes to actually producing plants that are medicinally reliable. As just a couple of examples . . .

While the reductionists want to standardize the plant for salvianolic acid B (SaB), there are in fact, at present count, salvianolic acids A, C, D, E, F, G, and K to take into account. These other salvianolic acids have highly synergistic effects with SaB and, in actuality, they form a complex interactive grouping that, together, produces the following medicinal effects: potent antioxidant actions, myocardial ischemic protection, antithrombotic activity, antifibrotic effects, inhibition of diabetes and its complications, and neuroprotection in the brain and central nervous system. Salvianolic acid A, for example, enhances the action of the herb in the treatment of Alzheimer's disease. It inhibits beta-amyloid self-aggregation and disaggregates preformed fibrils, reduces metal-induced aggregation by chelating metal ions, and blocks the formation of reactive oxygen species in the brain. The combined salvianolic compounds reduce leukocyte-endothelial adherence, inhibit inflammation, reduce metalloproteinase expression from aortic smooth muscle cells, and indirectly modulate immune function. These are some of the root reasons that the plant is so potent for heart disease. The isolated constituents, including SaB, are not as effective when used without the rest of the related compounds. And this still does not look at the effects of caffeic acid and its other derivatives on physiology.

Caffeic acid (and many of its non-salvianolic acid derivatives) produces a number of important biological activities, including antioxidant, anti-ischemia-reperfusion, antithrombosis, antihypertension, antifibrosis, antivirus, and antitumor actions. These actions are highly synergistic with the salvianolic acid compounds *and* the tanshinones (which possess strong antitumor actions among other things). The complex effects of the plant on circulatory disorders and heart disease comes from no isolated compound (SaB) but from the sophisticated interactivity and synergy of *all* the salvianolic acids *and* the caffeic acid and its derivatives *and* a great many other compounds not elucidated here.

And, finally, it should be recognized that the diterpenoid tanshionone IIA and cryptotanshinone are poorly bioavailable *unless* they are ingested along with the rest of the compounds in the plant. This includes the entire complex of phenolics and diterpenoids. Transfer across the GI tract membrane is eight- to tenfold higher *if* the other constituents are present. In other words, they act as P-glycoprotein inhibitors, allowing the "active" substances to bypass the GI tract efflux pumping mechanisms. As Kim et al. (2008) comment, "There are other unknown compounds in the [*Salvia miltiorrhiza*] extract that have a synergistic effect with tanshinone." And these "unknown" compounds enhance the effects of that constituent as well as facilitating its movement across the GI tract membrane.

To be clear, the exact identity, combination, and amounts of those other constituents, and the ones that most efficiently inhibit the P-glycoprotein response, have not been determined—and they probably never will be. The complexity of the synergy of so many compounds makes it impossible to actually identify what is doing what, what is crucial and what, if anything, is not. As Gao et al. (2012) put it, "Since there are more than twenty active compounds in Danshen, it is very difficult to predict that one compound will act the same way when it is combined with other compounds."

Protocatechuic aldehyde (PAL), another compound in the plant, generally considered to be irrelevant, and very much not a part of the standardization movement, has important impacts on the pharmacokinetics of the plant's other compounds. Chang et al. (2010) comment, "Complex, extensive pharmacokinetic interactions were observed among the major water-soluble constituents in the Danshen injection. The content variation of PAL had the most significant effect on the pharmacokinetic behaviors of the other major constituents."

Linearity, and the use of "an A then B" causality approach, begins to fail once you move past three interacting components. It is useless when dealing with whole systems . . . that is, if you want to gain any reliable understanding of what is actually occurring in living organisms. Actually, it is not even all that effective when dealing with simple physics. As Michael Crichton (1995) once put it . . .

> Do you realize the limits of our understanding? Mathematically, we can describe two things interacting, like two planets in space. Three things interacting—three planets in space—well, that becomes a problem. Four or five things interacting, we can't really do it. And inside the cell, there's one hundred thousand things interacting.

And to take that a bit further, inside the plant there are many more than 100,000 *cells* interacting. To reduce the plant compounds to one or two or three "active" constituents (and to ignore all the other constituents as irrelevant) is nineteenth-century thinking. It is based on inaccurate models of the world. The ramifications of that thinking for the health of living systems surrounds all of us every day of our lives—in the environmental devastation of our planet, in the increasing failure of our medical model. It does not present a pretty picture.

When working with plant medicines we are working with complex, nonlinear, self-organized living systems. Neither they nor their constituent elements can be viewed, or understood, in isolation. This is because at the moment of self-organization complexities that can't be found by the reductive mind come into play. Here is Michael Crichton again:

> It did not take long before the scientists began to notice that complex systems showed certain common behaviors. They started to think of these behaviors as characteristic of all complex systems. They realized that these behaviors could not be explained by analyzing the components of the systems. The time-honored scientific approach of reductionism—taking the watch apart to see how it worked—didn't get you anywhere with complex systems, because the interesting behavior seemed to arise from the spontaneous interaction of the components.

In other words, a complex synergy of interactions comes into play and it has nothing to do with "active" constituents. Every part is "active," every part is essential. So . . . your brain may be important but if you lose your heart, pancreas, kidneys, and intestinal tract it will do you no good. All components are crucial, none are extraneous, none are more important than any other.

A reductive reliance on a few compounds and an assertion that those compounds will produce the effects that the plant is noted for (in 2,000 years of practice, the span of *Salvia miltiorrhiza* use in China) is misleading in the extreme and will result, in the long run, in plant medicines that do not in fact do what they are being promoted as doing.

A MORE ACCURATE MAP

To be clear, the constituents that appear to the reductive mind as *the* active constituents should, in fact, be more properly thought of (if you must think this way) as analogous to plants that are "strong interactors" in ecosystems.

> *A plant's interior, viewed by itself, reveals an ecosystem*
> *in miniature. Its internal structure and relationships*
> *are a fractal pattern on a smaller scale of the larger*
> *structure and relationships we see in the larger scale of*
> *an ecosystem. And that ecosystem is itself only a reflection*
> *of the even larger scale of the Gaian system*
> *of which it is a part.*

To understand the complexity of plant chemicals acting as medicinals for us, we have to see them as an expressive element of a holistic system. To better understand the inextricable intertangling of plant chemicals within the individual plant-body ecosystem, it helps to understand just how ecosystems really *are*.

As researchers Eoin O'Gorman and Mark Emmerson (2009) observe, these "natural communities are finely structured, display-ing properties that promote stability despite complexity." As this per-tains to plant compounds, the entire complex of chemicals has to be seen as a finely structured community that displays certain properties when viewed as a whole. And those properties are essential to under-stand when approaching the plant as a healing herb. As O'Gorman and Emmerson continue . . . there is a "nonrandom arrangement of interaction strengths" between the living subunits of the system that "promotes community level stability." "Nonrandom" here meaning that there is something more than mere chance that is occurring; there is *meaning* in the system's subunits' associations. Further, the concept of interaction strengths is crucial. Medical herbal reductionists tend to see *only* the active compound—that is, they focus on what they consider to be the chemical that is most expressive of interaction strength. In typi-cal American fashion they focus on strength in isolation, not the more essential community interrelationships and interactivity.

In a forest ecosystem, as an example, the trees act as what are called "strong interactors," while other plants in the system are considered to be "weak" interactors. "Complex ecological networks," as O'Gorman and Emmerson comment, "are characterized by distributions of interaction strengths that are highly skewed, with many weak and a few strong interactors present."

O'Gorman and Emmerson conducted experiments in which they removed strong interactors from complex ecosystems and found, not surprisingly, that it "produced a dramatic trophic cascade" in the system. That is, the system immediately experienced a phase change, going from a state of high complexity to one much less sophisticated. They comment:

> Natural ecosystems are a complex tangle of interactions, with 95% of species typically no more than 3 links apart. This natural complexity persists against the odds because it is governed by fundamental laws and principles that confer stability. One of the most widely accepted of these principles is the pattern of species interactions. There is a tendency to consider biodiversity in terms of taxonomic identities or functional roles, yet every species can be considered as a node in a complex web of interactions. Each node contributes to the overall balance of interactions, whether it is a strong or weak interactor. Given the highly interconnected nature of food webs, any loss of biodiversity could contribute to a ripple effect, changing the pattern of interaction strengths and thus threatening to unbalance the stability conferred by this pattern. (O'Gorman and Emmerson, 2009)

The loss of a strong interactor in such circumstances was found to "have effects disproportionally large, relative to their abundance." But further . . .

> Fluctuations in population biomass are commonplace, and compensatory actions among species can maintain aggregate biomass.

The changes in primary and secondary production shown here are community-level responses however, suggesting that the insurance effect of community diversity is not sufficient to overwhelm the impacts of [removing] strong interactors. Trophic cascades such as these can alter energy flow, community composition, and habitat provision, and lead to secondary extinctions.

In other words, while the strong interactors remain relatively stable over long timelines (they do change, but very slowly), the weak interactors are in constant flux around them, increasing or decreasing their density, some moving out, others moving in, as the environment in which the system is located changes its nature and needs.

This is also true of the chemical composition of medicinal plants. Chemical innovations flow into and out of the plant over time in response to environmental inputs. There is no such thing as a "standard" chemical profile of a plant medicine, something that drives technological medicalists crazy. Every plant's chemical profile is different from season to season and from location to location. And it is supposed to be that way. If, prior to goldenseal's innovation of 5'-MHC, the plant had been standardized for a particular chemical profile, once bacteria developed resistance, that standardized profile would have become highly ineffective in use. Evolution is ongoing; it has not ended. The diseases we encounter are altering themselves all the time. They possess tremendous genetic flexibility. However, so do the plants. They alter their genome and their chemical relationships right along with the bacteria. The alterations in plant chemical profiles are essential for them to remain functional medicines.

The numbers and kinds of the weak interactors in an ecosystem change over time. This keeps the system homeodynamics intact. As the system responds to perturbations, the particular species that are present shift their numbers and their locations, and, sometimes, they move on and others take their place. New weak attractors, with different capacities and chemical production abilities, continually flow through the system over very long timelines in order to keep the system adaptable to altered environmental circumstances. These movements, called *asynchronous fluctuations* in system stability, are actually an element of the system remaining close to the boundary of self-organization. As new plants move into the system, they then *synchronize* their actions with the rest of the links in the system, much the same way human beings do when two people begin to walk together. Out of this synchronicity come patterns of self-organization that cannot be developed in any other way. The same is true of the plant chemicals that exist within a single plant medicine.

The plant responds to the environmental scenario in which it lives by producing a complex of compounds that it utilizes for a very large number of complex behaviors. Among these are its own, and its ecosystem's, healing. The complex of compounds alters its nature from moment to moment to moment in response to environmental inputs. The plants—and this is important—*never* produce the same complex of compounds in every location in which they grow and in any year in which they grow. As bacterial dynamics shift, the plants, *worldwide,* shift their chemical production and constituent spectrum in response.

While the removal of the "strong interactors" in an ecosystem has immediate, detrimental effects on the system, causing its complexity to collapse into a simpler state, the removal of "weak interactors" also has extremely deleterious effects. O'Gorman and Emmerson found that while removal of "weak" interactors did not have as extreme an effect in the short run, those plants play a crucial stabilizing role in the system. In other words, the strong interactors generate potent effects on the system but the weak interactors modulate those effects toward specific outcomes. More, if the weak interactors are removed, the ecosystem fails. As they note, "Crucially, when strong interactors were present in the community without a sufficient number of weakly interacting species around them," the ecosystem destabilized. Weak interactor loss led to "reductions in temporal and spacial stability of ecosystem process rates, community diversity, and resistance" (O'Gorman and Emmerson, 2009).

More dynamically (and more accurately), weak and strong interactors can be thought of as "links" (as some researchers have it) rather than "actors" in a communicatory network.

> *Though O'Gorman and Emmerson's concept of "nodes" is even better. A node is a point of concentration of matter, where the gravity well becomes strongest, and that "well" immediately generates "gravitational" links to all other nodes in the system. Everything is then connected in a web of stronger and weaker fields—what chaos theory aficionados refer to as strong and weak attractors. They are always to be found in nonlinear systems irrespective of their nature; this includes medicinal plants.*

In all healthy ecosystems, there exists a network of a few strong attractors embedded in a majority field of weak attractors. The strong exert more easily seen effects but they are held in a tightly coupled web of weak attractors that modulate their actions. This same pattern exists within herbal medicines. To understand herbal medicines, for true sophistication to occur in herbal practice, an understanding of this pattern is essential.

The whole interwoven network, with just this combination of attractors, produces a tremendously adaptable ecorange or zone in which each part contributes essential responses that, together, modulate the system's successful adaptation to perturbations. It is not just which species are present that is important, but rather the species' *behaviors,* their interactions with the other species in the network, that is crucial. All together, they make a *community* in which every organism's actions and presence are crucial to continued functionality. To slightly restate . . .

> *The whole interwoven plant network, with just this combination of chemicals, produces a tremendously adaptable medicinal plant in which each part contributes essential responses that, together, modulate the system's successful adaptation to the treatment of disease conditions. It is not just which chemicals are present, but rather the chemicals' behaviors, their interactions with the other chemicals in the network, that is crucial. All together, they make a community in which every chemical's actions and presence are crucial to continued functionality.*

To give this even a bit more definition, here is a relevant quotation from Iain McGilchrist.

> Water just falls in the way that water has to, and the landscape resists its path in the way it has to. The result of the amorphous water and the form of the landscape is a river. The river is not only passing across the landscape, but entering into it and changing it too, as the landscape has "changed" and yet not changes the water. . . . The river does not exist before the encounter. Only water exists before the encounter, and the river actually comes into being in the process of encountering the landscape. (McGilchrist, 2012)

In essence, they make each other. This same dynamic occurs in the creation of plant medicines inside plants. The world touches the plant, the plant touches back, and the chemicals that are produced are something that emerges out of that touching. The chemical dynamics in such a co-evolved community of chemicals inside a plant are so tightly coupled that they can't legitimately be viewed in isolation from each other. Or as Masanobu Fukuoka once put it:

> The living and holistic biosystem that is nature cannot be broken down or resolved into its parts. Once broken down it dies. Or rather, those who break off a piece of nature lay hold of something that is dead, and, unaware that what they are examining is no longer what they think it to be, claim to understand nature. . . . Because [man] starts out with misconceptions about nature and takes the wrong approach to understanding it, regardless of how rational his thinking, everything winds up all wrong. (Fukuoka, 1985)

To successfully adapt to the changes now present in our world, the old linear models, of necessity, must be abandoned. They are the source of many of the problems we face, including the emergence of stealth and resistant pathogens. The world, and many of the people within it, is changing. They see the writing on the wall. We in the United States, in the Western nations, must change as well.

Sources of Supply and a Few Good Practitioners

Ooooh, look! A flower.

FOUR-YEAR-OLD ON A WALK

The tree which moves some to tears of joy is in the eyes of others only a green thing that stands in the way.

WILLIAM BLAKE

Many of the herbs I have talked about in this book—and, of course, a great many others—grow wild. Even if you live in a city you can find many of them co-habitating with you or only a short drive away. Since many of these herbs are invasives, most people will be glad for you to take them away.

If you need to buy your herbs, the Internet is a good way to seek them. I suggest running a Web search for the herbs you are looking for to find the cheapest prices; if you are persistent you can often save half off normal retail.

If you are going to be buying a lot of herbs and you live in the United States it makes sense to buy a resale license from your state. The price is often minimal ($5.00 or so) and it will allow you to buy wholesale; most wholesalers will want a resale certificate before they will sell to you.

And, of course, you can grow them yourself. Once established most of the herbs in this book will provide medicine for you and your family forever.

Here are some of the best sources I know of for the herbs in this book. All of them are in the United States.

Elk Mountain Herbs

Wonderful tinctures from locally wildcrafted Western plants.

214 Ord Street
Laramie, WY 82070
(307) 742-0404
www.elkmountainherbs.com

1stChineseHerbs.com

Wonderful people with a very large selection of Chinese herbs, including most of those discussed in this book. Most herbs by the pound.

5018 View Ridge Drive
Olympia, WA 98501
(888) 842-2049; (360) 923-0486
www.1stchineseherbs.com

Healing Spirits Herb Farm

Matthias and Andrea Reisen have been growing wonderful medicinal plants for years. The plants just jump out of the bag and laugh when you open it up.

61247 Route 415
Avoca, NY 14809
(607) 566-2701
www.healingspiritsherbfarm.com

Horizon Herbs

Richo Cech has spent much of his life learning how to grow common and rare medicinals. He has seeds or young stock for most of the plants in this book as well as great information on how to grow them.

P.O. Box 69
Williams, OR 97544
(541) 846-6704
www.horizonherbs.com

Mountain Rose Herbs

A nice selection, sustainably produced.

P.O. Box 50220
Eugene, OR 97405
(800) 879-3337; (541) 741-7307
www.mountainroseherbs.com

Pacific Botanicals

This is perhaps the best wholesaler (they also sell retail) in the United States. Their herbs are magnificent. Normally, all are sold by the pound.

4840 Fish Hatchery Road
Grants Pass, OR 97527
(541) 479-7777
www.pacificbotanicals.com

Sage Woman Herbs

They have some herbs otherwise hard to get, especially isatis tincture (just the root though).

> 108 East Cheyenne Road
> Colorado Springs, CO 80906
> (888) 350-3911; (719) 473-8873
> www.sagewomanherbs.com

Woodland Essence

Kate and Don make wonderful tinctures and medicines and can sell you many of the herbal tinctures I discuss in this book; if they don't have them, they can probably point you in the right direction.

> 392 Teacup Street
> Cold Brook, NY 13324
> (315) 845-1515
> www.woodlandessence.com

Zack Woods Herb Farm

Melanie and Jeff are wonderful people and grow tremendously beautiful medicinal plants. Very, very high-quality herbs. Usually sold by the pound.

> 278 Mead Road
> Hyde Park, VT 05655
> (802) 888-7278
> www.zackwoodsherbs.com

A FEW GOOD PRACTITIONERS

Some time ago, a wonderful woman by the name of Julie Genser created a website about my work on Lyme disease and its coinfections. Julie herself has been struggling with a number of chronic conditions over the years but she still found the time to create a site that has helped a great many people. I don't, other than answering queries from time to time, have anything to do with that site, but it is a good source of information about practitioners who are knowledgeable about the protocols I suggest in my books on the Lyme group of infections. In addition to the practitioners on that site (buhnerhealinglyme.com; there is also a Facebook group from what I understand), I also highly recommend my partner Julie McIntyre (Silver City, NM, who also offers phone consultations), Tommy Priester (Bear Medicine Herbs, Lincoln, MA), Neil Nathan, M.D. (Gordon Medical Associates, Santa Rosa, CA), and Tim Scott, L.Ac. (Brattleboro, VT). All of them are very good, all are wonderful people who genuinely care about healing and their patients. Because contact information changes from time to time, I suggest googling them for current contact information.

Acronyms Used in This Book

ADP: adenosine diphosphate

ALT: alanine aminotransferase

AST: aspartate aminotransferase

ATP: adenosine triphosphate

ATPase: adenosine triphosphatase

CCL: CC chemokine ligand

CDK: cyclin-dependent kinases

CNS: central nervous system

COX: cyclooxygenase

CSF: colony-stimulating factor

CXCL: CXC chemokine ligand

CYP: cytochrome

DAMP: damage-associated molecular pattern

DC: dendritic cell

EGCG: epigallocatechin gallate

EGF: epidermal growth factor

ELISA: indirect enzyme-linked immunosorbent assay

ERK: extracelluar signal-regulated kinase

GI tract: gastrointestinal tract

HGA: human granulocytic anaplasmosis

HME: human monocytic ehrlichiosis

HMGB1: high-mobility group protein B

ICAM: intercellular adhesion molecule

IFA: indirect fluorescence assay

IFN: interferon

IgE: immunoglobulin E

IgG: immunoglobulin G

IgM: immunoglobulin M

IHC: immunohistochemistry

IL: interleukin

iNOS: inducible nitric oxide synthase

JAK: Janus kinase

JNK: c-Jun N-terminal kinase

LOX: lipoxygenase

LPS: lipopolysaccharide

MAPK: mitogen-activated protein kinase

MCP: monocyte chemoattractant protein

MHC: major histocompatibility complex

MIF: macrophage migration inhibitory factor

MIP: macrophage inflammatory protein

MMP: matrix metalloproteinase

MPO: myeloperoxidase

MRSA: methicillin-resistant *Staphylococcus aureus*

NAC: N-acetylcysteine

NADPH: nicotinamide adenine dinucleotide phosphate

NE: neutrophil elastase

NET: neutrophil extracellular trap

NF-κB: nuclear factor kappa-B

NGF: nerve growth factor

NK cell: natural killer cell

NO: nitric oxide

NOS: nitric oxide synthase

PAMP: pathogen-associated molecular pattern

PCR: polymerase chain reaction

PGE2: prostaglandin E2

PI3K: phosphatidylinositol 3-kinase

PKA: protein kinase A

PKB: protein kinase B

PKC: protein kinase C

PLCG2: phospholipase C gamma-2

PRR: pattern recognition receptor

RAGE: receptor for advanced glycation end-products

RANTES: regulated on activation, normal T cell expressed and secreted

RBC: red blood cell

ROS: reactive oxygen species

SOD: superoxide dismutase

STAT: signal transducer and activator of transcription

TGF: transforming growth factor

Th: T helper cell

TLR: toll-like receptor

TNF: tumor necrosis factor

VCAM: vascular cell adhesion molecule

VEGF: vascular endothelial growth factor

Works Cited

A book is the only place in which you can examine a fragile thought without breaking it, or explore an explosive idea without fear it will go off in your face.

EDWARD MORGAN

Addabbo, F., B. Ratliff, H. C. Park, et al. 2009. "The Krebs cycle and the mitochondrial mass are early victims of endothelial dysfunction: proteomic approach." *American Journal of Pathology* 174 (1): 34–43.

Ankrah, N.-A. 2010. "Treatment of falciparum malaria with a tea-bag formulation of *Cryptolepis sanguinolenta* root." Ghana Medical Journal 44 (1): 2.

Biksaktsis, C., B. Nandi, R. Racine, et al. (2007) "T-cell-independent humoral immunity is sufficient for protection against fatal intracellular ehrlichia infection." *Infection and Immunity* 75 (10): 4933–41.

Bosley, S. 2010. "Are you ready for a world without antibiotics?" *The Guardian*, August 12.

Brody, J. 2012. "Another tick-borne disease to guard against." *New York Times*, July 30.

Chan, K., S. A. E. Marras, and N. Parveen. 2013. "Sensitive multiplex PCR assay to differentiate Lyme spirochetes and emerging pathogens *Anaplasma phagocytophilum* and *Babesia microti*." *BMC Microbiology* 13: 295.

Chang, B., L. Zhang, W. Cao, et al. 2010. Pharmacokinetic interactions induced by content variation of major-water-soluble components of danshen preparation in rats." *Acta Pharmacologica Sinica* 31: 638–46.

Chauvin, A., E. Moreau, S. Bonnet, et al. 2009. "Babesia and its hosts: Adaptation to long-lasting interactions as a way to achieve efficient transmission." *Veterinary Research* 40 (2): 37–55.

Clark, I. A., L. M. Alleva, and W. B. Cowden. 2004. "Pathogenesis of malaria and clinically similar conditions." *Clinical Microbiology Reviews* 17 (3): 509–39.

Columbia University Medical Center. N.d. "Ehrlichiosis/anaplasmosis." http://columbia-lyme.org/patients/tbd_ehrli-anapla.html.

Crichton, M. 1995. *The Lost World*. New York: Knopf.

D. Gao, A. Mendoza, S. Lu, and D. A. Lawrence. 2012. "Immunomodulatory effects of danshen (*Salvia miltiorrhiza*) in BALB/c mice." *ISRN Inflammation* 2012, article ID 954032, doi:10.5402/2012/954032.

Dawson, J. E., C. D. Paddock, C. K. Warner, et al. 2001. "Tissue diagnosis of *Ehrlichia chaffeensis* in patients with fatal ehrlichiosis by use of immunohistochemistry, in situ hybridization, and polymerase chain reaction." *American Journal of Tropical Medicine and Hygiene* 65 (5): 603–9.

Dowling, D. P., M. Ilies, K. L. Olszewski, et al. 2010. "Crystal structure of arginase from *Plasmodium falciparum* and implications for L-arginine depletion in malarial infection." *Biochemistry* 49 (26): 5600–608.

Dumler, S. 2012. "The biological basis of severe outcomes in *Anaplasma phagocytophilum* infection." *FEMS Immunology and Medical Microbiology* 64 (1): 13–20.

Ekpo, M. A., and P. C. Elim. 2009. "Antimicrobial activity of ethanolic and aqueous extracts of *Sida acuta* of microorganisms from skin infections." *Journal of Medicinal Plants Research* 3 (9): 621–24.

Florescu, D., P. P. Sordillo, A. Glyptis, et al. 2008. "Splenic infarction in human babesiosis: Two cases and discussion." *Clinical Infectious Diseases* 46 (1): e8–11.

Francischetti, I. M., A. Sa-Nunes, B. J. Mans, et al. 2010. "The role of saliva in tick feeding." *Frontiers in Bioscience* 14: 2051–88.

Fukuoka, M. 1985. *The Natural Way of Farming*. Tokyo: Japan Publications.

Gaffar, F. R., F. F. Franssen, and E. de Vries. 2003. "*Babesia bovis* merozoites invade human ovine, equine, porcine, and caprine erythrocytes by a sialic acid-dependent mechanism followed by developmental arrest after a single round of cell fission." *International Journal for Parasitology* 33 (14): 1595–603.

Gao, D. A. Mendoza, S. Lu, D. A. Lawrence. 2012. "Immunomodulatory effects of Danshen (*Salva miltiorrhiza*) in BALB/c mice." *ISRN Inflammation* 2012, doi: 10.5402/2012/954032.

Graham, A. L., I. M. Cattadori, J. O. Lloyd-Smith, et al. 2007. "Transmission consequences of coinfection: Cytokines writ large?" *Trends in Parasitology* 23 (6): 284–91.

Griggs, B. 1991. *Green Pharmacy.* Rochester, Vt.: Healing Arts Press.

Hajdusek, O., R. Sima, N. Ayllon, et al. 2013. "Interaction of the tick immune system with transmitted pathogens." *Frontiers in Cellular and Infection Microbiology* 3 (26), doi:10.3389/fcimb.2013.00026.

Ismail, N., K. C. Bloch, and J. W. McBride. 2010. "Human ehrlichiosis and anaplasmosis." *Clinics in Laboratory Medicine* 30 (1): 261–92.

Jeong, Y.-I., S.-H. Hong, S.-H. Cho, et al. 2012. "Induction of IL-10-producing CD1d^{high}CD5$^+$ regulatory B cells following *Babesia microti*-infection." *PLOS One* 7 (10): e46553.

Johns, J. L., K. C. Macnamara, N. J. Walker, et al. 2009. "Infection with *Anaplasma phagocytophilum* induces multilineage alterations in hematopoietic progenitor cells and peripheral blood cells." *Infection and Immunity* 77 (9): 4070–80.

Kim, H. K., E. R. Woo, H. W. Lee, et al. 2008. "The correlation of *Salvia miltiorrhiza* extract-induced regulation of osteoclastogenesis with the amount of components tanshinone I, tanshinone IIA, cryptotanshinone, and dihydrotanshinone." *Immunopharmacology and Immunotoxicology* 30 (2): 347–64.

Krause, P. J., A. Spielman, S. R. Telford, et al. 1998. "Persistent parasitemia after acute babesiosis." *New England Journal of Medicine* 339 (3): 160–65.

Krugman, P. 2010. "The power of conventional wisdom." Blog post, *New York Times*, September 27, http://krugman.blogs.nytimes.com/2010/09/27/the-power-of-conventional-wisdom/?_php=true&_type=blogs&_r=0.

Kunz, S., K. Oberle, A. Sander, et al. 2008. "Lymphadenopathy in a novel mouse model of *Bartonella*-induced cat scratch disease results from lymphocyte immigration and proliferation and is regulated by interferon-alpha/beta." *American Journal of Pathology* 172 (4): 1005–18.

Levy, S. 1992. *The Antibiotic Paradox*. New York: Plenum Press.

Li, X. B., W. Wang, G. J. Zhou, et al. 2012. "Production of salvianolic acid B in roots of *Salvia miltiorrhiza* (Danshen) during the post-harvest drying process." *Molecules* 17 (3): 2388–407.

Lubin, A. S., D. R. Snydman, and K. B. Miller. 2011. "Persistent babesiosis in a stem cell transplant recipient." *Leukemia Research* 35 (6): e77–78.

MacNamara, K. C., R. Racine, M. Chatterjee, et al. 2009. "Diminished hematopoietic activity associated with alterations in innate and adaptive immunity in a mouse model of human monocytic ehrlichiosis." *Infection and Immunity* 77 (9): 4061–69.

Maskatia, Z. K., and K. Baker. 2010. "Hypereosinophilia associated with echinacea use." *Southern Medical Journal* 103 (11): 1173–74.

I. McGilchrist. 2012. *The Master and His Emissary: The Divided Brain and the Making of the Western World*. New Haven, Conn.: Yale University Press.

Moro, M. H., O. L. Zegarra-Moro, J. Bjornsson, et al. 2002. "Increased arthritis severity in mice coinfected with *Borrelia burgdorferi* and *Babesia microti*." *Journal of Infectious Diseases* 186: 428–31.

Mosqueda, J., A. Olvera-Ramirez, G. Aquilar-Tipacamu, and G. J. Canto. 2012. "Current advances in detection and treatment of babesiosis." *Current Medicinal Chemistry* 19: 1504–18.

O'Gorman, E. J., and M. C. Emmerson. 2009. "Perturbations to trophic interactions and the stability of complex food webs." *Proceedings of the National Academy of Sciences of the United States* 106 (32): 13393–98.

Paddock, C. D., and J. E. Childs. 2003. "*Ehrlichia chaffeensis*: A prototypical emerging pathogen." *Clinical Microbiology Reviews* 16 (1): 37–64.

Resto-Ruiz, S., A. Burgess, and B. E. Anderson. 2003. "The role of the host immune response in the pathogenesis of *Bartonella henselae*." *DNA and Cell Biology* 22 (6): 431–40.

Schnittger, L., A. E. Rodriguez, M. Florin-Christensen, and D. A. Morrison. 2012. "*Babesia*: A world emerging." *Infection, Genetics and Evolution* 12: 1788–809.

Shaio, M.-F., and P.-R. Lin. 1998. "A case study of cytokine profiles in acute human babesiosis." *American Journal of Tropical Medicine and Hygiene* 58 (3): 335–37.

Shoda, L. K., K. A. Kegerreis, C. E. Suarez, et al. 2001. "DNA from protozoan parasites *Babesia bovis, Trypanosoma cruzi,* and *T. brucei* is mitogenic for B lymphocytes and stimulates macrophage expression of interleukin-12, tumor necrosis factor alpha, and nitric oxide." *Infection and Immunity* 69 (4): 2162–71.

Shu, Q., X. Fang, Q. Chen, and F. Stuber. 2003. "IL-10 polymorphism is associated with increased incidence of severe sepsis." *Chinese Medical Journal* 116 (11): 1756–59.

Socolovschi, C., T. Kernif, D. Raoult, and P. Parola. 2012. "*Borrelia, Rickettsia,* and *Ehrlichia* species in bat ticks, France, 2010." *Emerging Infectious Diseases* 18 (12): 1966–76.

Song, J.-Z., C.-F. Qiao, S.-L. Li, et al. 2009. "Quality assessment of granule of danshen extract by high performance liquid chromatography." *Chinese Journal of Natural Medicines* 7 (5): 368–75.

Stevenson, H. 2009. "Ehrlichiosis: Understanding immune mechanisms that lead to the development of fatal disease." Ph.D. thesis, University of Texas at Galveston, 2009.

Telfer S., R. Birtles, M. Bennet, et al. 2008. "Parasite interactions in natural populations: Insights from longitudinal data." *Parasitology* 135 (7): 767–81.

Telfer, S., X. Lambin, R. Birtles, et al. 2010. "Species interactions in a parasite community drive infection risk in a wildlife population." *Science* 330 (6001): 342–46.

Thomas, R. J., J. S. Dumler, and J. A. Carlyon. 2009. "Current management of human granulocytic anaplasmosis, human monocytic ehrlichiosis and *Ehrlichia ewingii* ehrlichiosis." *Expert Review of Anti-Infective Therapy* 7 (6): 709–22.

Walsh, M. G. 2013. "The relevance of forest fragmentation on the incidence of human babesiosis: Investigating the landscape epidemiology of an emerging tick-borne disease." *Vector Borne Zoonotic Diseases* 13 (4): 250–55.

Waner, T. 2008. "Hematopathological changes in dogs infected with *Ehrlichia canis.*" *Israel Journal of Veterinary Medicine* 63 (1): 1–8.

Bibliography

The problem with digital books is that you can always find what you are looking for but you need to go to a bookstore to find what you weren't looking for.

PAUL KRUGMAN

The following are the books, journal papers, and various other articles I used as resources for this book.

BOOKS

Bone, Kerry, and Simon Mills. *Principles and Practice of Phytotherapy.* 2nd ed. Edinburgh: Churchill Livingstone, 2013. (A very nice piece of work.)

Buhner, Stephen Harrod. *Healing Lyme: Natural Healing and Prevention of Lyme Borreliosis and Its Coinfections.* Raven Press, 2005.

———. *Healing Lyme Disease Coinfections: Complementary and Holistic Treatments for Bartonella and Mycoplasma.* Rochester, Vt.: Healing Arts Press, 2013.

———. *Herbal Antibiotics: Natural Alternatives for Treating Drug-Resistant Bacteria.* 2nd ed. North Adams, Mass.: Storey Publishing, 2012.

———. *Herbal Antivirals: Natural Remedies for Emerging and Resistant Viral Infections.* North Adams, Mass.: Storey Publishing, 2013.

———. *The Lost Language of Plants: The Ecological Function of Plant Medicines for All Life on Earth*. White River Junction, Vt.: Chelsea Green, 2002.

———. *Plant Intelligence and the Imaginal Realm: Beyond the Doors of Perception into the Dreaming of Earth*. Rochester, Vt.: Bear & Co., 2014.

Chang, Hson-Mou, and Paul Pui-Hay But. *Pharmacology and Applications of Chinese Materia Medica*. 2 vols. River Edge, N.J.: World Scientific, 1987.

Felter, Harvey Wickes, and John Uri Lloyd. *King's American Dispensatory*. 2 vols. Sandy, Ore.: Eclectic Medical Publications, 1983.

Foster, Steven, and Yue Chongxi. *Herbal Emissaries*. Rochester, Vt.: Healing Arts Press, 1992.

Griggs, Barbara. *Green Pharmacy*. Rochester, Vt.: Healing Arts Press, 1991.

Grieve, Maude. *A Modern Herbal*. 2 vols. N.Y.: Dover, 1971.

Hobbs, Christopher. *Medicinal Mushrooms*. Loveland, Colo.: Interweave Press, 1995.

Lappé, Marc. *When Antibiotics Fail*. Berkeley, Calif.: North Atlantic Books, 1986.

Levy, Stuart. *The Antibiotic Paradox*. N.Y.: Plenum Press, 1992.

Manandhar, Narayan P. *Plants and People of Nepal*. Portland, Ore.: Timber Press, 2002.

Miller, Orson K. *Mushrooms of North America*. N.Y.: E. P. Dutton, 1972.

Moerman, Daniel. *Native American Ethnobotany*. Portland, Ore.: Timber Press, 1998.

Nadkarni, K. M., and A. K. Nadkarni. *Indian Materia Medica*. 3rd ed. Bombay: Popular Prakashan, 1954.

Schaller, James. *The Diagnosis and Treatment of Babesia*. Tampa, Fla.: Hope Academic Press, 2006.

———. *The Use of the Herb Artemisinin for Babesia, Malaria, and Cancer*. Tampa, Fla.: Hope Academic Press, 2006.

Scheld, W. Michael, Richard Whitley, and Christina M. Marra. *Infections of the Central Nervous System*. Philadelphia: Lippincott Williams and Wilkins, 2004.

Wu, Jing-Nuan. *An Illustrated Chinese Materia Medica*. N.Y.: Oxford University Press, 2005.

Zhu, You-Ping. *Chinese Materia Medica*. Amsterdam: Harwood Academic Publishers, 1998.

JOURNAL PAPERS AND ARTICLE REFERENCES

The following references are organized in five sections: Babesia, Ehrlichia/Anaplasma, *Salvia miltiorrhiza,* Miscellaneous Herbs, and Septic Shock.

Babesia

Abbas, H. M., R. A. Brenes, M. S. Ajemian, et al. "Successful conservative treatment of spontaneous splenic rupture secondary to babesiosis: A case report and literature review." *Connecticut Medicine* 75, no. 3 (2011): 143–46.

Aboge, G. O., H. Jia, M. A. Terkawi, et al. "Cloning, expression, and characterization of Babesia gibsoni dihydrofolate reductase-thymidylate synthase: Inhibitory effect of antifolates on its catalytic activity and parasite proliferation." *Antimicrobial Agents and Chemotherapy* 52, no. 11 (2008): 4072–80.

Aboulaila, M., T. Munkhjargal, T. Sivakumar, et al. "Apicoplast-targeting antibacterials inhibit the growth of Babesia parasites." *Antimicrobial Agents and Chemotherapy* 56, no. 6 (2012): 3196–206.

Aboulaila, M., K. Nakamura, Y. Govind, et al. "Evaluation of the in vitro growth-inhibitory effect of epoxomicin on Babesia parasites." *Veterinary Parasitology* 167, no. 1 (2010): 19–27.

Aboulaila, M., T. Sivakumar, N. Yokoyama, et al. "Inhibitory effect of terpene nerolidol on the growth of Babesia parasites." *Parasitology International* 59, no. 2 (2010): 278–82.

Aboulaila, M., N. Yokoyama, and I. Igarashi. "Inhibitory effects of (-)-epigallocatechin-3-gallate from green tea on the growth of Babesia parasites." *Parasitology* 137, no. 5 (2010): 785–91.

Abrams, Y. "Complications of coinfection with babesia and Lyme disease after splenectomy." *Journal of the American Board of Family Medicine* 21, no. 1 (2008): 75–77.

Acosta, M. E., P. T. Ender, E. M. Smith, et al. "Babesia microti infection, eastern Pennsylvania, USA." *Emerging Infectious Diseases* 19, no. 7 (2013): 1105–7.

Addabbo, F., B. Ratliff, H. C. Park, et al. "The Krebs cycle and mitochon-drial mass are early victims of endothelial dysfunction: Proteomic approach." *American Journal of Pathology* 174, no. 1 (2009): 34–43.

Aguilar-Delfin, I., M. J. Homer, P. J. Wettstein, et al. "Innate resistance to Babesia infection is influenced by genetic background and gender." *Infection and Immunity* 69, no. 12 (2001): 7955–58.

Aguilar-Delfin, I., P. J. Wettstein, and D. H. Persing. "Resistance to acute babesiosis is associated with interleukin-12- and gamma interferon-mediated responses and requires macrophages and natural killer cells." *Infection and Immunity* 71, no. 4 (2003): 2002–8.

Aktas, M. "A survey of ixodid tick species and molecular identification of tick-borne pathogens." *Veterinary Parasitology* 200, nos. 3–4 (2014): 276–83.

Asada, M., Y. Goto, K. Yahata, et al. "Gliding motility of Babesia bovis merozoites visualized by time-lapse video microscopy." *PLoS ONE* 7, no. 4 (2012): e35227.

Asman, M., M. Nowak, P. Cuber, et al. "The risk of exposure to Anaplasma phagocytophilum, Borrelia burgdorferi sensu lato, Babesia sp. and co-infections in Ixodes ricinus ticks on the territory of Niepolomice forest (southern Poland)." *Annals of Parasitology* 59, no. 1 (2013): 13–19.

Aysul, N., K. Ural, H. Cetinkaya, et al. "Doxycycline-chloroquine combination for the treatment of canine monocytic ehrlichiosis." *Acta Scientiae Veterinariae* 40, no. 2 (2012): 1031.

Bastos, R. G., W. C. Johnson, W. C. Brown, et al. "Differential response of splenic monocytes and DC from cattle to microbial stimulation with Mycobacterium bovis BCG and Babesia bovis merozoites." *Veterinary Immunology and Immunopathology* 115, nos. 3–4 (2007): 334–45.

Bastos, R. G., W. C. Johnson, W. Mwangi, et al. "Bovine NK cells acquire cytotoxic activity and produce IFN-gamma after stimulation by Mycobacterium bovis BCG- or Babesia bovis-exposed splenic dendritic cells." *Veterinary Immunology and Immunopathology* 124, nos. 3–4 (2008): 302–12.

Battsetseg, B., T. Matsuo, X. Xuan, et al. "Babesia parasites develop and are transmitted by the non-vector soft tick Ornithodoros moubata (Acari: Argasidae)." *Parasitology* 134, pt. 1 (2007): 1–8.

Begley, D. W., T. E. Edwards, A. C. Raymond, et al. "Inhibitor-bound complexes of dihydrofolate reductase-thymidylate synthase from Babesia bovis." *Acta crystallographica. Section F, Structural Biology and Crystallization Communications* 67, pt. 9 (2011): 1070–77.

Birkenheuer, A. J., M. G. Levy, and E. B. Breitschwerdt. "Efficacy of combined atovaquone and azithromycin for therapy of chronic Babesia gibsoni (Asian genotype) infections in dogs." *Journal of Veterinary Internal Medicine* 18, no. 4 (2004): 494–98.

Bitsaktsis, C., B. Nandi, R. Racine, et al. "T-cell-independent humoral immunity is sufficient for protection against fatal intracellular ehrlichia infection." *Infection and Immunity* 75, no. 10 (2007): 4933–41.

Blevins, S. M., R. A. Greenfield, and M. S. Bronze. "Blood smear analysis in babesiosis, ehrlichiosis, relapsing fever, malaria and Chagas disease." *Cleveland Clinic Journal of Medicine* 75, no. 7 (2008): 521–30.

Bork, S., S. Das, K. Okubo, et al. "Effects of protein kinase inhibitors on the in vitro growth of Babesia bovis." *Parasitology* 132, pt. 6 (2006): 775–79.

Bork, S., N. Yokoyama, Y. Ikehara, et al. "Growth-inhibitory effect of heparin on Babesia parasites." *Antimicrobial Agents and Chemotherapy* 48, no. 1 (2004): 236–41.

Bork, S., N. Yokoyama, T. Matsuo, et al. "Clotrimazole, ketoconazole, and clodinafop-propargyl as potent growth inhibitors of equine Babesia parasites during in vitro culture." *Journal of Parasitology* 89, no. 3 (2003): 604–6.

Bork, S., N. Yokoyama, T. Matsuo, et al. "Growth inhibitory effect of triclosan on equine and bovine Babesia parasites." *American Journal of Tropical Medicine and Hygiene* 68, no. 3 (2003): 334–40.

Bosman, A. M., M. C. Oosthuizen, E. H. Venter, et al. "Babesia lengau associated with cerebral and haemolytic babesiosis in two domestic cats." *Parasites and Vectors* 6 (2013): 128.

Brody, J. E. "Another tick-borne disease to guard against." Blog post for the *New York Times*, July 30, 2012, http://well.blogs.nytimes.com/2012/07/30/another-tick-borne-disease-to-guard-against/?_php=true&_type=blogs&_r=0.

Brooks, W. H. "Increased polyamines alter chromatin and stabilize autoantigens in autoimmune diseases." *Frontiers of Immunology* 4 (2013): 91.

Brown, W. C., T. F. McElwain, B. J. Ruef, et al. "Babesia bovis rhoptry-associated protein 1 is immunodominant for T helper cells of immune cattle and contains T-cell epitopes conserved among geographically distant B. bovis strains." *Infection and Immunity* 64, no. 8 (1996): 3341–50.

Brown, W. C, C. E. Suarez, L. K. Shoda, et al. "Modulation of host immune responses by protozoal DNA." *Veterinary Immunology and Immunopathology* 72, nos. 1–2 (1999): 87–94.

Cesta, M. F. "Normal structure, function, and histology of the spleen." *Toxic Pathology* 34, no. 5 (2006): 455–65.

Chauvin, A., E. Moreau, S. Bonnet, et al. "Babesia and its hosts: Adaptation to long-lasting interactions as a way to achieve efficient transmission." *Veterinary Research* 40, no. 2 (2009): 37.

Chan, K., S. A. Marras, and N. Parveen. "Sensitive multiplex PCR assay to differentiate Lyme spirochetes and emerging pathogens Anaplasma phagocytophilum and Babesia microti." *BMC Microbiology* 13 (2013): 295.

Chen, D., D. B. Copeman, J. Burnell, et al. "Helper T cell and antibody responses to infection of CBA mice with Babesia microti." *Parasite Immunology* 22, no. 2 (2000): 81–88.

Chong, A. J., A. Shimamoto, C. R. Hampton, et al. "Toll-like receptor 4 mediates ischemia/reperfusion injury of the heart." *Journal of Thoracic and Cardiovascular Surgery* 128, no. 2 (2004): 170–79.

Cichocka, A., and B. Skotarczak. "[Babesosis—difficulty of diagnosis]." *Wiadmości Parazytologiczne* 47, no. 3 (2001): 527–33.

Clark, I. A., L. M. Alleva, A. C. Mills, et al. "Pathogenesis of malaria and clinically similar conditions." *Clinical Microbiology Reviews* 17, no. 3 (2004): 509–39.

Clark, I. A., and L. S. Jacobson. "Do babesiosis and malaria share a common disease process?" *Annals of Tropical Medicine and Parasitology* 92, no. 4 (1998): 483–88.

Clark, I. A., J. E. Richmond, E. J. Wills, et al. "Intra-erythrocytic death of the parasite in mice recovering from infection with Babesia microti." *Parasitology* 72, no. 2 (1977): 189–96.

Clawson, M. L., N. Paciorkowski, T. V. Rajan, et al. "Cellular immunity, but not gamma interferon, is essential for resolution of Babesia microti infection in BALB/c mice." *Infection and Immunity* 70, no. 9 (2002): 5304–6.

Coipan, E. C., S. Jahfari, M. Fonville, et al. "Spatiotemporal dynamics of emerging pathogens in questing Ixodes ricinus." *Frontiers in Cellular and Infection Microbiology* 3 (2013): 36.

Coleman, J. L., D. LeVine, C. Thill, et al. "Babesia microti and Borrelia burgdorferi follow independent courses of infection in mice." *Journal of Infectious Diseases* 192, no. 9 (2005): 1634–41.

Conrad, P. A., A. M. Kjemtrup, R. A. Carreno, et al. "Description of Babesia duncani n.sp. (Apicomplexa: Babesiidae) from humans and its differentiation from other piroplasms." *International Journal for Parasitology* 36, no. 7 (2006): 779–89.

Cornillot, E., A. Daaouli, A. Garg, et al. "Whole genome mapping and re-organization of the nuclear and mitochondrial genomes of Babesia microti isolates." *PLoS ONE* 8, no. 9 (2013): e72657.

Csiszar, A., M. Wang, E. G. Lakatta, et al. "Inflammation and endothelial dysfunction during aging: Role of NF-kappaB." *Journal of Applied Physiology* 105, no. 4 (2008): 1333–41.

Cunha, B. A., S. Nausheen, and D. Szalda. "Pulmonary complications of babesiosis: Case report and literature review." *European Journal of Clinical Microbiology and Infectious Diseases* 26, no. 7 (2007): 505–8.

Cursino-Santos, J. R., A. Alhassan, M. Singh, et al. "Babesia: Impact of cold storage on the survival and the viability of parasites in blood bags." *Transfusion* 54, no. 3 (2014): 585–91. Published electronically ahead of print July 28, 2013.

Dandawate, S., L. Williams, N. Joshee, et al. "Scutellaria extract and wogonin inhibit tumor-mediated induction of T(reg) cells via inhibition of TGF-β1 activity." *Cancer Immunology, Immunotherapy* 61, no. 5 (2012): 701–11.

Danilchuk, B., and S. J. Leclair. "Hemolytic anemia accelerated by Babesia spp. infection in splenectomized patient." *Clinical Laboratory Science* 25, no. 4 (2012): 194–98.

de Caires, S., and V. Steenkamp. "Use of yokukansan (TJ-54) in the treatment of neurological disorders: A review." *Phytotherapy Research* 24, no. 9 (2010): 1265–70.

Dkhil, M. A., A. S. Abdel-Baki, S. Al-Quraishy, et al. "Hepatic oxidative stress in Mongolian gerbils experimentally infected with Babesia divergens." *Ticks and Tick-Borne Diseases* 4, no. 4 (2013): 346–51.

Dkhil, M. A., S. Al-Quraishy, and A. S. Abdel-Baki. "Hepatic tissue damage induced in Meriones ungliculatus due to infection with Babesia divergens-infected erythrocytes." *Saudi Journal of Biological Sciences* 17, no. 2 (2010): 129–32.

Dowling, D. P., M. Iles, K. L. Olszewski, et al. "Crystal structure of arginase from Plasmodium falciparum and implications for L-arginine depletion in malarial infection." *Biochemistry* 49, no. 26 (2010): 5600–608.

Duh, D., M. Jelovsek, and T. Avsic-Zupanc. "Evaluation of an indirect fluorescence immunoassay for the detection of serum antibodies against Babesia divergens in humans." *Parasitology* 134, pt. 2 (2007): 179–85.

Edelhofer, R., A. Muller, M. Schuh, et al. "Differentiation of Babesia bigemina, B. bovis, B. divergens and B. major by Western blotting—first report of B. bovis in Austrian cattle." *Parasitology Research* 92, no. 5 (2004): 433–35.

Eskow, E. S., P. J. Krause, A. Spielman, et al. "Southern extension of the range of human babesiosis in the eastern United States." *Journal of Clinical Microbiology* 37, no. 6 (1999): 2051–52.

Esmaeilnejad, B., M. Tavassoli, S. Asri-Rezaei, et al. "Evaluation of antioxidant status and oxidative stress in sheep naturally infected with Babesia ovis." *Veterinary Parasitology* 185, nos. 2–4 (2012): 124–30.

Falagas, M. E., and M. S. Klempner. "Babesiosis in patients with AIDS: A chronic infection presenting as fever of unknown origin." *Clinical Infectious Diseases* 22, no. 5 (1996): 809–12.

Florescu, D., P. P. Sordillo, A. Glyptis, et al. "Splenic infarction in human babesiosis: Two cases and discussion." *Clinical Infectious Diseases* 46, no. 1 (2008): e8–11.

Franssen, F. F., F. R. Gaffar, A. P. Yatsuda, et al. "Characterisation of erythrocyte invasion by Babesia bovis merozoites efficiently released from their host cell after high-voltage pulsing." *Microbes and Infection* 5, no. 5 (2003): 365–72.

Fritzen, C., E. Mosites, R. Applegate, et al. "Environmental investigation following the first human case of babesiosis in Tennessee." *Journal of Parasitology* 100, no. 1 (2014): 106–9.

Gaffar, F. R., F. F. Franssen, and E. deVries. "Babesia bovis merozoites invade human, ovine, equine, porcine and caprine erythrocytes by sialic acid-dependent mechanism followed by developmental arrest after a single round of cell fission." *International Journal for Parasitology* 33, no. 14 (2003): 1595–603.

Gallager, L. G., S. Chau, A. S. Owaisi, et al. "An 84-year-old woman with fever and dark urine." *Clinical Infectious Diseases* 49, no. 2 (2009): 310–11.

Gimenez, G., M. L. Belaunzaran, C. V. Poncini, et al. "Babesia bovis: Lipids from virulent S2P and attenuated R1A strains trigger differential signalling and inflammatory responses in bovine macrophages." *Parasitology* 140, no. 4 (2013): 530–40.

Goddard, A., B. Wiinberg, A. P. Schoeman, et al. "Mortality in virulent canine babesiosis is associated with a consumptive coagulopathy." *Veterinary Journal* 196, no. 2 (2013): 213–17.

Goff, W. L., R. G. Bastos, W. C. Brown, et al. "The bovine spleen: Interactions among splenic cell populations in the innate immunologic control of hemoparasitic infections." *Veterinary Immunology and Immunopathology* 138, nos. 1–2 (2010): 1–14.

Goff, W. L., W. C. Johnson, R. H. Horn, et al. "The innate immune response in calves to Boophilus microplus tick transmitted Babesia bovis involves type-1 cytokine induction and NK-like cells in the spleen." *Parasite Immunology* 25, no. 4 (2003): 185–88.

Goff, W. L., W. C. Johnson, S. M. Parish, et al. "IL-4 and IL-10 inhibition of IFN-gamma- and TNF-alpha-dependent nitric oxide production from bovine mononuclear phagocytes exposed to Babesia bovis merozoites." *Veterinary Immunology and Immunopathology* 84, nos. 3–4 (2002): 237–51.

Goff, W. L., W. C. Johnson, S. M. Parish, et al. "The age-related immunity in cattle to Babesia bovis infection involves the rapid induction of interleukin-12, interferon-gamma and inducible nitric oxide synthase mRNA expression in the spleen." *Parasite Immunology* 23, no. 9 (2001): 463–71.

Goff, W. L., W. C. Johnson, W. Tuo, et al. "Age-related innate immune response in calves to Babesia bovis involves IL-12 induction and IL-10 modulation." *Annals of the New York Academy of Sciences* 969, no. 1 (2002): 164–68.

Goff, W. L., A. K. Storset, W. C. Johnson, et al. "Bovine splenic NK cells synthesize IFN-gamma in response to IL-12-containing supernatants from Babesia bovis-exposed monocyte cultures." *Parasite Immunology* 28, no. 5 (2006): 221–28.

Goo, Y. K., A. Ueno, M. A. Terkawi, et al. "Actin polymerization mediated by Babesia gibsoni aldolase is required for parasite invasion." *Experimental Parasitology* 135, no. 1 (2013): 42–49.

Guan, G., A. Chauvin, H. Yin, et al. "Course of infection by Babesia sp BQ1 (Lintan) and B. divergens in sheep depends on the production of IFN-gamma and IL10." *Parasite Immunology* 32, no. 2 (2010): 143–52.

Guijarro-Muñoz, I., M. Compte, A. Alvarez-Cienfuegos, et al. "Lipoolysaccharide activates toll-like receptor 4 (TLR4)-mediated NF-kB signaling pathway and proinflammatory response in human pericytes." *Journal of Biological Chemistry* 289, no. 4 (2014): 2457–68.

Guillemi, E., P. Ruybal, V. Lia, et al. "Multi-locus typing scheme for Babesia bovis and Babesia bigemina reveals high levels of genetic variability in strains from northern Argentina." *Infection Genetics and Evolution* 14 (2013): 214–22.

Haapasalo, K., P. Suomalainen, A. Sukura, et al. "Fatal babesiosis in man, Finland, 2004." *Emerging Infectious Diseases* 16, no. 7 (2010): 1116–18.

Hagiwara, S., H. Iwasaka, S. Hidaka, et al. "Neutrophil elastase inhibitor (sivelestat) reduces the levels of inflammatory mediators by inhibiting NF-kB." *Inflammation Research* 58, no. 4 (2009): 198–203.

Hajdusek, O., R. Sima, N. Ayollon, et al. "Interaction of the tick immune system with transmitted pathogens." *Frontiers in Cellular and Infection Microbiology* 3 (2013): 26.

Hatcher, J. C., P. D. Greenberg, J. Antique, et al. "Severe babesiosis in Long Island: Review of 34 cases and their complications." *Clinical Infectious Diseases* 32, no. 8 (2001): 1117–25.

Hefeneider, S. H., K. A. Cornell, L. E. Brown, et al. "Nucleosomes and DNA bind to specific cell-surface molecules on murine cells and induce cytokine production." *Clinical Immunology and Immunopathology* 63, no. 3 (1992): 245–51.

Hemmer, R. M., D. A. Ferrick, and P. A. Conrad. "Role of T cells and cytokines in fatal and resolving experimental babesiosis: Protection in

TNFRp55-/- mice infected with the human Babesia WA1 parasite." *Journal of Parasitology* 86, no. 4 (2000): 736–42.

Hemmer, R. M., D. A. Ferrick, and P. A. Conrad. "Up-regulation of tumor necrosis factor-alpha and interferon-gamma expression in the spleen and lungs of mice infected with the human Babesia isolate WA1." *Parasitology Research* 86, no. 2 (2000): 121–28.

Hemmer, R. M., E. J. Wozniak, L. J. Lowenstine, et al. "Endothelial cell changes are associated with pulmonary edema and respiratory distress in mice infected with the WA1 human Babesia parasite." *Journal of Parasitology* 85, no. 3 (1999): 479–89.

Hersh, M. H., M. Tibbetts, M. Strauss, et al. "Reservoir competence of wildlife host species for Babesia microti." *Emerging Infectious Diseases* 18, no. 12 (2012): 1951–57.

Hildebrandt, A., J. S. Gray, and K. P. Hunfeld. "Human babesiosis in Europe: What clinicians need to know." *Infection* 41, no. 6 (2013): 1057–72.

Hirano, T. "Interleukin-6 and its relation to inflammation and disease." *Clinical Immunology and Immunopathology* 62, no. 1, pt. 2 (1992): S60–65.

Hirano, T., T. Taga, T. Matsuda, et al. "Interleukin 6 and its receptor in the immune response and hematopoiesis." *International Journal of Cell Cloning* 8, suppl. 1 (1990): 155–66.

Hossain, M. A., O. Yamato, M. Yamasaki, et al. "Inhibitory effect of pyrimidine and purine nucleotides on the multiplication of Babesia gibsoni: Possible cause of low parasitemia and simultaneous reticulocytosis in canine babesiosis." *Journal of Veterinary Medical Science* 66, no. 4 (2004): 389–95.

Hwang, S. J., M. Yamasaki, K. Nakamura, et al. "Development and characterization of a strain of Babesia gibsoni resistant to diminazene aceturate in vitro." *Journal of Veterinary Medical Science* 72, no. 6 (2010): 765–71.

Igarashi, I., R. Suzuki, S. Waki, et al. "Roles of CD4+ T cells and gamma interferon in protective immunity against Babesia microti infection in mice." *Infection and Immunity* 67, no. 8 (1999): 4143–48.

Ishihara, K., and T. Hirano. "IL-6 in autoimmune disease and chronic inflammatory proliferative disease." *Cytokine Growth Factor Reviews* 13, nos. 4–5 (2002): 357–68.

Jeong, Y. I., S. H. Hong, S. H. Cho, et al. "Induction of IL-10-producing CD1d^{high}CD5$^+$ regulatory B cells following Babesia microti-infection." *PLoS ONE* 7, no. 10 (2012): e46553.

Johns, J. L., K. C. MacNamara, N. J. Walker, et al. "Infection with Anaplasma phagocytophilum induces multilineage alterations in hematopoietic progenitor cells and peripheral blood cells." *Infection and Immunity* 77, no. 9 (2009): 4070–80.

Johnson, S. T., R. G. Cable, L. Tonnetti, et al. "Seroprevalence of Babesia microti in blood donors from Babesia-endemic areas of the northeastern United States: 2000 through 2007." *Transfusion* 49, no. 12 (2009): 2574–82.

Joseph, J. T., K. Purtill, S. J. Wong, et al. "Vertical transmission of Babesia microti, United States." *Emerging Infectious Diseases* 18, no. 8 (2012): 1318–21.

Kania, S. A., D. R. Allred, and A. F. Barbet. "Babesia bigemina: Host factors affecting the invasion of erythrocytes." *Experimental Parasitology* 80, no. 1 (1995): 76–84.

Kawahara, M., Y. Rikihisa, E. Isogai, et al. "Ultrastructure and phylogenetic analysis of 'Candidatus Neoehrlichia mikurensis' in the family Anaplasmataceae, isolated from wild rats and found in Ixodes ovatus ticks." *International Journal of Systematic and Evolutionary Microbiology* 54, pt. 5 (2004): 1837–43.

Kelly, P. J., C. Xu, H. Lucas, et al. "Ehrlichiosis, babesiosis, anaplasmosis and hepatozoonosis in dogs from St. Kitts, West Indies." *PLoS ONE* 8, no. 1 (2013): e53450.

Kjemtrup, A. M., and P. A. Conrad. "Human babesiosis: An emerging tick-borne disease." *International Journal of Parasitology* 30, nos. 12–13 (2000): 1323–37.

Koh, Y. S., J. E. Koo, A. Biswas, et al. "MyD88-dependent signaling contributes to host defense against ehrlichial infection." *PLoS ONE* 5, no. 7 (2010): e11758.

Krause, P. J., B. E. Gewurz, D. Hill, et al. "Persistent and relapsing babesiosis in immunocompromised patients." *Clinical Infectious Diseases* 46, no. 3 (2008): 370–76.

Krause, P. J., K. McKay, J. Gadbaw, et al. "Increasing health burden of human babesiosis in endemic sites." *American Journal of Tropical Medicine and Hygiene* 68, no. 4 (2003): 431–36.

Krause, P. J., K. McKay, C. A. Thompson, et al. "Disease-specific diagnosis of coinfecting tickborne zoonoses: Babesiosis, human granulocytic ehrlichiosis, and Lyme disease." *Clinical Infectious Diseases* 34, no. 9 (2002): 1184–91.

Krause, P. J., R. Ryan, S. Telford III, et al. "Efficacy of immunoglobulin M serodiagnostic test for rapid diagnosis of acute babesiosis." *Journal of Clinical Microbiology* 34, no. 8 (1996): 2014–16.

Krause, P. J., S. R. Telford III, R. J. Pollack, et al. "Babesiosis: An underdiagnosed disease of children." *Pediatrics* 89, no. 6 (1992): 1045–48.

Krause, P. J., S. R. Telford III, R. Ryan, et al. "Diagnosis of babesiosis: Evaluation of a serologic test for the detection of Babesia microti antibody." *Journal of Infectious Diseases* 169, no. 4 (1994): 923–26.

Krause, P. J., S. R. Telford III, A. Spielman, et al. "Comparison of PCR with blood smear and inoculation of small animals for diagnosis of Babesia microti parasitemia." *Journal of Clinical Microbiology* 34, no. 11 (1996): 2791–94.

Kuwayama, D. P., and R. J. Briones. "Spontaneous splenic rupture caused by Babesia microti infection." *Clinical Infectious Diseases* 46, no. 9 (2008): e92–95.

Lau, A. O., M. J. Pedroni, and P. Bhanot. "Target specific-trisubstituted pyrrole inhibits Babesia bovis erythrocytic growth." *Experimental Parasitology* 133, no. 3 (2013): 365–68.

Lederberg, J. "Infectious disease as an evolutionary paradigm." *Emerging Infectious Diseases* 3, no. 4 (1997): 417–23.

Leiby, D. A. "Transfusion-transmitted Babesia spp.: Bull's-eye on Babesia microti." *Clinical Microbiology Reviews* 24, no. 1 (2011): 14–28.

Leiby, D. A., A. P. Chung, J. E. Gill, et al. "Demonstrable parasitemia among Connecticut blood donors with antibodies to Babesia microti." *Transfusion* 45, no. 11 (2005): 1804–10.

Lobo, C. A. "Babesia divergens and Plasmodium falciparum use common receptors, glycophorins A and B, to invade the human red blood cell." *Infection and Immunity* 73, no. 1 (2005): 649–51.

Lobo, C. A., J. R. Cursino-Santos, A. Alhassan, et al. "Babesia: An emerg-

Babesia 359

ing infectious threat in transfusion medicine." *PLoS Pathogens* 9, no. 7 (2013): e1003387.

Lobo, C. A., M. Rodriguez, and J. R. Cursino-Santos. "Babesia and red cell invasion." *Current Opinion in Hematology* 19, no. 3 (2012): 170–75.

Lu, C. Y., P. D. Winterberg, J. Chen, et al. "Acute kidney injury: A conspiracy of toll-like receptor 4 on endothelia, leukocytes, and tubules." *Pediatric Nephrology* 27, no. 10 (2012): 1847–54.

Lu, P., C. P. Sodhi, and D. J. Hackam. "Toll-like receptor regulation of intestinal development and inflammation in the pathogenesis of necrotizing enterocolitis." *Pathophysiology* 21, no. 1 (2014): 81–93. Published electronically ahead of print December 22, 2013.

Lubin, A. S., D. R. Snydman, and K. B. Miller. "Persistent babesiosis in a stem cell transplant recipient." *Leukemia Research* 35, no. 6 (2011): e77–78.

Luciano, R. L., G. Moeckel, M. Palmer, et al. "Babesiosis-induced acute kidney injury with prominent urinary macrophages." *American Journal of Kidney Diseases* 62, no. 4 (2013): 801–5.

Maamun, J. M., M. A. Suleman, M. Akinyi, et al. "Prevalence of Babesia microti in free-ranging baboons and African green monkeys." *Journal of Parasitology* 97, no. 1 (2011): 63–67.

Maeda, H., D. Boldbaatar, K. Kusakisako, et al. "Inhibitory effect of cyclophilin A from the hard tick Haemaphysalis longicornis on the growth of Babesia bovis and Babesia bigemina." *Parasitology Research* 112, no. 6 (2013): 2207–13.

Magnarelli, L. A., S. C. Williams, S. J. Norris, et al. "Serum antibodies to Borrelia burgdorferi, Anaplasma phagocytophilum, and Babesia microti in recaptured white-footed mice." *Journal of Wildlife Diseases* 49, no. 2 (2013): 294–302.

Malandrin, L., M. Jouglin, E. Moreau, et al. "Individual heterogeneity in erythrocyte susceptibility to Babesia divergens is a critical factor for the outcome of experimental spleen-intact sheep infections." *Veterinary Research* 40, no. 4 (2009): 25.

Mao, Y. W., H. W. Tseng, W. L. Liang, et al. "Anti-inflammatory and free radial scavenging activities of the constituents isolated from Machilus zuihoensis." *Molecules* 16, no. 11 (2011): 9451–66.

Martinot, M., M. M. Zadeh, Y. Hansmann, et al. "Babesiosis in immuno-competent patients, Europe." *Emerging Infectious Diseases* 17, no. 1 (2011): 114–16.

Matsuu, A., Y. Koshida, M. Kawahara, et al. "Efficacy of atovaquone against Babesia gibsoni in vivo and in vitro." *Veterinary Parasitology* 124, nos. 1–2 (2004): 9–18.

Mayne, P. J. "Emerging incidence of Lyme borreliosis, babesiosis, bartonel-losis, and granulocytic ehrlichiosis in Australia." *International Journal of General Medicine* 4 (2011): 845–52.

Mócsai, A. "Diverse novel functions of neutrophils in immunity, inflamma-tion, and beyond." *Journal of Experimental Medicine* 210, no. 7 (2013): 1283–99.

Montero, E., M. Rodriguez, Y. Oksov, et al. "Babesia divergens apical mem-brane antigen 1 and its interaction with the human red blood cell." *Infec-tion and Immunity* 77, no. 11 (2009): 4783–93.

Moro, M. H., O. L. Zegarra-Moro, J. Bjornsson, et al. "Increased arthri-tis severity in mice coinfected with Borrelia burgdorferi and Babesia microti." *Journal of Infectious Diseases* 186, no. 3 (2002): 428–31.

Mosqueda, J., A. Olvera-Ramirez, G. Aguilar-Tipacamu, et al. "Current advances in detection and treatment of babesiosis." *Current Medicinal Chemistry* 19, no. 10 (2012): 1504–18.

Muller, I. B., R. D. Walter, and C. Wrenger. "Structural metal dependency of the arginase from the human malaria parasite Plasmodium falciparum." *Biological Chemistry* 386, no. 2 (2005): 117–26.

Munkhjargal, T., M. AbouLaila, M. A. Terkawi, et al. "Inhibitory effects of pepstatin A and mefloquine on the growth of babesia parasites." *American Journal of Tropical Medicine and Hygiene* 87, no. 4 (2012): 681–88.

Nakamura, K., N. Yokoyama, and I. Igarashi. "Cyclin-dependent kinase inhibitors block erythrocyte invasion and intraerythrocytic development of Babesia bovis in vitro." *Parasitology* 134, pt. 10 (2007): 1347–53.

Norimine, J., J. Mosqueda, C. Suarez, et al. "Stimulation of T-helper cell gamma interferon and immunoglobulin G responses specific for Babe-sia bovis rhoptry-associated protein 1 (RAP-1) or a RAP-1 protein lacking the carboxy-terminal repeat region is insufficient to provide protective immunity against virulent B. bovis challenge." *Infection and Immunity* 71, no. 9 (2003): 5021–32.

Okamura, M., N. Yokoyama, N. Takabatake, et al. "Babesia bovis: Subcellular localization of host erythrocyte membrane components during their asexual growth." *Experimental Parasitology* 116, no. 1 (2007): 91–94.

Okamura, M., N. Yokoyama, N. P. Wickramathilaka, et al. "Babesia caballi and Babesia equi: Implications of host sialic acids in erythrocyte infection." *Experimental Parasitology* 110, no. 4 (2005): 406–11.

Okubo, K., P. Wilawan, S. Bork, et al. "Calcium-ions are involved in erythrocyte invasion by equine Babesia parasites." *Parasitology* 133, pt. 3 (2006): 289–94.

Pantanowitz, L., E. Ballesteros, and P. De Girolami. "Laboratory diagnosis of babesiosis." *Laboratory Medicine* 32, no. 4 (2001): 184–87.

Prince, H. E., M. Lape-Nixon, H. Patel, et al. "Comparison of the Babesia duncani (WA1) IgG detection rates among clinical sera submitted to a reference laboratory for WA1 IgG testing and blood donor specimens from diverse geographic areas of the United States." *Clinical and Vaccine Immunology* 17, no. 11 (2010): 1729–33.

Poisnel, E., M. Ebbo, Y. Berda-Haddad, et al. "Babesia microti: An unusual travel-related disease." *BMC Infectious Diseases* 13 (2013): 99.

Quick, R. E., B. L. Herwaldt, J. W. Thomford, et al. "Babesiosis in Washington State: A new species of Babesia?" *Annals of Internal Medicine* 119, no. 4 (1993): 284–90.

Rao, N. V., B. Argyle, X. Xu, et al. "Low anticoagulant heparin targets multiple sites of inflammation, suppresses heparin-induced thrombocytopenia, and inhibits interaction of RAGE with its ligands." *American Journal of Physiology. Cell Physiology* 299, no. 1 (2010): C97–110.

Rosenblatt, J. E. "Laboratory diagnosis of infections due to blood and tissue parasites." *Clinical Infectious Diseases* 49, no. 7 (2009): 1103–8.

Rosenblatt-Bin, H., Y. Kalechman, A. Vonsover, et al. "The immunomodular AS101 restores T(H1) type of response suppressed by Babesia rodhaini in BALB/c mice." *Cellular Immunology* 184, no. 1 (1998): 12–25.

Ryan, R., P. J. Krause, J. Radolf, et al. "Diagnosis of babesiosis using an immunoblot serologic test." *Clinical and Diagnostic Laboratory Immunology* 8, no. 6 (2001): 1177–80.

Sa-Nunes, A., A. Bafica, D. A. Lucas, et al. "Prostaglandin E2 is a major inhibitor of dendritic cell maturation and function in Ixodes scapularis saliva." *Journal of Immunology* 179, no. 3 (2007): 1497–505.

Sakuma, M., A. Setoguchi, and Y. Endo. "Possible emergence of drug-resistant variants of Babesia gibsoni in clinical cases treated with atovaquone and azithromycin." *Journal of Veterinary Internal Medicine* 23, no. 3 (2009): 493–98.

Sasaki, M., Y. Fujii, M. Iwamoto, et al. "Effect of sex steroids on Babesia microti infection in mice." *American Journal of Tropical Medicine and Hygiene* 88, no. 2 (2013): 367–75.

Saukkonen, K., P. Lakkisto, M. Varpula, et al. "Association of cell-free plasma DNA with hospital mortality and organ dysfunction in intensive care unit patients." *Intensive Care Medicine* 33, no. 9 (2007): 1624–27.

Scheepers, E., A. L. Leisewitz, P. N. Thompson, et al. "Serial haematology results in transfused and non-transfused dogs naturally infected with Babesia rossi." *Journal of the South African Veterinary Association* 82, no. 3 (2011): 136–43.

Schneider, D. A., H. Yan, R. G. Bastos, et al. "Dynamics of bovine spleen cell populations during the acute response to Babesia bovis infection: An immunohistological study." *Parasite Immunology* 33, no. 1 (2011): 34–44.

Schnittger, L., A. E. Rodriguez, M. Florin-Christensen, et al. "Babesia: A world emerging." *Infection, Genetics and Evolution* 12, no. 8 (2012): 1788–809.

Shaio, M. F., and P. R. Lin. "A case study of cytokine profiles in acute human babesiosis." *American Journal of Tropical Medicine and Hygiene* 58, no. 3 (1998): 335–37.

Shimamoto, Y., M. Sasaki, H. Ikadai, et al. "Downregulation of hepatic cytochrome P450 3A in mice infected with Babesia microti." *Journal of Veterinary Medical Science/Japanese Society of Veterinary Science* 74, no. 2 (2012): 241–45.

Shoda, L. K., K. A. Kegerreis, C. E. Suarez, et al. "DNA from protozoan parasites Babesia bovis, Trypanosoma cruzi, and T. brucei is mitogenic for B lymphocytes and stimulates macrophage expression of interleukin-12, tumor necrosis factor alpha, and nitric oxide." *Infection and Immunity* 69, no. 4 (2001): 2162–71.

Shoda, L. K., G. H. Palmer, J. Florin-Christensen, et al. "Babesia bovis-stimulated macrophages express interleukin-1beta, interleukin-12, tumor necrosis factor alpha, and nitric oxide and inhibit parasite replication in vitro." *Infection and Immunity* 68, no. 9 (2000): 5139–45.

Smith, F. D., and L. E. Wall. "Prevalence of Babesia and Anaplasma in ticks infesting dogs in Great Britain." *Veterinary Parasitology* 198, nos. 1–2 (2013): 18–23.

Sondgeroth, K. S., T. F. McElwain, A. J. Allen, et al. "Loss of neurovirulence is associated with reduction of cerebral capillary sequestration during acute Babesia bovis infection." *Parasites and Vectors* 6, no. 1 (2013): 181.

Sousse, L. E., S. Wells, P. Enkhbaatar, et al. "Analysis of arginase and nitric oxide synthase (NOS) to excess collagen deposition in inhalation injury." *FASEB Journal* 23, no. 1 (2009): 1025.6.

Stempin, C. C., L. R. Dulgerian, V. V. Garrido, et al. "Arginase in parasitic infections: Macrophage activation, immunosuppression, and intracellular signals." *Journal of Biomedicine and Biotechnology*, 2010: 683485.

Stitch, R. W., L. K. Shoda, M. Dreewes, et al. "Stimulation of nitric oxide production in macrophages." *Infection and Immunity* 66, no. 9 (1998): 4130–36.

Sun, Y., E. Moreau, A. Chauvin, et al. "The invasion process of bovine erythrocyte by Babesia divergens: Knowledge from an in vitro assay." *Veterinary Research* 42 (2011): 62.

Taiwo, B., C. Lee, D. Venkat, et al. "Can tumor necrosis factor alpha blockade predispose to severe babesiosis?" *Arthritis and Rheumatism* 57, no. 1 (2007): 179–81.

Takabatake, N., M. Okamura, N. Yokoyama, et al. "Glycophorin A-knockout mice, which lost sialoglycoproteins from the red blood cell membrane, are resistant to lethal infection of Babesia rodhaini." *Veterinary Parasitology* 148, no. 2 (2007): 93–101.

Takabatake, N., M. Okamura, N. Yokoyama, et al. "Involvement of a host erythrocyte sialic acid content in Babesia bovis infection." *Journal of Veterinary Medical Science* 69, no. 10 (2007): 999–1004.

Tian, Z. C., G. Y. Liu, H. Yin, et al. "RPS8—a new informative DNA marker for phylogeny of Babesia and Theileria parasites in China." *PLoS ONE* 8, no. 11 (2013): e79860.

Tobler, W. D. Jr., D. Cotton, T. Lepore, et al. "Case report: Successful non-operative management of spontaneous splenic rupture in a patient with babesiosis." *World Journal of Emergency Surgery* 6 (2011): 4.

Tone, A., K. Shikata, M. Sasaki, et al. "Erythromycin ameliorates renal injury via anti-inflammatory effects in experimental diabetic rats." *Diabetologia* 48, no. 11 (2005): 2402–11.

Tonnetti, L., A. M. Thorp, B. Deisting, et al. "Babesia microti seroprevalence in Minnesota blood donors." *Transfusion* 53, no. 8 (2013): 1698–705.

Tsuji, M., Q. Wei, A. Zamato, et al. "Human babesiosis in Japan: Epizootiologic survey of rodent reservoir and isolation of new type of Babesia microti-like parasite." *Journal of Clinical Microbiology* 39, no. 12 (2001): 4316–22.

Tsuji, N., B. Battsetseg, D. Boldbaatar, et al. "Babesial vector tick defensin against Babesia sp. parasites." *Infection and Immunity* 75, no. 7 (2007): 3633–40.

Uesugi, T., M. Froh, G. E. Arteel, et al. "Toll-like receptor 4 is involved in the mechanism of early alcohol-induced liver injury in mice." *Hepatology* 34, no. 1 (2001): 101–8.

Ueti, M. W., J. O. Reagan, Jr., D. P. Knowles, Jr., et al. "Identification of midgut and salivary glands as specific and distinct barriers to efficient tick-borne transmission of Anaplasma marginale." *Infection and Immunity* 75, no. 6 (2007): 2959–64.

Umemiya, R., T. Hatta, M. Liao, et al. "Haemaphysalis longicornis: Molecular characterization of a homologue of the macrophage migration inhibitory factor from the partially fed ticks." *Experimental Parasitology* 115, no. 2 (2007): 135–42.

Usmani-Brown, S., J. J. Halperin, and P. J. Krause. "Neurological manifestations of human babesiosis." *Handbook of Clinical Neurology* 114 (2013): 199–203.

Vannier, E., B. E. Gewurz, and P. J. Krause. "Human babesiosis." *Infectious Disease Clinics of North America* 22, no. 3 (2008): 469–88.

Vannier, E., and P. J. Krause. "Update on babesiosis." *Interdisciplinary Perspectives on Infectious Diseases*, 2009: 984568.

Velickovic, K., M. Markelic, I. Golic, et al. "Long-term dietary L-arginine supplementation increases endothelial nitric oxide synthase and vasoactive intestinal peptide immunoexpression in rat small intestine." *European Journal of Nutrition* 53, no. 3 (2014): 813–21. Published electronically ahead of print October 8, 2013.

Vial, H. J., and Gorenflot, A. "Chemotherapy against babesiosis." *Veterinary Parasitology* 138, nos. 1–2 (2006): 147–60.

Walsh, M. G. "The relevance of forest fragmentation on the incidence of human babesiosis: Investigating the landscape epidemiology of an emerging tick-borne disease." *Vector Borne and Zoonotic Diseases* 13, no. 4 (2013): 250–55.

Wattanachaiyingcharoen, R., K. Komatsu, S. Zhu, et al. "Authentication of Coscinium fenestratum among the other Menispermaceae plants prescribed in Thai folk medicines." *Biological and Pharmaceutical Bulletin* 33, no. 1 (2010): 91–94.

Welc-Faleciak, R., J. Werszko, K. Cydzik, et al. "Co-infection and genetic diversity of tick-borne pathogens in roe deer from Poland." *Vector Borne and Zoonotic Diseases* 13, no. 5 (2013): 277–88.

Welch, D. F., K. C. Carroll, E. K. Hofmeister, et al. "Isolation of a new subspecies, Bartonella vinsonii subsp. arupensis, from a cattle rancher: Identity with isolates found in conjunction with Borrelia burgdorferi and Babesia microti among naturally infected mice." *Journal of Clinical Microbiology* 37, no. 8 (1999): 2598–601.

Wells, G. A., I. B. Muller, C. Wrenger, et al. "The activity of Plasmodium falciparum arginase is mediated by a novel inter-monomer salt-bridge between Glu295-Arg404." *FEBS Journal* 276, no. 13 (2009): 3517–30.

White, D. J., J. Talarico, H. G. Chang, et al. "Human babesiosis in New York State: Review of 139 hospitalized cases and analysis of prognostic factors." *Archives of Internal Medicine* 158, no. 19 (1998): 2149–54.

Wormser, G. P., R. J. Dattwyler, E. D. Shapiro, et al. "The clinical assessment, treatment, and prevention of Lyme disease, human granulocytic anaplasmosis, and babesiosis: Clinical practice guidelines by the Infectious Diseases Society of America." *Clinical Infectious Diseases* 43, no. 9 (2006): 1089–134.

Wormser, G. P., A. Prasad, E. Neuhaus, et al. "Emergence of resistance to azithromycin-atovaquone in immunocompromised patients with Babesia microti infection." *Clinical Infectious Diseases* 50, no. 3 (2010): 381–86.

Wozniak, E. J., L. J. Lowenstine, R. Hemmer, et al. "Comparative patho-genesis of human WA1 and Babesia microti isolates in a Syrian hamster model." *Laboratory Animal Science* 46, no. 5 (1996): 507–15.

Yamasaki, M., A. Takada, O. Yamato, et al. "Inhibition of Na, K-ATPase activity reduces Babesia gibsoni infection of canine erythrocytes with inherited high K, low Na concentrations." *Journal of Parasitology* 91, no. 6 (2005): 1287–92.

Yamasaki, M., N. Tamura, K. Nakamura, et al. "Effects and mechanisms of action of polyene macrolide antibiotic nystatin on Babesia gibsoni in vitro." *Journal of Parasitology* 97, no. 6 (2011): 1190–92.

Yang, F., X. Li, L. K. Wang, et al. "Inhibitions of NF-κB and TNF-α result in differential effects in rats with acute on chronic liver failure induced by D-Gal and LPS." *Inflammation* 37, no. 3 (2014): 848–57.

Yang, Y. S., B. Murciano, K. Moubri, et al. "Structural and functional char-acterization of Bc28.1, major erythrocyte-binding protein from Babesia canis merozoite surface." *Journal of Biological Chemistry* 287, no. 12 (2012): 9495–508.

Yokoyama, N., S. Bork, M. Nishisaka, et al. "Roles of the Maltese cross form in the development of parasitemia and protection against Babesia microti infection in mice." *Infection and Immunity* 71, no. 1 (2003): 411–17.

Yokoyama, N., M. Okamura, and I. Igarashi. "Erythrocyte invasion by Babe-sia parasites: Current advances in the elucidation of the molecular inter-actions between the protozoan ligands and host receptors in the invasion stage." *Veterinary Parasitology* 138, nos. 1–2 (2006): 22–32.

Zamoto-Niikura, A., M. Tsuji, W. Qiang, et al. "Detection of two zoonotic Babesia microti lineages, the Hobetsu and U.S. lineages, in two sympatric tick species, Ixodes ovatus and Ixodes persulcatus, respectively, in Japan." *Applied and Enviornmental Microbiology* 78, no. 9 (2012): 3424–30.

Zintl, A., C. Westbrook, H. E. Skerrett, et al. "Chymotrypsin and neuramin-idase treatment inhibits host cell invasion by Babesia divergens (Phylum Apicomplexa)." *Parasitology* 125, pt. 1 (2002): 45–50.

Ehrlichia/Anaplasma

Akkoyunlu, M., and E. Fikrig. "Gamma interferon dominates the murine cytokine response to the agent of human granulocytic ehrlichiosis and helps to control the degree of early rickettsemia." *Infection and Immunity* 68, no. 4 (2000): 1827–33.

Akkoyunlu, M., S. E. Malawista, J. Anguita, et al. "Exploitation of interleukin-8-induced neutrophil chemotaxis by the agent of human granulocytic ehrlichiosis." *Infection and Immunity* 69, no. 9 (2001): 5577–88.

Bayard-Mc Neeley, M., A. Bansal, I. Chowdhury, et al. "In vivo and in vitro studies on Anaplasma phagocytophilum infection of the myeloid cells of a patient with chronic myelogenous leukaemia and human granulocytic ehrlichiosis." *Journal of Clinical Pathology* 57, no. 5 (2004): 499–503.

Beatriz Silva, A., S. Pina Canseco, P. Gabriel de la Torre Mdel, et al. "[Asymptomatic human infection from contact with dogs: A case of human ehrlichiosis]." *Gaceta Medica de Mexico* 150, no. 2 (2014): 171–74.

Bitsaktis, C., J. Huntington, and G. Winslow. "Production of IFN-gamma by CD4 T cells is essential for resolving ehrlichia infection." *Journal of Immunology* 172, no. 11 (2004): 6894–901.

Bogdan, C. "Nitric oxide and the immune response." *Nature Immunology* 2, no. 10 (2001): 907–16.

Brown, W. C. "Adaptive immunity to anaplasma pathogens and immune dysregulation: Implication for bacterial persistence." *Comparative Immunology, Microbiology and Infectious Diseases* 35, no. 3 (2012): 241–52.

Cheng, Z. "Transcriptional regulators of Ehrlichia chaffeensis during intracellular development and the roles of OmpA in the bacterial infection and survival." PhD diss., Ohio State University, 2008, http://rave.ohiolink.edu/etdc/view?acc_num=osu1227561447.

Cheng, Z., Y. Kumagai, M. Lin, et al. "Intra-leukocyte expression of two-component systems in Ehrlichia chaffeensis and Anaplasma phagocytophilum and effects of the histidine kinase inhibitor closantel." *Cellular Microbiology* 8, no. 8 (2006): 1241–52.

Chmielewska-Badora, J., A. Moniuszko, W. Zukiewicz-Sobczak, et al. "Serological survey in persons occupationally exposed to tick-borne pathogens in cases of co-infections with Borrelia burgdorferi, Anaplasma phagocytophilum, Bartonella spp. and Babesia microti." *Annals of Agricultural and Environmental Medicine* 19, no. 2 (2012): 271–74.

Choi, K. S., D. J. Grab, and J. S. Dumler. "Anaplasma phagocytophilum infection induces protracted neutrophil degranulation." *Infection and Immunity* 72, no. 6 (2004): 3680–83.

Choi, K. S., J. T. Park, and J. S. Dumler. "Anaplasma phagocytophilum delay neutrophil apoptosis through the p38 mitogen-activated protein kinase signal pathway." *Infection and Immunity* 73, no. 12 (2005): 8209–18.

Choi, K. S., T. Webb, M. Oelke, et al. "Differential innate immune cell activation and proinflammatory response in Anaplasma phagocytophilum infection." *Infection and Immunity* 75, no. 6 (2007): 3124–30.

Cruz, A. C., E. Zweygarth, M. F. Ribeiro, et al. "New species of Ehrlichia isolated from Rhipicephalus (Boophilus) microplus shows an ortholog of the E. canis major immunogenic glycoprotein gp36 with a new sequence of tandem repeats." *Parasites and Vectors* 5 (2012): 291.

Dahlgren, F. S., E. J. Mandel, and J. W. Krebs. "Increasing incidence of Ehrlichia chaffeensis and Anaplasma phagocytophilum in the United States, 2000–2007." *American Journal of Tropical Medicine and Hygiene* 85, no. 1 (2011): 124–31.

Dawson, J. E., C. D. Paddock, C. K. Warner, et al. "Tissue diagnosis of Ehrlichia chaffeensis in patients with fatal ehrlichiosis by use of immuno-histochemistry, in situ hybridization, and polymerase chain reaction." *American Journal of Tropical Medicine and Hygiene* 65, no. 5 (2001): 603–9.

Dedonder, S. E., C. Cheng, L. H. Willard, et al. "Transmission electron microscopy reveals distinct macrophage- and tick cell-specific morphological stages of Ehrlichia chaffeensis." *PLoS ONE* 7, no. 5 (2012): e36749.

de la Fuente, J., A. Lew, H. Lutz, et al. "Genetic diversity of anaplasma species major surface proteins and implications for anaplasmosis serodiagnosis and vaccine development." *Animal Health Research Reviews* 6, no. 1 (2005): 75–89.

de la Fuente, J., P. Ruybal, M. S. Mtshali, et al. "Analysis of world strains of Anaplasma marginale using major surface protein 1a repeat sequences." *Veterinary Microbiology* 119, nos. 2–4 (2007): 382–90.

Dumler, J. S. "The biological basis of severe outcomes in Anaplasma phagocytophilum infection." *FEMS Immunology and Medical Microbiology* 64, no. 1 (2012): 13–20.

Dumler, J. S., and J. S. Bakken. "Human granulocytic ehrlichiosis in Wisconsin and Minnesota: A frequent infection with the potential for persistence." *Journal of Infectious Diseases* 173, no. 4 (1995): 1027–30.

Dumler, J. S., E. R. Trigiani, J. S. Bakken, et al. "Serum cytokine responses during acute human granulocytic ehrlichiosis." *Clinical and Diagnostic Laboratory Immunology* 7, no. 1 (2000): 6–8.

Dumler, J. S., J. E. Madigan, N. Pusterla, et al. "Ehrlichioses in humans: Epidemiology clinical presentation, diagnosis, and treatment." *Clinical Infectious Diseases* 45, suppl. 1 (2007): S45–51.

Dumler, J. S., N. C. Barat, C. E. Barat, et al. "Human granulocytic anaplasmosis and macrophage activation." *Clinical Infectious Diseases* 45, no. 2 (2007): 199–204.

Foley, J. E., N. C. Nieto, and P. Foley. "Emergence of tick-borne granulocytic anaplasmosis associated with habitat type and forest change in northern California." *American Journal of Tropical Medicine and Hygiene* 81, no. 6 (2009): 1132–40.

Francischetti, I. M., T. N. Mather, and J. M. Ribeiro. "Cloning of a salivary gland metalloprotease and characterization of gelatinase and fibrin(ogen)lytic activities in the saliva of the Lyme disease tick vector Ixodes scapularis." *Biochemical and Biophysical Research Communications* 305, no. 4 (2003): 869–75.

Ganguly, S., and S. K. Mukhopadhayay. "Tick-borne ehrlichiosis infection in human beings." *Journal of Vector Borne Diseases* 45, no. 4 (2008): 273–80.

Ganta, R. R., C. Cheng, E. C. Miller, et al. "Differential clearance and immune responses to tick cell-derived versus macrophage culture-derived Ehrlichia chaffeensis in mice." *Infection and Immunity* 75, no. 1 (2007): 135–45.

Ganta, R. R., M. J. Wilkerson, C. Cheng, et al. "Persistent Ehrlichia chaffeensis infection occurs in the absence of functional major histocompatibility complex class II genes." *Infection and Immunity* 70, no. 1 (2002): 380–88.

Gao, Y., J. Deng, X. F. Yu, et al. "Ginsenoside Rg1 inhibits vascular intimal hyperplasia in balloon-injured rat carotid artery by down-regulation of extracellular signal-regulated kinase 2." *Journal of Ethnopharmacology* 138, no. 2 (2011): 472–78.

Ge, Y., K. Yoshiie, F. Kuribayashi, et al. "Anaplasma phagocytophilum inhibits human neutrophil apoptosis via upregulation of bfl-1, maintenance of mitochondrial membrane potential and prevention of caspase 3 activation." *Cellular Microbiology* 7, no. 1 (2005): 29–38.

Ghose, P., A. Q. Ali, R. Fang, et al. "The interaction between IL-18 and IL-18 receptor limits the magnitude of protective immunity and enhances pathogenic responses following infection with intracellular bacteria." *Journal of Immunology* 187, no. 3 (2011): 1333–46.

Harrus, S., T. Waner, H. Bark, et al. "Recent advances in determining the pathogenesis of canine monocytic ehrlichiosis." *Journal of Clinical Microbiology* 37, no. 9 (1999): 2745–49.

Harrus, S., T. Waner, A. Keysary, et al. "Investigation of splenic functions in canine monocytic ehrlichiosis." *Veterinary Immunology and Immunopathology* 62, no. 1 (1998): 15–27.

Havens, N. S., B. R. Kinnear, and S. Mato. "Fatal ehrlichial myocarditis in a healthy adolescent: A case report and review of the literature." *Clinical Infectious Diseases* 54, no. 8 (2012): e113–14.

Iqbal, Z., and Y. Rikihisa. "Reisolation of Ehrlichia canis from blood and tissues of dogs after doxycycline treatment." *Journal of Clinical Microbiology* 32, no. 7 (1994): 1644–49.

Ismail, N., K. C. Bloch, and J. W. McBride. "Human ehrlichiosis and anaplasmosis." *Clinics in Laboratory Medicine* 30, no. 1 (2010): 261–92.

Ismail, N., E. C. Crossley, H. L. Stevenson, et al. "Relative importance of T-cell subsets in monocytotropic ehrlichiosis: A novel effector mechanism involved in Ehrlichia-induced immunopathology in murine ehrlichiosis." *Infection and Immunity* 75, no. 9 (2007): 4608–20.

Ismail, N., L. Soong, J. W. McBride, et al. "Overproduction of TNF-apha by CD8+ type 1 cells and down-regulation of IFN-gamma production by CD4+ Th1 cells contribute to toxic shock-like syndrome in an animal model of fatal monocytotropic ehrlichiosis." *Journal of Immunology* 172, no. 3 (2004): 1786–800.

Ismail, N., H. L. Stevenson, and D. H. Walker. "Role of tumor necrosis factor alpha (TNF-alpha) and interleukin-10 in the pathogenesis of severe murine monocytotropic ehrlichiosis: Increased resistance of TNF receptor p55- and p75-deficient mice to fatal ehrlichial infection." *Infection and Immunity* 74, no. 3 (2006): 1846–56.

Ismail, N., D. H. Walker, P. Ghose, and Y.-W. Tang. "Immune mediators of protective and pathogenic immune responses in patients with mild and fatal human monocytotropic ehrlichiosis." *BMC Immunology* 13 (2012): 26.

Jahangir, A., C. Kolbert, W. Edwards, et al. "Fatal pancarditis associated with human granulocytic ehrlichiosis in a 44-year-old man." *Clinical Infectious Diseases* 27, no. 6 (1998): 1424–27.

Katavolos, P., P. M. Armstrong, J. E. Dawson, et al. "Duration of tick attachment required for transmission of granulocytic ehrlichiosis." *Journal of Infectious Diseases* 177, no. 5 (1998): 1422–25.

Kim, H. Y., J. Mott, N. Zhi, et al. "Cytokine gene expression by peripheral blood leukocytes in horses experimentally infected with Anaplasma phagocytophila." *Clinical and Diagnostic Laboratory Immunology* 9, no. 5 (2002): 1079–84.

Kim, H. Y., and Y. Rikihisa. "Expression of interleukin-1beta, tumor necrosis factor alpha, and interleukin-6 in human peripheral blood leukocytes exposed to human granulocytic ehrlichiosis agent or recombinant major surface protein P44." *Infection and Immunity* 68, no. 6 (2000): 3394–402.

Kim, H. Y., and Y. Rikihisa. "Roles of p38 mitogen-activated protein kinase, NF-κB, and protein kinase C in proinflammatory cytokine mRNA expression by human peripheral blood leukocytes, monocytes, and neutrophils in response to Anaplasma phagocytophila." *Infection and Immunity* 70, no. 8 (2002): 4132–41.

Klein, M. B., S. Hu, C. C. Chao, et al. "The agent of human granulocytic ehrlichiosis induces the production of myelosuppressing chemokines without induction of proinflammatory cytokines." *Journal of Infectious Diseases* 182, no. 1 (2000): 200–205.

Klien, M. B., J. S. Miller, C. M. Nelson, et al. "Primary bone marrow progenitors of both granulocytic and monocytic lineages are susceptible to infection with the agent of human granulocytic ehrlichiosis." *Journal of Infectious Diseases* 176, no. 5 (1997): 1405–9.

Kotsyfakis, M., A. Sa-Nunes, I. M. Francischetti, et al. "Antiinflammatory and immunosuppressive activity of sialostatin L, a salivary cystatin from the tick Ixodes scapularis." *Journal of Biological Chemistry* 281, no. 36 (2006): 26298–307.

Kumagai, Y., Z. Cheng, M. Lin, et al. "Biochemical activities of three pairs of Ehrlichia chaffeensis two-component regulatory system proteins involved in inhibition of lysosomal fusion." *Infection and Immunity* 74, no. 9 (2006): 5014–22.

Lee, E. H., and Y. Rikihisa. "Absence of tumor necrosis factor alpha, interleukin-6 (IL-6), and granulocyte-macrophage colony-stimulating factor expression but presence of IL-1beta, IL-8, and IL-10 expression in human monocytes exposed to viable or killed Ehrlichia chaffeensis." *Infection and Immunity* 64, no. 10 (1996): 4211–19.

Lepidi, H., J. E. Bunnell, M. E. Martin, et al. "Comparative pathology and immunohistology associated with clinical illness after Ehrlichia phagocytophila-group infections." *American Journal of Tropical Medicine and Hygiene* 62, no. 1 (2000): 29–37.

Lester, S. J., E. B. Breitschwerdt, C. D. Collis, et al. "Anaplasma phagocytophilum infection (granulocytic anaplasmosis) in a dog from Vancouver Island." *Canadian Veterinary Journal* 46, no. 9 (2005): 825–27.

Li, H., Y. Zhou, W. Wang, et al. "The clinical characteristics and outcomes of patients with human granulocytic anaplasmosis in China" *International Journal of Infectious Diseases* 15, no. 12 (2011): e859–66.

Lin, M., and Y. Rikihisa. "Ehrlichia chaffeensis downregulates surface toll-like receptors 2/4, C14 and transcription factors PU.1 and inhibits lipopolysaccharide activation of NF-kappa B, ERK 1/2 and p38 MAPK in host monocytes." *Cellular Microbiology* 6, no. 2 (2004): 175–86.

Lin, M., M. X. Zhu, and Y. Rikihisa. "Rapid activation of protein tyrosine kinase and phospholipase C-gamma2 and increase in cytosolic free calcium are required by Ehrlichia chaffeensis for internalization and growth in THP-1 cells." *Infection and Immunity* 70, no. 2 (2002): 889–98.

Lin, T., Y. H. Kwak, F. Sammy, et al. "Synergistic inflammation is induced by blood degradation products with microbial toll-like receptor agonists and is blocked by hemopexin." *Journal of Infectious Diseases* 202, no. 4 (2010): 624–32.

Liu, Y., Z. Zhang, Y. Jiang, et al. "Obligate intracellular bacterium Ehrlichia inhibiting mitochondrial activity." *Microbes and Infection* 13, no. 3 (2011): 232–38.

Louw, M., M. T. Allsopp, and E. C. Meyer. "Ehrlichia ruminantium, an emerging human pathogen—a further report." *South African Medical Journal* 95, no. 12 (2005): 948.

Macció, A., and C. Madeddu. "Management of anemia of inflammation in the elderly." *Anemia*, 2012: 563251.

Machado, R. J., N. K. Monteiro, L. Migliolo, et al. "Characterization and pharmacological properties of a novel multifunctional Kunitz inhibitor from Erythrina velutina seeds." *PLoS ONE* 8, no. 5 (2013): e63571.

MacNamara, K. C., R. Racine, M. Chatterjee, et al. "Diminished hematopoietic activity associated with alterations in innate and adaptive immunity in a mouse model of human monocytic ehrlichiosis." *Infection and Immunity* 77, no. 9 (2009): 4061–69.

Martin, M. E., J. E. Bunnell, and J. S. Dumler. "Pathology, immunohistology, and cytokine responses in early phases of human granulocytic ehrlichiosis in a murine model." *Journal of Infectious Diseases* 181, no. 1 (2000): 374–78.

Mavrimatis, K., C. K. Doyle, A. Lykidis, et al. "The genome of the obligately intracellular bacterium Ehrlichia canis reveals themes of complex membrane structure and immune evasion strategies." *Journal of Bacteriology* 188, no. 11 (2006): 4015–23.

McBride, J. W., and D. H. Walker. "Molecular and cellular pathobiology of Ehrlichia infection: Targets for new therapeutics and immunomodulation strategies." *Expert Reviews in Molecular Medicine* 13 (2011): e3.

McBride, J. W., and D. H. Walker. "Progress and obstacles in vaccine development for the ehrlichioses." *Expert Review of Vaccines* 9, no. 9 (2010): 1071–82.

Munder, M. "Arginase: An emerging key player in the mammalian immune system." *British Journal of Pharmacology* 158, no. 3 (2009): 638–51.

Neelakanta, G., H. Sultana, D. Fish, et al. "Anaplasma phagocytophilum induces Ixodes scapularis ticks to express an antifreeze glycoprotein gene that enhances their survival in the cold." *Journal of Clinical Investigation* 120, no. 9 (2010): 3179-90.

Niu, H., V. Kozjak-Pavlovic, T. Rudel, et al. "Anaplasma phagocytophilum Ats-1 is imported into host cell mitochondria and interferes with apoptosis induction." *PLoS Pathogens* 6, no. 2 (2010): e1000774.

Ojogun, N., B. Barnstein, B. Huang, et al. "Anaplasma phagocytophilum infects mast cells via alpha1,3-fucosylated but not sialylated glycans and inhibits IgE-mediated cytokine production and histamine release." *Infection and Immunity* 79, no. 7 (2011): 2717–26.

Paddock, C. D., and J. E. Childs. "Ehrlichia chaffeensis: A prototypical emerging pathogen." *Clinical Microbiology Reviews* 16, no. 1 (2003): 37–64.

Palomar, A. M., L. García-Álvarez, S. Santibáñez, et al. "Detection of tickborne 'Candidatus Neoehrlichia mikurensis' and Anaplasma phagocytophilum in Spain in 2013." *Parasites & Vectors* 7, no. 57 (2014): 57.

Park, J., K. S. Choi, D. J. Grab, et al. "Divergent interactions of Ehrlichia chaffeensis- and Anaplasma phagocytophilum-infected leukocytes with endothelial cell barriers." *Infection and Immunity* 71, no. 12 (2003): 6728–33.

Park, J., K. J. Kim, K. S. Choi, et al. "Anaplasma phagocytophilum AnkA binds to granulocyte DNA and nuclear proteins." *Cellular Microbiology* 6, no. 8 (2004): 743–51.

Park, S. J., and H. S. Youn. "Suppression of homodimerization of toll-like receptor 4 by isoliquiritigenin." *Phytochemistry* 71, nos. 14–15 (2010): 1736–40.

Perez, M., M. Bodor, C. Zhang, et al. "Human infection with Ehrlichia canis accompanied by clinical signs in Venezuela." *Annals of the New York Academy of Sciences* 1078 (2006): 110–17.

Perez, M., Y. Rikihisa, and B. Wen. "Ehrlichia canis-like agent isolated from a man in Venezuela: Antigenic and genetic characterization." *Journal of Clinical Microbiology* 34, no. 9 (1996): 2133–39.

Popov, V. L., E. L. Korenberg, V. V. Nefedova, et al. "Ultrastructural evidence of the ehrlichial developmental cycle in naturally infected Ixodes persulcatus ticks in the course of coinfection with Rickettsia, Borrelia, and a flavivirus." *Vector Borne and Zoonotic Diseases* 7, no. 4 (2007): 699–716.

Pritt, B. S., L. M. Sloan, D. K. H. Johnson, et al. "Emergence of a new pathogenic ehrlichia species, Wisconsin and Minnesota, 2009." *New England Journal of Medicine* 365, no. 5 (2011): 422–29.

Rikihisa, Y. "Molecular events involved in cellular invasion by Ehrlichia chaffensis and Anaplasma phagocytophilum." *Veterinary Parasitology* 167, nos. 2–4 (2010): 155.

Rikihisa, Y., and M. Lin. "Anaplasma phagocytophilum and Ehrlichia chaffeensis type IV secretion and Ank proteins." *Current Opinion in Microbiology* 13, no. 1 (2010): 59–66.

Rikihisa, Y., Y. Zhang, and J. Park. "Inhibition of infection of macrophages with Ehrlichia risticii by cytochalasins, monodansylcadaverine, and taxol." *Infection and Immunity* 62, no. 11 (1994): 5126–32.

Rymaszewska, A., and S. Grenda. "Bacteria of the genus Anaplasma—characteristics of Anaplasma and their vectors: A review." *Veterinarni Medicina* 53, no. 11 (2008): 573–84.

Sehdev, A. E., and S. Dumler. "Hepatic pathology in human monocytic ehrlichiosis. Ehrlichia chaffeensis infection." *American Society for Clinical Pathology* 119, no. 6 (2003): 859–65.

Shah, S. S., and J. P McGowan. "Rickettsial, ehrlichial and bartonella infections of the myocardium and pericardium." *Frontiers in Bioscience* 8 (2003): e197–201.

Sharma, L., J. Wu, V. Patel, et al. "Partially-desulfated heparin improves survival in Pseudomonas pneumonia by enhancing bacterial clearance and ameliorating lung injury." *Journal of Immunotoxicology* 11, no. 3 (2014): 260–67. Published electronically ahead of print October 7, 2013.

Socolovschi, C., T. Kernif, D. Raoult, et al. "Borrelia, Rickettsia, and Ehrlichia species in bat ticks, France, 2010." *Emerging Infectious Diseases* 18, no. 12 (2012): 1966–75.

Stevenson, H. L., M. D. Estes, N. R. Thirumalapura, et al. "Natural killer cells promoted tissue injury and systemic inflammatory responses during fatal Ehrlichia-induced toxic shock-like syndrome." *American Journal of Pathology* 177, no. 2 (2010): 766–76.

Stevenson, H., J. M. Jordan, Z. Peerwani, et al. "An intradermal environment promotes a protective type-1 response against lethal systemic monocytotropic ehrlichial infection." *Infection and Immunity* 74, no. 8 (2006): 4856–64.

Stitch, R. W., J. J. Schaefer, W. G. Bremer, et al. "Host surveys, ixodid tick biology and transmission scenarios as related to the tick-borne pathogen, Ehrlichia canis." *Veterinary Parasitology* 158, no. 4 (2008): 256–73.

Stone, J. H., K. Dierberg, G. Aram, et al. "Human monocytic ehrlichiosis."

Journal of the American Medical Association 292, no. 18 (2004): 2263–70.

Stuen, S., E. G. Granquist, and C. Silaghi. "Anaplasma phagocytophilum—a widespread multi-host pathogen with highly adaptive strategies." *Frontiers in Cellular and Infection Microbiology* 3, no. 31 (2013).

Talsness, S. R., S. K. Shukla, J. J. Mazza, et al. "Rhabdomyolysis-induced acute kidney injury secondary to Anaplasma phagocytophilum and concomitant statin use." *WMJ* 110, no. 2 (2011): 82–84.

Thirumalapura, N. R., H. L. Stevenson, D. H. Walker, et al. "Protective heterologous immunity against fatal ehrlichiosis and lack of protection following homologous challenge." *Infection and Immunity* 76, no. 5 (2008): 1920–30.

Thomas, R. J., J. S. Dumler, and J. A. Carlyon. "Current management of human granulocytic anaplasmosis, human monocytic ehrlichiosis and Ehrlichia ewingii ehrlichiosis." *Expert Review of Anti-Infective Therapy* 7, no. 6 (2009): 709–22.

Thomas, S., V. L. Popov, and D. H. Walker. "Exit mechanisms of the intracellular bacterium Ehrlichia." *PLoS ONE* 5, no. 12 (2010): e15775.

Thring, T. S., P. Hili, and D. P. Naughton. "Anti-collagenase, anti-elastase and anti-oxidant activities of extracts from 21 plants." *BMC Complementary and Alternative Medicine* 9 (2009): 27.

Torina, A., A. Alongi, V. Naranjo, et al. "Characterization of anaplasma infections in Sicily, Italy." *Annals of the New York Academy of Sciences* 1149 (2008): 90–93.

Torina, A., V. Blanda, F. Antoci, et al. "A molecular survey of Anaplasma spp., Rickettsia spp., Ehrlichia canis and Babesia microti in foxes and fleas from Sicily." *Transbound Emerging Diseases* 60, suppl. 2 (2013): 125–30.

Troese, M. J., A. Kahlon, S. A. Ragland, et al. "Proteomic analysis of Anaplasma phagocytophilum during infection of human myeloid cells identifies a protein that is pronouncedly upregulated on the infectious dense-cored cell." *Infection and Immunity* 79, no. 11 (2011): 4696–707.

Tuo, W., G. H. Palmer, T. C. McGuire, et al. "Interleukin-12 as an adjuvant promotes immunoglobulin G and type 1 cytokine recall responses to major surface protein 2 of the ehrlichial pathogen Anaplasma marginale." *Infection and Immunity* 68, no. 1 (2000): 270–80.

Unver, A., H. Huang, and Y. Rikihisa. "Cytokine gene expression by peripheral blood leukocytes in dogs experimentally infected with a new virulent strain of Ehrlichia canis." *Annals of the New York Academy of Sciences* 1078 (2006): 482–86.

Vezzani, A., M. Maroso, S. Balosso, et al. "IL-1 receptor/toll-like receptor signaling in infection, inflammation, stress and neurodegeneration couples hyperexcitability and seizures." *Brain, Behavior and Immunity* 25, no. 7 (2011): 1281–89.

Vieira, R. F., T. S. Vieira, and A. Nascimento Ddo. "Serological survey of Ehrlichia species in dogs, horses and humans: Zoonotic scenery in a rural settlement from southern Brazil." *Revista do Instituto de Medicina Tropical de São Paulo* 55, no. 5 (2013): 335–40.

Wakeel, A., B. Zhu, X. J. Yu, et al. "New insights into molecular Ehrlichia chaffeensis-host interactions." *Microbes and Infections* 12, no. 5 (2010): 337–45.

Walker, D. H. "Ehrlichia under our noses and no one notices." *Archives of Virology. Supplementum*, no. 19 (2005): 147–56.

Walker, D. H., N. Ismail, J. P. Olano, et al. "Ehrlichia chaffeensis: A prevalent, life-threatening, emerging pathogen." *Transactions of the American Clinical and Climatological Association* 115 (2004): 375–84.

Waner, T. "Hematopathological changes in dogs infected with Ehrlichia canis." *Israel Journal of Veterinary Medicine* 63, no. 1 (2008).

Weil, A. A., E. L. Baron, C. M. Brown, et al. "Clinical findings and diagnosis in human granulocytic anaplasmosis: A case series from Massachusetts." *Mayo Clinic Proceedings* 87, no. 3 (2012): 233–39.

Xiong, Q., W. Bao, Y. Ge, et al. "Ehrlichia ewingii infection delays spontaneous neutrophil apoptosis through stabilization of mitochondria." *Journal of Infectious Diseases* 197, no. 8 (2008): 1110–18.

Xiong, Q., X. Wang, and Y. Rikihisa. "High-cholesterol diet facilitates Anaplasma phagocytophilum infection and up-regulates macrophage inflammatory protein-2 and CXCR2 expression in apolipoprotein E-deficient mice." *Journal of Infectious Diseases* 195 (2007): 1497–503.

Yager, E., C. Bitsaktsis, B. Nandi, et al. "Essential role for humoral immunity during Ehrlichia infection in immunocompetent mice." *Infection and Immunity* 73, no. 12 (2005): 8009–16.

Yoshie, K., H. Y. Kim, J. Mott, et al. "Intracellular infection by the human granulocytic ehrlichiosis agent inhibits human neutrophil apoptosis." *Infection and Immunity* 68, no. 3 (2000): 1125–33.

Zhang, J. Z., M. Sinha, B. A. Luxon, et al. "Survival strategy of obligately intracellular Ehrlichia chaffeensis: Novel modulation of immune response and host cell cycles." *Infection and Immunity* 72, no. 1 (2004): 498–507.

Zhang, Y., and Y. Rikihisa. "Tyrosine phosphorylation is required for ehrlichial internalization and replication in P388D1 cells." *Infection and Immunity* 65, no. 7 (1997): 2959–64.

Zhu, B., J. A. Kuriakose, T. Luo, et al. "Ehrlichia chaffeensis TRP120 binds a G+C-rich motif in host cell DNA and exhibits eukaryotic transciptional activator function." *Infection and Immunity* 79, no. 11 (2011): 4370–81.

Zhu, B., K. A. Nethery, J. A. Kuriakose, et al. "Nuclear translocated Ehrlichia chaffeensis ankyrin protein interacts with a specific adenine-rich motif of host promoter and intronic Alu elements." *Infection and Immunity* 77, no. 10 (2009): 4243–55.

Salvia miltiorrhiza

Ai, C. B., and L. N. Li. "Salvianolic acids D and E: Two new depsides from Salvia miltiorrhiza." *Planta Medica* 58, no. 2 (1992): 197–99.

Bao, Y., L. Wang, Y. Xu, et al. "Salvianolic acid B inhibits macrophage uptake of modified low density lipoprotein (mLDL) in a scavenger receptor CD36-dependent manner." *Atherosclerosis* 223, no. 1 (2012): 152–59.

Cao, J., Y. J. Wei, L. W. Qi, et al. "Determination of fifteen bioactive components in radix et rhizoma salviae miltiorrhizae by high-performance liquid chromatography with ultraviolet and mass spectrometric detection." *Biomedical Chromatography* 22, no. 2 (2008): 164–72.

Cao, Y. G., J. G. Chai, Y. C. Chen, et al. "Beneficial effects of danshensu, an active component of Salvia miltiorrhiza, on homocysteine metabolism via the trans-sulphuration pathway in rats." *British Journal of Pharmacology* 157, no. 3 (2009): 482–90.

Cao, Y. Y., L. Wang, H. Ge, et al. "Salvianolic acid A, a polyphenolic derivative from Salvia miltiorrhiza Bunge, as a multifunctional agent for the treatment of Alzheimer's disease." *Molecular Diversity* 17, no. 3 (2013): 515–24.

Chan, K., S. H. Chui, D. Y. Wong, et al. "Protective effects of danshensu from the aqueous extract of Salvia miltiorrhiza (danshen) against homocysteine-induced endothelial dysfunction." *Life Sciences* 75, no. 26 (2004): 3157–71.

Chang, B. B., L. Zhang, W. W. Cao, et al. "Pharmacokinetic interactions induced by content variation of major water-soluble components of danshen preparation in rats." *Acta Pharmacologica Sinica* 31, no. 5 (2010): 638–46.

Chen, J., F. Wang, F. S. Lee, et al. "Separation and identification of water-soluble salvianolic acids from Salvia miltiorrhiza Bunge by high-speed counter-current chromatography and ESI-MS analysis." *Talanta* 69, no. 1 (2006): 172–79.

Chen, M. K., Z. X. Chen, J. C. Han, et al. "[Effects of Salvia miltiorrhiza on Chlamydia trachomatis mice of salpingitis.]" *Zhongguo Zhong Yao Za Zhi* 32, no. 6 (2007): 523–25.

Chen, Y. S., S. M. Lee, Y. J. Lin, et al. "Effects of danshensu and salvianolic acid B from Salvia miltiorrhiza Bunge (Lamiaceae) on cell proliferation and collagen and melanin production." *Molecules* 19, no. 2 (2014): 2029–41.

Choi, H. S., and K. M. Kim. "Tanshinones inhibit mast cell degranulation by interfering with IgE receptor-mediated tyrosine phosphorylation of PLCgamma2 and MAPK." *Planta Medica* 70, no. 2 (2004): 178–80.

Chumming, J., Z. Miao, S. Cheng, et al. "Tanshinone IIA attenuates peritoneal fibrosis through inhibition of fibrogenic growth factors expression in peritoneum in a peritoneal dialysis rat model." *Renal Failure* 33, no. 3 (2011): 355–62.

Cui, L., T. Li, Y. Liu, et al. "Salvianolic acid B prevents bone loss in prednisone-treated rats through stimulation of osteogenesis and bone marrow angiogenesis." *PLoS ONE* 7, no. 4 (2012): e34647.

Cui, Y., B. Bhandary, A. Marahatta, et al. "Characterization of Salvia miltiorrhiza ethanol extract as an anti-osteoporotic agent." *BMC Complementary and Alternative Medicine* 11 (2011): 120.

Dai, H., X. Li, X. Li, et al. "Coexisted components of Salvia miltiorrhiza enhance intestinal absorption of cryptotanshinone via inhibition of the intestinal P-gp." *Phytomedicine* 19, no. 14 (2012): 1256–62.

Dai, H., C. Xiao, H. Liu, et al. "Combined NMR and LC-MS analysis reveals the metabonomic changes in Salvia miltiorrhiza Bunge induced by water depletion." *Journal of Proteome Research* 9, no. 3 (2010): 1460–75.

Dasgupta, A., E. Kang, M. Olsen, et al. "New enzyme-linked chemiluminescent immunosorbent digoxin assay is free from interference of Chinese medicine danshen." *Therapeutic Drug Monitoring* 28, no. 6 (2006): 775–78.

De Palma, A., R. Rossi, M. Carai, et al. "Pharmaceutical and biomedical analysis of terpene constituents in Salvia miltiorrhiza." *Current Pharmaceutical Analysis* 4, no. 4 (2008): 249–57.

Ding, M., T. X. Ye, G. R. Zhao, et al. "Aqueous extract of Salvia miltiorrhiza attenuates increased endothelial permeability induced by tumor necrosis factor alpha." *International Immunopharmacology* 5, no. 11 (2005): 1641–51.

Ding, M., G. R. Zhao, Y. J. Yuan, et al. "Aqueous extract of Salvia miltiorrhoza regulates adhesion molecule expression of tumor necrosis factor alpha-induced endothelial cells by blocking activation of nuclear factor kappaB." *Journal of Cardiovascular Pharmacology* 45, no. 6 (2005): 516–24.

Dong, J., Y. Liu, Z. Liang, et al. "Investigation on ultrasound-assisted extraction of salvianolic acid B from Salvia miltiorrhiza root." *Ultrasonics Sonochemistry* 17, no. 1 (2010): 61–65.

Dong, Y., S. L. Morris-Natschke, and K. H. Lee. "Biosynthesis, total syntheses, and antitumor activity of tanshinones and their analogs as potential therapeutic agents." *Natural Product Reports* 28, no. 3 (2011): 529–42.

Gao, D., A. Mendoza, S. Lu, et al. "Immunomodulatory effects of danshen (Salvia miltiorrhiza) in BALB/c mice." *ISRN Inflammation*, 2012: 954032.

Han, J. Y., J. Y. Fan, Y. Horie, et al. "Ameliorating effects of compounds derived from Salvia miltiorrhiza root extract on microcirculatory disturbance and target organ injury by ischemia and reperfusion." *Pharmacology and Therapeutics* 117, no. 2 (2008): 280–95.

Hatfield, M. J., L. G. Tsurkan, J. L. Hyatt, et al. "Modulation of esterified drug metabolism by tanshinones from Salvia miltiorriza ('danshen')." *Journal of Natural Products* 76, no. 1 (2013): 36–44.

Ho, J. H., and C. Y. Hong. "Salvianolic acids: Small compounds with multiple mechanisms for cardiovascular protection." *Journal of Biomedical Science* 18 (2011): 30.

Jang, S. I., S. I Jeong, K. J. Kim, et al. "Tanshinone IIA from Salvia miltiorrhiza inhibits inducible nitric oxide synthase expression and production of TNF-alpha, IL-1beta and IL-6 in activated RAW 264.7 cells." *Planta Medica* 69, no. 11 (2003): 1057–59.

Ji, K. T., J. D. Chai, C. Xing, et al. "Danshen protects endothelial progenitor cells from oxidized low-density lipoprotein induced impairment." *Journal of Zhejiang University. Science. B* 11, no. 8 (2010): 618–26.

Jia, Y., F. Huang, S. Zhang, et al. "Is danshen (Salvia miltiorrhiza) dripping pill more effective than isosorbide dinitrate in treating angina pectoris? A systematic review of randomized controlled trials." *International Journal of Cardiology* 157, no. 3 (2012): 330–40.

Jiang, B., D. Li, Y. Deng, et al. "Salvianolic acid A, a novel matrix metalloproteinase-9 inhibitor, prevents cardiac remodeling in spontaneously hypertensive rats." *PLoS ONE* 8, no. 3 (2013): e59621.

Jiang, R. W., K. M. Lau, P. M. Hon, et al. "Chemistry and biological activities of caffeic acid derivatives from Salvia miltiorrhiza." *Current Medicinal Chemistry* 12, no. 2 (2005): 237–46.

Jin, H. J., X. L. Xie, J. M. Ye, et al. "TanshinoneIIA and cryptotanshinone protect against hypoxia-induced mitochondrial apoptosis in H9c2 cells." *PLoS ONE* 8, no. 1 (2013): e51720.

Joe, Y., M. Zheng, H. J. Kim, et al. "Salvianolic acid B exerts vasoprotective effects through the modulation of heme oxygenase-1 and arginase activities." *Journal of Pharmocology and Experimental Therapeutics* 341, no. 3 (2012): 850–58.

Kim, H. K., E. R. Woo, H. W. Lee, et al. "The correlation of Salvia miltiorrhiza extract-induced regulation of osteoclastogenesis with the amount of components tanshinone I, tanshinone IIA, cryptotanshinone, and dihydrotanshinone." *Immunopharmacology and Immunotoxicology* 30, no. 2 (2008): 347–64.

Kim, J. S., A. S. Narula, and C. Jobin. "Salvia miltiorrhiza water-soluble extract, but not its constituent salvianolic acid B, abrogates LPS-induced NF-kappaB signalling in intestinal epithelial cells." *Clinical and Experimental Immunology* 141, no. 2 (2005): 288–97.

Lee, D. S., and S. H. Lee. "Biological activity of dihydrotanshinone I: Effect on apoptosis." *Journal of Bioscience and Bioengineering* 89, no. 3 (2000): 292–93.

Lee, D. S., S. H. Lee, J. G. Noh, et al. "Antibacterial acitivities of crypto-tanshinone and dihydrotanshinone I from a medicinal herb, Salvia miltiorrhiza Bunge." *Bioscience, Biotechnology and Biochemistry* 63, no. 12 (1999): 2236–39.

Lee, J. C., J. H. Park, O. K. Park, et al. "Neuroprotective effects of tanshinone I from danshen extract in a mouse model of hypoxia ischemia." *Anatomy and Cell Biology* 46, no. 3 (2013): 183–90.

Lee, J. W., Y. J. Ji, S. O. Lee, et al. "Effect of Salvia miltiorrhiza Bunge on antimicrobial activity and resistant gene regulation against methicillin-resistant Staphylococcus aureus (MRSA)." *Journal of Microbiology* 45, no. 4 (2007): 350–57.

Lee, K. M., J. H. Bang, J. S. Han, et al. "Carditonic pill attenuates white matter and hippocampal damage via inhibiting microglial activation and downregulating ERK and p38 MAPK signaling in chronic cerebral hypoperfused rat." *BMC Complementary and Alternative Medicine* 13 (2013): 334.

Li, C. G., S. J. Sheng, E. C. Pang, et al. "HPLC profiles and biomarker contents of Australian-grown Salvia miltiorrhiza f. alba roots." *Chemistry and Biodiversity* 6, no. 7 (2009): 1077–86.

Li, C. G., S. J. Sheng, E. C. Pang, et al. "Plant density-dependent variations in bioactive markers and root yield in Australian-grown Salvia miltiorrhiza Bunge." *Chemistry and Biodiversity* 8, no. 4 (2011): 699–709.

Li, F. L., R. Xu, Q. C. Zeng, et al. "Tanshinone IIA inhibits growth of keratinocytes through cell cycle arrest and apoptosis: Underlying treatment mechanism of psoriasis." *Evidence-Based Complementary and Alternative Medicine*, 2012: 927658.

Li, M. H., Q. Q. Li, Y. Z. Liu, et al. "Pharmacophylogenetic study on plants of genus Salvia L. from China." *Chinese Herbal Medicines* 5, no. 3 (2013): 164–81.

Li, X. B., W. Weng, G. J. Zhou, et al. "Production of salvianolic acid B in roots of Salvia miltiorrhiza (danshen) during the post-harvest drying process." *Molecules* 17, no. 3 (2012): 2388–407.

Li, Y. G., L. Song, M. Liu, et al. "Advancement in analysis of salviae miltior-rhizae radix et rhizoma (danshen)." *Journal of Chromatography. A* 1216, no. 11 (2009): 1941–53.

Lin, T. S., and C. L. Hsieh. "Pharmacological effects of Salvia miltiorrhiza (danshen) on cerebral infarction." *Chinese Medicine* 5 (2010): 22

Liu, M., Y. G. Li, F. Zhang, et al. "Chromatographic fingerprinting analysis of danshen root (Salvia miltiorrhiza radix et rhizoma) and its prepara-tions using high performance liquid chromatography with diode array detection and electrospray mass spectrometry (HPLC-DAD-ESI/MS)." *Journal of Separation Science* 30, no. 14 (2007): 2256–67.

Lu, L., Y. Liu, Z. Zhang, et al. "Analysis of danshen and twelve related Salvia species." *Natural Product Communications* 7, no. 1 (2012): 59–60.

Luo, Y., W. Chen, H. Zhou, et al. "Cryptotanshinone inhibits lymphatic endothelial cell tube formation by supressing VEGFR-3/ERK and small GTPase pathways." *Cancer Prevention Research* (Philadelphia) 4, no. 12 (2011): 2083–91.

Lv, Z., and L. Xu. "Salvianolic acid B inhibits ERK and p38 MAPK sig-naling in TGF-beta1-stimulated human hepatic stellate cell line (LX-2) via distinct pathways." *Evidence-Based Complementary and Alternative Medicine*, 2012: 960128.

Ma, H. L., M. J. Qin, L. W. Qi, et al. "Improved quality evaluation of radix Salvia miltiorrhiza through simultaneous quantification of seven major active components by high-performance liquid chromatography and principal component analysis." *Biomedical Chromatog*raphy 21, no. 9 (2007): 931–39.

Moon, S., S. Shing, S. Kim, et al. "Role of Salvia miltiorrhiza for modulation of Th2-derived cytokines in the resolution of inflammation." *Immune Network* 11, no. 5 (2011): 288–98.

Nosrati, H., and A. Nostrati. "A survey on the genus Salvia as the largest genus of plants." *Agriculture Science Developments* 2, no. 1 (2013): 1–3.

Pan, T. L., and P. W. Wang. "Explore the molecular mechanism of apop-tosis induced by tanshinone IIA on activated rat hepatic stellate cells." *Evidence-Based Complementary and Alternative Medicine*, 2012: 734987.

Qiu, F., G. Wang, R. Zhang, et al. "Effect of danshen extract on the activity of CYP3A4 in healthy volunteers." *British Journal of Clinical Pharmacology* 69, no. 6 (2010): 656–62.

Qiu, F., G. Wang, Y. Zhao, et al. "Effect of danshen extract on pharmacokinetics of theophylline in healthy volunteers." *British Journal of Clinical Pharmacology* 65, no. 2 (2007): 270–74.

Qiu, F., R. Zhang, J. Sun, et al. "Inhibitory effects of seven components of danshen extract on catalytic activity of cytochrome P450 enzyme in human liver microsomes." *Drug Metabolism and Disposition* 36, no. 7 (2008): 1308–14.

Sferra, R., A. Vetuschi, V. Catitti, et al. "Boswellia serrata and Salvia miltiorrhiza extracts reduce DMN-induced hepatic fibrosis in mice by TGF-beta1 downregulation." *European Review for Medical and Pharmocological Sciences* 16, no. 11 (2012): 1484–98.

Shen, Y., X. Wang, L. Xu, et al. "Characterization of metabolites in rat plasma after intravenous administration of salvianolic acid A by liquid chromatography/time-of-flight mass spectrometry and liquid chromatography/ion trap mass spectrometry." *Rapid Communications in Mass Spectrometry* 23, no. 12 (2009): 1810–16.

Sheng, S. J., E. C. Pang, C. C. Xue, et al. "Seasonal variation in bioactive marker contents in Australian-grown Salvia miltiorrhiza roots." *Chemistry and Biodiversity* 6, no. 4 (2009): 551–60.

Shu, T., M. Pang, L. Rong, et al. "Effects of Salvia miltiorrhiza on neural differentiation of induced pluripotent stem cells." *Journal of Ethnopharmacology* 153, no. 1 (2014): 233–41.

Song, J. Z., C. F. Qiao, S. L. Li, et al. "Quality assessment of granule of danshen extract by high performance liquid chromatography." *Chinese Journal of Natural Medicines* 7, no. 5 (2009): 368–75.

Song, M., T. J. Hang, Z. Zhang, et al. "Effects of the coexisting diterpenoid tanshinones on the pharmacokinetics of cryptotanshinone and tanshinone IIA in rat." *European Journal of Pharmaceutical Sciences* 32, nos. 4–5 (2007): 247–53.

Song, Y. H., Q. Liu, Z. P. Lv, et al. "Protection of a polysaccharide from Salvia miltiorrhiza, a Chinese medicinal herb, against immunological liver injury in mice." *International Journal of Biological Macromolecules* 43, no. 2 (2008): 170–75.

Sung, H. J., S. M. Choi, Y. Yoon, et al. "Tanshinone IIA, an ingredient of Salvia miltiorrhiza Bunge, induces apoptosis in human leukemia cell lines through the activation of caspase-3." *Experimental and Molecular Medicine* 31, no. 4 (1999): 174–78.

Tsai, H. H., H. W. Lin, Y. H. Lu, et al. "A review of potential harmful interactions between anticoagulant/antiplatelet agents and Chinese herbal medicines." *PLoS ONE* 8, no. 5 (2013): e64255.

Wan, J. M., W. H. Sit, C. L. Lee, et al. "Protection of lethal toxicity of endotoxin by Salvia miltiorrhiza Bunge is via reduction in tumor necrosis factor alpha release and liver injury." *International Immunopharmacology* 6, no. 5 (2006): 750–58.

Wang, J., X. Xiong, and B. Feng. "Cardiovascular effects of salvianolic acid B." *Evidence-Based Complementary and Alternative Medicine*, 2013: 247948.

Wang, X., W. Y. Lee, X. Zhou, et al. "A pharmacodynamic-pharmacokinetic (PD-PK) study on the effects of danshen (Salvia miltiorrhiza) on midazolam, a model CYP3A probe substrate, in the rat." *Phytomedicine* 17, no. 11 (2010): 876–83.

Wang, X., S. L. Morris-Natschke, and K. H. Lee. "New developments in the chemistry and biology of the bioactive constituents of tanshen." *Medical Research Reviews* 27, no. 1 (2007): 133–48.

Wang, X., and J. H. Yeung. "Effects of Salvia miltiorrhiza extract on the liver CYP3A activity in humans and rats." *Phytotherapy Research* 25, no. 11 (2011): 1653–59.

Wang, X., and J. H. Yeung. "Investigation of cytochrome P450 1A2 and 3A inhibitory properties of danshen tincture." *Phytomedicine* 19, nos. 3–4 (2012): 348–54.

Wang, Y., H. Peng, Y. Shen, et al. "The profiling of bioactive ingredients of differently aged Salvia miltiorrhiza roots." *Microscopy Research and Technique* 76, no. 9 (2013): 947–54.

Wang, Y. S., L. N. Zhao, G. W. Song, et al. "Effect of different growth periods on tanshinone IIA and crypto-tanshinone contents in Salvia miltiorrhiza of Yu canton." *Food, Agriculture and Environment* 11, nos. 3–4 (2013): 448–50.

Won, S. H., H. J. Lee, S. J. Jeong, et al. "Tanshinone IIA induces mitochondria dependent apoptosis in prostate cancer cells in association with an inhibition of phosphoinositide 3-kinase/AKT pathway." *Biological and Pharmaceutical Bulletin* 33, no. 11 (2010): 1828–34.

Wong, C. K., Y. X. Bao, E. L. Wong, et al. "Immunomodulatory activities of yunzhi and danshen in post-treatment breast cancer patients." *American Journal of Chinese Medicine* 33, no. 3 (2005): 381–95.

Wong, C. K., P. S. Tse, E. L. Wong, et al. "Immunomodulatory effects of yun zhi and danshen capsules in health subjects—a randomized, double-blind, placebo-controlled, crossover study." *International Immunopharmacology* 4 (2004): 201–11.

Woo, K. S., T. W. Yip, S. K. Kwong, et al. "Cardiovascular protective effects and adjunctive alternative medicine (Salvia miltiorrhiza and Pueraria lobata) in high-risk hypertension." *Evidence-Based Complementary Alternative Medicine*, 2013: 132912.

Wu, S. J., S. J. Lee, C. H. Su, et al. "Bioactive constituents and anti-proliferative properties of supercritical carbon dioxide Salvia miltiorrhiza extract in 3T3-L1 adipocytes." *Process Biochemistry* 47, no. 2 (2012): 216–24.

Wu, W., Y. Zhu, L. Zhang, et al. "Extraction, preliminary structural characterization, and antioxidant activities of polysaccharides from Salvia miltiorrhiza Bunge." *Carbohydrate Polymers* 87, no. 2 (2012): 1348–53.

Xing, H. C., L. J. Li, K. J. Xu, et al. "Effects of Salvia miltiorrhiza on intestinal microflora in rats with ischemia/reperfusion liver injury." *Hepatobiliary and Pancreatic Diseases International* 4, no. 2 (2005): 274–80.

Xiping, Z., L. Chuyang, Z. Jie, et al. "Protection of Salvia miltiorrhizae to the spleen and thymus of rats with severe acute pancreatitis or obstructive jaundice." *Mediators of Inflammation*, 2009: 186136.

Xiping, Z., Z. Jie, Y. Shuyun, et al. "Influence of Salvia miltiorrhizae on the mesentric lymph node of rats with severe acute pancreatitis or obstructive jaundice." *Mediators of Inflammation*, 2009: 675195.

Yao, F., D. W. Zhang, G. W. Qu, et al. "New abietane norditerpenoid from Salvia miltiorrhiza with cytotoxic activities." *Journal of Asian Natural Product Research* 14, no. 9 (2012): 913–17.

Yin, X., Y. Yin, F. L. Cao, et al. "Tanshinone IIA attenuates the inflammatory response and apoptosis after traumatic injury of the spinal cord in adult rats." *PLoS ONE* 7, no. 7 (2012): e38381.

Yu, P. F., W. Y. Wang, G. Eerdun, et al. "The role of P-glycoprotein in transport of danshensu across the blood-brain barrier." *Evidence-Based Complementary Alternative Medicine*, 2011: 713523.

Yu, X., L. Zhang, X. Yang, et al. "Salvianolic acid A protects the peripheral nerve function in diabetic rats through regulation of the AMPK-PGC1alpha-Sirt3 axis." *Molecules* 17, no. 9 (2012): 11216–28.

Yu, X. Y., S. G. Lin, X. Chen, et al. "Transport of cryptotanshinone, a major active triterpenoid in Salvia miltiorrhiza Bunge widely used in the treatment of stroke and Alzheimer's disease, across the blood-brain barrier." *Current Drug Metabolism* 8, no. 4 (2007): 365–78.

Yuan, J., X. Wang, T. Chen, et al. "Salvia miltiorrhiza depresses plasminogen activator inhibitor-1 production through inhibition of angiotension II." *American Journal of Chinese Medicine* 36, no. 5 (2008): 1005–15.

Yuan, Y., H. Zhang, W. Ma, et al. "Influence of compound danshen tablet on the pharmacokinetics of losartan and its metabolite EXP3174 by liquid chromatography coupled with mass spectrometry." *Biomedical Chromatography* 27, no. 9 (2013): 1219–24.

Zelenak, C., V. Pasham, K. Jilani, et al. "Tanshinone IIA stimulates erythrocyte phosphatidylserine exposure." *Cellular Physiology and Biochemistry* 30, no. 1 (2012): 282–94.

Zeng, G., H. Xiao, J. Liu, et al. "Identification of phenolic constituents in radix Salvia miltiorrhizae by liquid chromatography/electrospray ionization mass spectrometry." *Rapid Communications in Mass Spectrometry* 20, no. 3 (2006): 499–506.

Zhang, D. W., X. Liu, D. Xie, et al. "Two new diterpenoids from cell cultures of Salvia miltiorrhiza." *Chemical and Pharmaceutical Bulletin* 61, no. 5 (2013): 576–80.

Zhang, L., W. Zhang, Y. Zhao, et al. "[Research progress of salvianolic acid A]." *Zhongguo Zhong Yao Za Zhi* 36, no. 19 (2011): 2603–9.

Zhang, L., H. X. Zhao, X. Fan, et al. "Genetic diversity among Salvia miltiorrhiza Bunge and related species inferred from nrDNA ITS sequences." *Turkish Journal of Biology* 36 (2012): 319–26.

Zhang, Y., P. Jiang, M. Ye, et al. "Tanshinones: Sources, pharmacokinetics and anti-cancer activities." *International Journal of Molecular Sciences* 13, no. 10 (2012): 13621–66.

Zhao, J., J. Lou, Y. Mou, et al. "Diterpenoid tanshinones and phenolic acids from cultured hairy roots of Salvia miltiorrhiza Bunge and their antimicrobial activities." *Molecules* 16, no. 3 (2011): 2259–67.

Zhong, G. X., P. Li, L. J. Zeng, et al. "Chemical characteristics of Salvia miltiorrhiza (danshen) collected from different locations in China." *Journal of Agricultural and Food Chemistry* 57, no. 15 (2009): 6879–87.

Zhou, H. Z., T. M. Lv, P. Shen, et al. "[Protective effects of nerve growth factor vs danshen on hippocampal neuron against global ischemia-reperfusion injury in gerbils]." *Nan Fang Yi Ke Da Xue Xue Bao* 31, no. 6 (2011): 965–69.

Zhou, L., W. K. Chan, N. Xu, et al. "Tanshinone IIA, an isolated compound from Salvia miltiorrhiza Bunge, induces apoptosis in HeLa cells through mitotic arrest." *Life Sciences* 83, nos. 11–12 (2008): 394–403.

Zhou, L., S. Wang, Z. Zhang, et al. "Pharmacokinetic and pharmacodynamic interaction of danshen-gegan extract with warfarin and aspirin." *Journal of Ethnopharmacology* 143, no. 2 (2012): 648–55.

Zhou, X., K. Chan, and J. H. Yeung. "Herb-drug interactions with danshen (Salvia miltiorrhiza): A review on the role of cytochrome P450 enzymes." *Drug Metabolism and Drug Interactions* 27, no. 1 (2012): 9–18.

Zhou, Z. H., Q. Weng, J. H. Zhou, et al. "Extracts of Salvia miltiorrhiza Bunge on the cytokines of rats endometriosis models." *African Journal of Traditional, Complementary and Alternative Medicine* 9, no. 3 (2012): 303–14.

Miscellaneous Herbs

Abdollah, G. P., G. M. Reza, M. Hasan, et al. "The effect of some of the Iranian medicinal plants on Brucella abortus on in-vitro and in-vivo." *Journal of Herbal Drugs* 1, no. 1 (2010): 21–29.

Adams, M. R., C. J. Forsyth, W. Jessup, et al. "Oral L-arginine inhibits platelet aggregation but does not enhance endothelium-dependent dilation in healthy young men." *Journal of the American College of Cardiology* 26, no. 4 (1995): 1054–61.

Adams, M. R., R. McCredie, W. Jessup, et al. "Oral L-arginine improves endothelium-dependent dilatation and reduces monocyte adhesion to endothelial cells in young men with coronary artery disease." *Atherosclerosis* 129, no. 2 (1997): 261–69.

Agarwal, C., R. P. Singh, S. Dhanalakshmi, et al. "Silibinin upregulates the expression of cyclin-dependent kinase inhibitors and causes cell cycle arrest and apoptosis in human colon carcinoma HT-29 cells." *Oncogene* 22, no. 51 (2003): 8271–82.

Ahmad, N., P. Cheng, and H. Mukhtar. "Cell cycle dysregulation by green tea polyphenol epigallocatechin-3-gallate." *Biochemical and Biophysical Research Communications* 275, no. 2 (2000): 328–34.

Ahn, S. I., J. K. Lee, and H. S. Youn. "Inhibition of homodimerization of toll-like receptor 4 by 6-shogaol." *Molecules and Cells* 27, no. 2 (2009): 211–15.

Ajayi, A. F., R. E Akhigbe, O. M. Adewumi, et al. "Haematological evaluation of Cryptolepis sanguinolenta stem ethanolic extract in rats." *International Journal of Medicine and Biomedical Research* 1, no. 1 (2012): 56–61.

Allan, B. F., H. P. Humberto, L. S. Goessling, et al. "Invasive honeysuckle eradication reduces tick-borne disease risk by altering host dynamics." *Proceedings of the National Academy of Sciences USA* 107, no. 43 (2010): 18523–27.

Al-Mariri, A., and M. Safi. "The antibacterial activity of selected Labiatae (Lamiaceae) essential oils against Brucella melitensis." *Iranian Journal of Medical Sciences* 38, no. 1 (2013): 44–50.

Al-Mariri, A., G. Saour, and R. Hamoud. "In vitro antibacterial effects of five volatile oil extracts against intramacrophage Brucella abortus 544." *Iranian Journal of Medical Sciences* 37, no. 2 (2012): 119–125.

Amirghofran, Z. "Herbal medicines for immunosuppression." *Iranian Journal of Allergy, Asthma, and Immunology* 11, no. 2 (2012): 111–19.

Bani, S., M. Gautam, F. A. Sheikh, et al. "Selective Th1 up-regulating activity of Withania somnifera aqueous extract in an experimental system using flow cytometry." *Journal of Ethnopharmacology* 107, no. 1 (2006): 107–15.

Banjerdpongchai, R., and P. Kongtawelert. "Ethanolic extract of fermented Thunb induces human leukemic HL-60 and Molt-4 cell apoptosis via oxidative stress and a mitochondrial pathway." *Asian Pacific Journal of Cancer Prevention* 12, no. 11 (2011): 2871–74.

Bi, C. W., H. Q. Xie, L. Xu, et al. "Fo shou san, an ancient herbal decoction prepared from rhizoma chuanxiong and radix angelicae sinensis, stimulates the production of hemoglobin and erythropoietin in cultured cells." *Planta Medica* 76, no. 14 (2010): 1525–29.

Bickford, P. C., J. Tan, R. D. Shytle, et al. "Nutraceuticals synergistically promote proliferation of human stem cells." *Stem Cells and Development* 15, no. 1 (2006): 118–23.

Blum, A., L. Hathaway, R. Mincemoyer, et al. "Effects of oral L-arginine on endothelium-dependent vasodilation and markers of inflammation in healthy postmenopausal women." *Journal of the American College of Cardiology* 35, no. 2 (2000): 271–76.

Borrelli, F., G. Aviello, B. Romano, et al. "Cannabidiol, a safe and non-psychotropic ingredient of the marijuana plant Cannibis sativa, is protective in a murine model of colitis." *Journal of Molecular Medicine* (Berlin) 87, no. 11 (2009): 1111–21.

Bose, A., K. Chakraborty, K. Sarkar, et al. "Neem leaf glycoprotein directs T-bet-associated type 1 immune commitment." *Human Immunology* 70, no. 1 (2009): 6–15.

Braga, P. C., M. Dal Sasso, M. Culici, et al. "Anti-inflammatory activity of thymol: Inhibitory effect on the release of human neutrophil elastase." *Pharmacology* 77, no. 3 (2006): 130–36.

Burnett, B. P., L. Pillai, A. Bitto, et al. "Evaluation of CYP450 inhibitory effects and steady-state pharmacokinetics of genistein in combination with cholecalciferol and citrated zinc bisglycinate in postmenopausal women." *International Journal of Women's Health* 3 (2011): 139–50. Published electronically ahead of print May 9, 2011.

Cai, T. G. and Y. Cai. "Triterpenes from the fungus Poria cocos and their inhibitory activity on nitric oxide production in mouse macrophages via blockade of activating protein-1 pathway." *Chemistry and Biodiversity* 8, no. 11 (2011): 2135–43.

Calixto, J. B., M. M. Campos, M. F. Otuki, et al. "Anti-inflammatory compounds of plant origin. Part II. Modulation of pro-inflammatory cytokines chemokines and adhesion molecules." *Planta Medica* 70, no. 2 (2004): 93–103.

Chao, W. W., Y. H. Kuo, W. C. Li, et al. "The production of nitric oxide and prostaglandin E2 in peritoneal macrophages is inhibited by Andrographis paniculata, Angelica sinensis and Morus alba ethyl acetate fractions." *Journal of Ethnopharmacology* 122, no. 1 (2009): 68–75.

Chen, C. C., T. H. Hung, Y. H. Wang, et al. "Wogonin improves histological and functional outcomes, and reduces activation of TLR4/NF-kappaB signaling after experimental traumatic brain injury." *PLoS ONE* 7, no. 1 (2012): e30294.

Chen, D., et al. "[Experimental study on expressing GM-CSF in human bone marrow stromal cells by total saponins of Panax ginseng (TSPG)]." *Journal of Chongqing Medical University* 2003-04. http://en.cnki.com.cn/Article_en/CJFDTOTAL-ZQYK200304000.htm.

Chen, T., et al."[Effect of total saponins of Panax ginseng on K562 cells in expressing clusters of differentiation antigen and hematopoietic growth factor recepters]." *Journal of Chongqing Medical University* 2003-05. http://en.cnki.com.cn/Article_en/CJFDTOTAL-ZQYK200305003.htm.

Chen, X., J. Chen, P. Zhang, and J. Du. "Angelica stimulates proliferation of murine bone marrow mononuclear cells by the MAPK pathway." *Blood Cells, Molecules and Diseases* 36, no. 3 (2006): 402–5. Published electronically ahead of print May 9, 2006.

Chen, Y. C., S. C. Shen, W. R. Lee, et al. "Emodin induces apoptosis in human promyeloleukemic HL-60 cells accompanied by activation of caspase 3 cascade but independent of reactive oxygen species production." *Biochemical Pharmacology* 64, no. 12 (2002): 1713–24.

Chen, Z., M. Y. Soon, N. Srinivasan, et al. "Activation of macrophages by polysaccharide-protein complex from Lycium barbarum L." *Phytotherapy Research* 23, no. 8 (2009): 1116–22.

Cheng, A. S., Y. H. Cheng, and T. L. Chang. "Scopoletin attenuates allergy by inhibiting Th2 cytokines production in EL-4 T cells." *Food and Function* 3, no. 8 (2012): 886–90.

Chiu, J. H., C. H. Ju, L. H. Wu, et al. "Cordyceps sinensis increases the expression of major histocompatibility complex class II antigens on human hepatoma cell line HA22T/VGH cells." *American Journal of Chinese Medicine* 26, no. 2 (1998): 159–70.

Chouhan, H. S., and S. K. Singh. "A review of plants of genus Leucas." *Journal of Pharmacognosy and Phytotherapy* 3, no. 3 (2011): 13–26.

Chu, F., L. Huoliang, L. Gui, et al. "[Protection of nucleated bone marrow cells of mice against effect of radiation-induced micronucleus formation with using polysaccharides extracted from 'Zi Zhi', a ganoderma]." *Radialization Protection* 1988-01. http://en.cnki.com.cn/Article_en/CJFDTOTAL-FSFH198801003.htm.

Chun, J. N., S. Y. Kim, E. J. Park, et al. "Schisandrin B suppresses TGF beta1-induced stress fiber formation by inhibiting myosin light chain phosphorylation." *Journal of Ethnopharmacology* 152, no. 2 (2014): 364–71.

Cruz, Ede M.., E. R. da Silva, C. Maquiaveli Cdo, et al. "Leishmanicidal activity of Cecropia pachystachya flavonoids: Arginase inhibition and altered mitochondrial DNA arrangement." *Phytochemistry* 89 (2013): 71–77.

Cruz-Silva, I., C. Neuhof, A. J. Gozzo, et al. "Using a Caesalpinia echinata Lam. protease inhibitor as a tool for studying the roles of neutrophil elastase, cathepsin G and proteinase 3 in pulmonary edema." *Phytochemistry* 96 (2013): 235–43.

Dai, Q., Y. P. Wang, K. Z. Zhao, et al. "[Effect of ginseng polysaccharide on the proliferation and differentiation of granulocyte-monocyte progenitor cells]." *Basic Medical Sciences and Clinics* 2004-01. http://en.cnki.com.cn/Article_en/CJFDTOTAL-JCYL200401013.htm.

Dai, Z. J., X. J. Wang, Z. F. Li, et al. "Scutellaria barbate extract induces apoptosis of hepatoma H22 cells via the mitochondrial pathway involving caspase-3." *World Journal of Gastroenterology* 14, no. 48 (2008): 7321–28.

Dalrymple, B. P., and J. M. Peters. "Characterization of a cDNA clone from the haemoparasite Babesia bovis encoding a protein containing an 'HMG-box'." *Biochemical and Biophysical Research Community* 184, no. 1 (1992): 31–35.

Demirci, B., O. Demir, T. Dost, et al. "Treated effect of silymarin on vascular function of aged rats: Dependant on nitric oxide pathway." *Pharmaceutical Biology*. Published electronically ahead of print November 5, 2013.

Demirci, B., T. Dost, F. Gokalp, et al. "Silymarin improves vascular function of aged ovariectomized rats." *Phytotherapy Research* 28, no. 6 (2014): 868–72. Published electronically ahead of print September 30, 2013.

Diaz-Perez, F., C. Radojkovic, V. Aguilera, et al. "L-arginine transport and nitric oxide synthesis in human endothelial progenitor cells." *Journal of Cardiovascular Pharmacology* 60, no. 5 (2012): 439–49.

Dold, A. P., and M. L. Cocks. "Traditional veterinary medicine in the Alice district of the Easter Cape Province, South Africa." *South African Journal of Science* 97, no. 9/10 (2001): 375–79.

dos Reis, M. B., L. C. Manjolin, C. do C. Maquiaveli, et al. "Inhibition of Leishmania (Leishmania) amazonensis and rat arginases by green tea EGCG, (+)-catechin and (-)-epicatechin: A comparative structural analysis of enzyme-inhibitor interactions." *PLoS ONE* 8, no. 11 (2013): e78387.

Du, J. X., M. Y. Sun, G. L. Du, et al. "Ingredients of huangqi decoction slow biliary fibrosis progression by inhibiting the activation of the transforming growth factor-beta signaling pathway." *BMC Complementary and Alternative Medicine* 12 (2012): 33.

Ehrman, T. M., D. J. Barlow, and P. J. Hylands. "Virtual screening of Chinese herbs with Random Forest." *Journal of Chemical Information and Modeling* 47, no. 2 (2007): 264–78.

El Daly, A. A., "The protective effect of green tea extract against enrofloxacin action on the rat liver: Histological, histochemical and ultrastructural studies." *Journal of American Science* 7, no. 4 (2011): 669–79.

Elisabetsky, E. "Phytotherapy and the new paradigm of drugs mode of action." *Scientia et Technica* 12, no. 33 (2007): 459–64.

Elkady, A., O. A., Abuzinadah, N. A. Baeshen, et al. "Differential control of growth, apoptotic activity, and gene expression in human breast cancer cells by extracts derived from medicinal herbs Zingiber officinale." *Journal of Biomedicine and Biotechnology*, 2012: 614356.

Elkhateeb, A., Subeki, K. Takahashi, et al. "Anti-babesial ellagic acid rhamnosides from the bark of Elaeocarpus parvifolius." *Phytochemistry* 66, no. 21 (2005): 2577–80.

Fook, J. M., L. L. Macedo, G. E. Moura, et al. "A serine proteinase inhibitor isolated from Tamarindus indica seeds and its effects on the release of human neutrophil elastase." *Life Sciences* 76, no. 25 (2005): 2881–91.

Friedl, R., T. Moeslinger, B. Kopp, et al. "Stimulation of nitric oxide synthesis by the aqueous of Panax ginseng root in RAW 264.7 cells." *British Journal of Pharmacology* 134, no. 8 (2001): 1663–70.

Fu, X., S. Li, G. Jia, et al. "Protective effect of the nitric oxide pathway in L-citruline renal ischaemia-reperfusion injury in rats." *Folia Biologica* 59, no. 6 (2013): 225–32.

Fu, Y., B. Liu, N. Zhang, et al. "Magnolol inhibits lipopolysaccharide-induced inflammatory response by interfering with TLR4 mediated NF-kB and MAPKs signaling pathways." *Journal of Ethnopharmacology* 145, no. 1 (2013): 193–99.

Fujii, Y., M. Imamura, M. Han, et al. "Recipient-mediated effect of a traditional Chinese herbal medicine, ren-shen-yang-rong-tang (Japanese name: ninjin-youei-to), on hematopoietic recovery following lethal irradiation and syngeneic bone marrow transplantation." *International Journal of Immunopharmacology* 16, no. 8 (1994): 615–22.

Galay, R. L., H. Maeda, K. M. Aung, et al. "Anti-babesial activity of a potent peptide fragment derived from longicin of Haemaphysalis longicornis." *Tropical Animal Health and Production* 44, no. 2 (2012): 343–48.

Gao, Y., J. Deng, X. F. Yu, et al. "Ginsenoside Rg1 inhibits vascular intimal hyperplasia in balloon-injured rat carotid artery by down-regulation of extracellular signal-regulated kinase 2." *Journal of Ethnopharmacology*-138, no. 2 (2011): 472–78.

Goo, Y. K., M. A. Terkawi, H. Jia, et al. "Artesunate, a potential drug for treatment of Babesia infection." *Parasitology International* 59, no. 3 (2010): 481–86.

Gou, L., L. Zhang, C. Yin, et al. "Protective effect of L-citrulline against acute gastric mucosal lesions induced by ischemia-reperfusion in rats." *Canadian Journal of Physiology and Pharmacology* 89, no. 5 (2011): 317–27.

Gradé, J. T., J. R. Tabuti, and P. Van Damme. "Ethnoveterinary knowledge in pastoral Karamoja, Uganda." *Journal of Ethnopharmacology* 122, no. 2 (2009): 273–93.

Guo, P., J. F. Wang, S. Q. Wang, et al. "[Effects of paeoniflorin on Epo and G-CSF gene expression in bone marrow of irradiated blood deficiency mice]." *Journal of Shandong University of Traditional Chinese Medicine* 2005-02. http://en.cnki.com.cn/Article_en/CJFDTOTAL-SDYX200503026.htm.

Gupta, S., N. Ahmad, A. L. Nieminen, et al. "Growth inhibition, cell-cycle dysregulation, and induction of apoptosis by green tea constituent (-)-epigallocatechin-3-gallate in androgen-sensitive and androgen-insensitive human prostate carcinoma cells." *Toxicology and Applied Pharmacology* 164, no. 1 (2000): 82–90.

Gupta, S., T. Hussain, and H. Mukhtar. "Molecular pathway for (-)-epigallocatechin-3-gallate-induced cell cycle arrest and apoptosis of human prostate carcinoma cells." *Archives of Biochemistry and Biophysics* 410, no. 1 (2003): 177–85.

Halder, B., S. Das Gupta, and A. Gomes. "Black tea polyphenols induce human leukemic cell cycle arrest by inhibiting Akt signaling: Possible involvement of Hsp90, Wnt/beta-catenin signaling and FOXO1." *FEBS Journal* 279, no. 16 (2012): 2876–91.

Han, E. H., J. H. Park, J. Y. Kim, et al. "Houttuynia cordata water extract suppresses anaphylactic reaction and IgE-mediated allergic response by inhibiting multiple steps of FcepsilonRI signaling in mast cells." *Food and Chemical Toxicology* 47, no. 7 (2009): 1659–66.

Han, J. M., H. G. Kim, M. K. Choi, et al. "Artemisia capillaris extract protects against bile-duct ligation-induced liver fibrosis in rats." *Experimental and Toxicologic Pathology* 65, no. 6 (2013): 837–44.

Han, J. M., H. G. Kim, M. K. Choi, et al. "Aqueous extract of Artemisia iwayomogi Kitamura attenuates cholestatic liver fibrosis in a rat model of bile duct ligation." *Food and Chemical Toxicology* 50, no. 10 (2012): 3505–13.

He, X., X. Li, B. Liu, et al. "Down-regulation of Treg cells and up-regulation of Th1/Th2 cytokine ratio were induced by polysaccharide from radix glycyrrhizae in H22 hepatocarcinoma bearing mice." *Molecules* 16, no. 10 (2011): 8343–52.

He, X., X. Niu, J. Li, et al. "Immunomodulatory activities of five clinically used Chinese herbal polysaccharides." *Journal of Experimental and Integrative Medicine* 2, no. 1 (2012): 15–27.

Heffernan, K. S., C. A. Fahs, S. M. Ranadive, et al. "L-arginine as a nutritional prophylaxis against vascular endothelial dysfunction with aging." *Journal of Cardiovascular Pharmacology and Therapeutics* 15, no. 1 (2010): 17–23.

Hisha, H., H. Yamada, M. H. Sakurai, et al. "Isolation and identification of hematopoietic stem cell-stimulating substances from kampo (Japanese herbal) medicine, juzen-taiho-to." *American Society of Hematology* 90, no. 3 (1997): 1022–30.

Hosseinimehr, S., S. Ahmadashrafi, F. Naghshvar, et al. "Chemoprotective effects of Zataria multiflora against genotoxicity induced by cyclophosphamide in mice bone marrow cells." *Integrative Cancer Therapies* 9, no. 2 (2010): 219–23.

Hou, H., Y. Z. Bao, L. Qian, et al. "[Establishment of blood-deficient model and research of Chinese angelica on hemopoiesis]." *Progress in Veterinary Medicine* 2009-12. http://en.cnki.com.cn/Article_en/CJFDTOTAL -DYJZ200912016.htm.

Huang, D. F., Y. F. Tang, S. P. Nie, et al. "Effect of phenylethanoid glycosides and polysaccharides from the seed of Plantago asiatica L. on the maturation of murine bone marrow-derived dendritic cells." *European Journal of Pharmacology* 620, nos. 1–3 (2009): 105–11.

Huang, J., M. Nasr, Y. Kim, et al. "Genistein inhibits protein histidine kinase." *Journal of Biological Chemistry* 267, no. 22 (1992): 15511–15.

Huang, M., X. Mei, and S. Zhang. "Mechanism of nitric oxide production in macrophages treated with medicinal mushroom extracts (review)." *International Journal of Medicinal Mushrooms* 13, no. 1 (2011): 1–6.

Huang, Y., L. Chen, L. Feng, et al. "Characterization of total phenolic constituents from the stems of Spatholobus suberectus using LC-DAD-MS(n) and their inhibitory effect on human neutrophil elastase activity." *Molecules* 18, no. 7 (2013): 7549–56.

Ignarro, L. J., R. E. Burns, D. Sumi, et al. "Pomegranate juice protects nitric oxide against oxidative destruction and enhances the biological actions of nitric oxide." *Nitric Oxide* 15, no. 2 (2006): 93–102.

Ikadai, H., T. Tetsuya, N. Shibahara, et al. "Short report: Inhibitory effect of lactoferrin on in vitro growth of Babesia caballi." *American Journal of Tropical Medicine and Hygiene* 73, no. 4 (2005): 710–12.

Im, J. H., Y. R. Jin, J. J. Lee, et al. "Antiplatelet activity of beta-carboline alkaloids from Perganum harmala: A possible mechanism through inhibiting PLCgamma2 phosphorylation." *Vascular Pharmacology* 50, nos. 5–6 (2009): 147–52.

Jiang, W. L., F. H. Fu, B. M. Xu, et al. "Cardioprotection with forsythoside B in rat myocardial ischemia-reperfusion injury: Relation to inflammation response." *Phytomedicine* 17, nos. 8–9 (2010): 635–39.

Jiao, L., D. Wan, X. Zhang, et al. "Characterization and immunostimulating effects on murine peritoneal macrophages of oligosaccharide isolated from Panax ginseng C.A. Meyer." *Journal of Ethnopharmacology* 144, no. 3 (2012): 490–96.

Joh, E. H., I. A. Lee, S. J. Han, et al. "Lancemaside A ameliorates colitis by inhibiting NF-kappaB activation in TNBS-induced colitis mice." *International Journal of Colorectal Disease* 25, no. 5 (2010): 545–51.

Joshi, J. V., R. A. Vaidya, S. N. Pandey, et al. "Plasma levels of genistein following a single dose of soy extract capsule in Indian women." *Indian Journal of Medical Research* 125, no. 4 (2007): 534–41.

Kacem, R., and Z. Meraihi. "Effects of essential oil extracted from Nigella sativa (L.) seeds and its main components on human neutrophil elastase activity." *Yakugaku Zasshi* 126, no. 4 (2006): 301–5.

Kamaraj, C., N. K. Kaushik, A. A. Rahuman, et al. "Antimalarial activities of medicinal plants traditionally used in the villages of Dharmapuri regions of South India." *Journal of Ethnopharmacology* 141, no. 3 (2012): 796–802.

Kaneko, M., T. Kawakita, Y. Kumazawa, et al. "Accelerated recovery from cyclophosphamide-induced leukopenia in mice administered a Japanese ethical herbal drug, hochu-ekki-to." *Immunopharmacology* 44, no. 3 (1999): 223–31.

Katiyar, S. K. "Treatment of silymarin, a plant flavonoid, prevents ultraviolet light-induced immune suppression and oxidative stress in mouse skin." *International Journal of Oncology* 21, no. 6 (2002): 1213–22.

Kawabata, K., T. Hagio, and S. Matsuoka. "[Pharmacological profile of a specific neutrophil elastase inhibitor, sivelestat sodium hydrate]." *Nihon Yakurigaku Zasshi* 122, no. 2 (2003): 151–60.

Kempuraj, D., B. Madhappan, S. Christodoulou, et al. "Flavonols inhibit proinflammatory mediator release, intracellular calcium ion levels and protein kinase C theta phosphorylation in human mast cells." *British Journal of Pharmacology* 145, no. 7 (2005): 934–34.

Khan, S., F. Malik, K. A. Suri, et al. "Molecular insight into the immune up-regulatory properties of the leaf extract of ashwagandha and identification of Th1 immunostimulatory chemical entity." *Vaccine* 27, no. 43 (2009): 6080–87.

Khoo, K. S., and P. T. Ang. "Extract of Astragalus membranaceus and Ligustrum lucidum does not prevent cyclophosphamide-induced myelosuppression." *Singapore Medical Journal* 36, no. 4 (1995): 387–90.

Kikuchi, T., E. Uchiyama, M. Ukiya, et al. "Cytotoxic and apoptosis-inducing activities of triterpene acids from Poria cocos." *Journal of Natural Products* 74, no. 2 (2011): 137–44.

Kim, E. K., K. B. Kwon, M. J. Han, et al. "Induction of G1 arrest and apoptosis by Scutellaria barbata in the human promyelocytic leukemia HL-60 cell line." *International Journal of Molecular Medicine* 20, no. 1 (2007): 123–28.

Kim, H. J., B. Y. Cha, I. S. Park, et al. "Dehydroglyasperin C, a component of liquorice, attenuates proliferation and migration induced by platelet-derived growth factor in human arterial smooth muscle cells." *British Journal of Nutrition* 110, no. 3 (2013): 391–400.

Kim, H. J., M. H. Kim, Y. Y. Byon, et al. "Radioprotective effects of an acidic polysaccharide of Panax ginseng on bone marrow cells." *Journal of Veterinary Science* 8, no. 1 (2007): 39–44.

Kim, K., N. Jung, K. Lee, et al. "Dietary omega-3 polyunsaturated fatty acids attenuate hepatic ischemia/reperfusion injury in rats by modulating toll-like receptor recruitment into lipid rafts." *Clinical Nutrition* 32, no. 5 (2013): 855–62.

Kim, N. Y., H. O. Pae, G. S. Oh, et al. "Butein, a plant polyphenol, induces apoptosis concomitant with increased caspase-3 activity, decreased Bcl-2 expression and increased Bax expression in HL-60 cells." *Pharmacology & Toxicology* 88, no. 5 (2001): 261–66.

Kim, S. J., H. Y. Min, E. J. Lee, et al. "Growth inhibition and cell cycle arrest in the G0/G1 schizandrin, a dibenzocyclooctadiene lignan isolated from Schisandra chinensis, on T47D human breast cancer cells." *Phytotherapy Research* 24, no. 2 (2010): 193–97.

Kim, S. W., T. D. Cuong, T. M. Hung, et al. "Arginase II inhibitory activity of flavonoid compounds from Scutellaria indica." *Archives of Pharmacal Research* 36, no. 8: 922–26.

Kim, Y. G., M. Sumiyoshi, K. Kawahira, et al. "Effects of red ginseng extract on ultraviolet B-irradiated skin change in C57BL mice." *Phytotherapy Research* 22, no. 11 (2008): 1423–27.

Kim, Y., Y. H. Choi, Y. W. Chin, et al. "Effect of plant matrix and fluid ethanol concentration on supercritical fluid extraction efficiency of schisandrin derivatives." *Journal of Chromatographic Science* 37, no. 12 (1999): 457–61.

Kim, Y. S., D. H. Jung, N. H. Kim, et al. "Effect of magnolol on TGF-beta1 fibronectin expression in human retinal pigment epithelial cells under diabetic conditions." *European Journal of Pharmacology* 562, nos. 1–2 (2007): 12–19.

Kiss, A. K., A. Filipek, M. Czerwinska, et al. "Oenothera paradoxa defatted seeds extract and its bioactive component penta-O-galloyl-beta-D-glucose decreased production of reactive oxygen species and inhibited release of leukotriene B4, interleukin-8, elastase, and myeloperoxidase in human neutrophils." *Journal of Agriculture Food Chemistry* 58, no. 18 (2010): 9960–66.

Koga, Y., Y. Akita, N. Junko, et al. "Endothelial dysfunction in MELAS improved by l-arginine supplementation." *Neurology* 66, no. 11 (2006): 1766–69.

Kohnen, S., T. Franck, P. Van Antwerpen, et al. "Resveratrol inhibits the activity of equine neutrophil myeloperoxidase by a direct interaction with the enzyme." *Journal of Agricultural and Food Chemistry* 55, no. 20 (2007): 8080–87.

Korokin, M. V., M. V. Pokrovsky, O. O. Novikov, et al. "Effect of L-arginine, vitamin B6 and folic acid on parameters of endothelial dysfunction and microcirculation in the placenta in modeling of L-NAME-induced NO deficiency." *Bulletin of Experimental Biology and Medicine* 152, no. 1 (2011): 70–72.

Lai, K. C., Y. J. Chiu, Y. J. Tang, et al. "Houttuynia cordata Thunb extract inhibits cell growth and induced apoptosis in human primary colorectal cancer cells." *Anticancer Research* 30, no. 9 (2010): 3549–56.

Latella, G., R. Sferra, A. Vetuschi, et al. "Prevention of colonic fibrosis by Boswellia and Scutellaria extracts in rats with colitis induced by 2,4,5-trinitrobenzene sulphonic acid." *European Journal of Clinical Investigation* 38, no. 6 (2008): 410–20.

Lee, C. L., T. L. Hwang, C. Y. Peng, et al. "Anti-neutrophilic inflammatory secondary metabolites from the traditional Chinese medicine, tiankuizi." *Natural Products Communications* 7, no. 12 (2012): 1623–26.

Lee, D. C., C. L. Yang, S. C. Chik, et al. "Bioactivity-guided identification and cell signaling technology to delineate the immunomodulatory effects of Panax ginseng on human promonocytic U937 cells." *Journal of Translational Medicine* 7 (2009): 34.

Lee, J. H., J. Y. Lee, J. H. Park, et al. "Immunoregulatory activity by daucosterol, a beta-sitosterol glycoside, induces protective Th1 immune response against disseminated candidiasis in mice." *Vaccine* 25, no. 19 (2007): 3834–40.

Lee, S. J., H. M. Kim, Y. H. Cho, et al. "Aqueous extract of Magnolia officinalis mediates proliferative capacity, p21WAF1 expression and TNF-alpha-induced NF-kappaB activity in human urinary bladder cancer 5637 cells; involvement of p38 MAP kinase." *Oncolology Reports* 18, no. 3 (2007): 729–36.

Lee, S. J., W. G. Ko, J. H. Kim, et al. "Induction of apoptosis by a novel intestinal metabolite of ginseng saponin via cytochrome c-mediated activation of caspase-3 protease." *Biochemical Pharmacology* 60, no. 5 (2000): 677–85.

Lee, W., S. K. Ku, J. S. Bae. "Barrier protective effects of rutin in LPS-induced inflammation in vitro and in vivo." *Food and Chemical Toxicology* 50, no. 9 (2012): 3048–55.

Lekakis, J. P., S. Papathanassiou, T. G. Papaioannou, et al. "Oral L-arginine improves endothelial dysfunction in patients with essential hypertension." *International Journal of Cardiology* 86, nos. 2–3 (2002): 317–23.

Li, C. Y., C. S. Chiang, M. L. Tsai, et al. "Two-sided effect of Cordyceps sinensis on dendritic cells in different physiological stages." *Journal of Leukocyte Biology* 85, no. 6 (2009): 987–95.

Li, J., and Y. P. Wang. "[Effect of angelica polysaccharide on bone marrow macrophage and its relationship to hematopoietic regulation]." *Chinese Traditional and Herbal Drugs* 2005-01. http://en.cnki.com.cn/Article_en/CJFDTOTAL-ZCYO200501031.htm.

Li, J., Y. Zhong, H. Li, et al. "Enhancement of Astragalus polysaccharide on the immune responses in pigs inoculated with foot-and-mouth disease virus vaccine." *International Journal of Biological Macromolocules* 49, no. 3 (2011): 362–68.

Li, J. Z., J. H. Wu, S. Y. Yu, et al. "Inhibitory effects of paeoniflorin on lysophosphatidylcholine-induced inflammatory factor production in human umbilical vein endothelial cells." *International Journal of Molecular Medicine* 31, no. 2 (2013): 493–97.

Li, Y. S., J. L. Jiang, and T. Li. "[Effects of traditional ShengBaiYin on immune and hematopoietic function of leukopenia animal model in mice]." *Journal of Hubei Institute for Nationalities (Medical Edition)* 2006-03. http://en.cnki.com.cn/Article_en/CJFDTOTAL-FBMZ200603002.htm.

Li, Y., F. Liang, W. Jiang, et al. "DH334, a beta-carboline anti-cancer drug, inhibits the CDK activity of budding yeast." *Cancer Biology and Therapy* 6, no. 8 (2007): 1193–99.

Liang, Q., Q. Wu, J. Jiang, et al. "Characterization of sparstolonin B, a Chinese herb-derived compound, as a selective toll-like receptor antagonist with potent anti-inflammatory properties." *Journal of Biological Chemistry* 286, no. 30 (2011): 26470–79.

Lim, C. J., T. D. Cuong, T. M. Hung, et al. "Arginase II inhibitory activity of phenolic compounds from Saururus chinensis." *Bulletin of the Korean Chemical Society* 33, no. 9 (2012): 3079–82.

Lin, F. Y., Y. H. Chen, Y. L. Chen, et al. "Ginkgo biloba extract inhibits endotoxin-induced human aortic smooth muscle cell proliferation via suppression of toll-like receptor 4 expression and NADPH oxidase activation." *Journal of Agricultural and Food Chemistry* 55, no. 5 (2007): 1977–84.

Lin, Z., J. Gu, J. Xiu, et al. "Traditional Chinese medicine for senile dementia." *Evidence-Based Complementary and Alternative Medicine*, 2012: 692621.

Lin, Z., D. Zhu, Y. Yan, et al. "An antioxidant phytotherapy to rescue neuronal oxidative stress." *Evidence-Based Complementary and Alternative Medicine*, 2011: 519517.

Lin, Z., D. Zhu, Y. Yan, and B. Yu. "Herbal formula FBD extracts prevented brain injury and inflammation induced by cerebral ischemia-reperfusion." *Journal of Ethnopharmacology* 118, no. 1 (2008): 140–47.

Liou, C. J., and J. Tseng. "A Chinese herbal medicine, fu-ling, regulates interleukin-10 production by murine spleen cells." *American Journal of Chinese Medicine* 30, no. 4 (2002): 551–60.

Liu, B., W. J. Liu, Q. L. Guo, et al. "[Effect of ganiclovir (GCV) and Astragalus membranaceus on proliferation of megakaryocyte progenitors after HCMV infection in vitro]." *Journal of Pediatric Pharmacy* 2003-06. http://en/cnki.com.cn/Article_en/CJFDTOTAL-EKYX200306000 .htm.

Liu, C., J. Li, F. Y. Meng, et al. "Polysaccharides from the root of Angelica sinensis promotes hematopoiesis and thrombopoiesis through the PI3K/AKT pathway." *BMC Complementary and Alternative Medicine* 10 (2010): 79.

Liu, J. J., R. W. Huang, D. J. Lin, et al. "Ponicidin, an ent-kaurane diterpenoid derived from a constituent of the herbal supplemement PC-SPES, Rabdosia rubescens, induces apoptosis by activation of caspase-3 and mitochondrial events in lung cancer cells in vitro." *Cancer Investigation* 24, no. 2 (2006): 136–48.

Liu, Q. Y., Y. M. Yao, S. W. Zhang, et al. "Astragalus polysaccharides regulate T cell-mediated immunity via CD11c(high)CD45RB(low) DCs in vitro." *Journal of Ethnopharmacology* 136, no. 3 (2011): 457–64.

Liu, S. Q., J. P. Yu, H. L. Chen, et al. "Therapeutic effects and molecular mechanism of Ginkgo biloba extract on liver fibrosis in rats." *American Journal of Chinese Medicine* 34, no. 1 (2006): 99–114.

Liu, S. Q., J. P. Yu, L. He, et al. "[Effects of nuclear factor kappaB and transforming growth factor beta1 in the anti-liver fibrosis process using Ginkgo biloba extract]." *Zhonghua gan zang bing za zhi* [Chinese Journal of Hepatology] 13, no. 12 (2005): 903–7.

Liu, W. C., S. C. Wang, M. L. Tsai, et al. "Protection against radiation-induced bone marrow and intestinal injuries by Cordyceps sinensis, a Chinese herbal medicine." *Radiation Research* 166, no. 6 (2006): 900–907.

Lou, X., B. Zhang, J. Song, et al. "[Effect of astragalus polysaccharide in stimulating the secretion of hematopoietic growth factors from activated human PBMC]." *Traditional Chinese Drug Research and Clinical Pharmacology* 2003-05. http://en.cnki.com.cn/Article_en/CJFDTOTAL -ZYXY200305006.htm.

Lu, Y., W. Chen, W. Ke, et al. "Chinese medicinal herb therapy for the rehabilitation of peripheral facial palsy." *Journal of Medicinal Plants Research* 4, no. 6 (2010): 455–58.

Lucotti, P., L. Monti, E. Setola, et al. "Oral L-arginine supplementation improves endothelial function and ameliorates insulin sensitivity and inflammation in cardiopathic nondiabetic patients after an aortocoronary bypass." *Metabolism* 58, no. 9 (2009): 1270–76.

Lv, Y., X. Feng, and B. Zhu. "[Study on effect of Astragalus membranaceus injection on hematopoiesis in anemic mice with myelosuppression]." *Zhong Yao Cai* 28, no. 9 (2005): 791–93.

Machado, R. J., N. K. Monteiro, L. Migliolo, et al. "Characterization and pharmacological properties of a novel multifuntional Kunitz inhibitor from Erythrina velutina seeds." *PLoS ONE* 8, no. 5 (2013): e63571.

Malik, F., J. Singh, A. Khajuria, et al. "A standardized root extract of Withania somnifera and its major constituent withanolide-A elicit humoral and cell-mediated immune responses by up regulation of Th1-dominant polarization in BALB/c mice." *Life Sciences* 80, no. 16 (2007): 1525–38.

Martina, V., A. Masha, V. R. Gigliardi, et al. "Long-term N-acetylcysteine and L-arginine administration reduces endothelial activation and systolic blood pressure in hypertensive patients with type 2 diabetes." *Diabetes Care* 31, no. 5 (2008): 940–44.

Materska, M. "Evaluation of the lipophilicity and stability of phenolic compounds in herbal extracts." *Acta Scientiarum Polonorum, Technologia Alimentaria* 9, no. 1 (2010): 61–69.

Mazuz, M. L., J. Golenser, L. Fish, et al. "Artemisone inhibits in vitro and in vivo propagation of Babesia bovis and B. bigemina parasites." *Experimental Parasitology* 135, no. 4 (2013): 690–94.

Meeran, S. M., and S. K. Katiyar. "Grape seed proanthocyanidins promote apoptosis in human epidermoid carcinoma A431 cells through alterations in Cdki-Cdk-cyclin cascade, and caspase-3 activation via loss of mitochondrial membrane potential." *Experimental Dermatology* 16, no. 5 (2007): 405–15.

Metzner, J. E., T. Frank, I. Kunz, et al. "Study on the pharmacokinetics of synthetic genistein after multiple oral intake in post-menopausal women." *Arzneimittelforschung* 59, no. 10 (2009): 513–20.

Miao, Z., L. Wenli, S. Hanying, et al. "[Gui Qi oral liquor promoting the hematopoietic recovery in bone marrow of acute irraditation injured mice and mechanism]." *Acta Universitatis Medictnae Tangji* 2005-04. http://en.cnki.com.cn/Article_en/CJFDTOTAL-TJYX200504017 .htm.

Misha, L. C., B. B. Singh, and S. Dagenais. "Scientific basis for the therapeutic use of Withania somnifera (ashwagandha): A review." *Alternative Medicine Review* 5, no. 4 (2000): 334–46.

Miura, S., I. Kawamura, A. Yamada, et al. "Effect of a traditional Chinese herbal medicine ren-shen-yang-rong-tang (Japanese name: ninjin-youei-to) on hematopoietic stem cells in mice." *International Journal of Immunopharmacology* 11, no. 7 (1989): 771–80.

Monti, L. D., M. C. Casiraghi, E. Setola, et al. "L-arginine enriched biscuits improve endothelial function and glucose metabolism: A pilot study in healthy subjects and a cross-over study in subjects with impaired glucose tolerance and metabolic syndrome." *Metabolism* 62, no. 2 (2013): 255–64.

Moskaug, J. Ø., G. I. Borge, A. M. Fagervoll, et al. "Dietary polyphenols identified as intracellular protein kinase A inhibitors." *European Journal of Nutrition* 47, no. 8 (2008): 460–69.

Motaharinia, Y., M. A. Rezaee, M. S. Hazhir, et al. "Evaluation of the antibacterial activity of Zataria multiflora Boiss., Rhus coriaria L. (sumac), Mentha piperita L., and Ocimum basilicum L. extracts on Brucella strains isolated from brucellosis patients." *Turkish Journal of Medical Sciences* 42, no. 5 (2012): 816–22.

Motamedi, H., E. Darabpour, M. Gholipour, et al. "In vitro assay for the anti-brucella activity of medicinal plants against tetracycline-resistant Brucella melitensis." *Journal of Zhejian University* 11, no. 7 (2010): 506–11.

Murnigsih, T., H. Matsuura, K. Takahashi, et al. "Evaluation of the inhibitory activities of the extracts of Indonesian traditional medicinal plants against Plasmodium falciparum and Babesia gibsoni." *Journal of Veterinary Medical Science* 67, no. 8 (2005): 829–31.

Nagai, A., N. Yokoyama, T. Matsuo, et al. "Growth-inhibitory effects of artesunate, pyrimethamine, and pamaquine against Babesia equi and Babesia caballi in in vitro cultures." *Antimicrobial Agents and Chemotherapy* 47, no. 2 (2003): 800–803.

Naghshvar, F., S. M. Abianeh, S. Ahmadashrafi, et al. "Chemoprotective effects of carnosine against genotoxicity induced by cyclophosphamide in mice bone marrow cells." *Cell Biochemistry and Function* 30, no. 7 (2012): 569–73.

Naidoo, V., E. Zweygarth, J. N. Eloff, et al. "Identification of anti-babesial activity for four ethnoveterinary plants in vitro." *Veterinary Parasitology*-130, nos. 1–2 (2005): 9–13.

Nair, N., S. Mahanjan, R. Chawda, et al. "Grape seed extract activates Th1 cells in vitro." *Clinical and Diagnostic Laboratory Immunology* 9, no. 2 (2002): 470–76.

Nakao, R., C. Mizukami, Y. Kawamura, et al. "Evaluation of efficacy of bruceine A, a natural quassinoid compound extracted from a medicinal plant, Brucea javanica, for canine babesiosis." *Journal of Veterinary Medical Science* 71, no. 1 (2009): 33–41.

Nanyingi, M. O., J. M. Mbaria, A. L. Lanyasunya, et al. "Ethnopharmacological survey of Samburu district, Kenya." *Journal of Ethnobiology and Ethnomedicine* 4 (2008): 14.

Narayanan, B. A., N. K. Narayanan, G. G. Re, et al. "Differential expression of genes induced by resveratrol in LNCaP P53-mediated molecular targets." *International Journal of Cancer* 104, no. 2 (2003): 204–12.

Narendhirakannan, R. T., and T. P. Limmy. "Anti-inflammatory and antioxidant properties of Sida rhombifolia stems and roots in adjuvant induced arthritic rats." *Immunopharmacology and Immunotoxicology* 34, no. 2 (2012): 326–36.

Ni, Y. F., T. Jiang, Q. S. Cheng, et al. "Protective effect of magnolol on lipopolysaccharide-induced acute lung injury in mice." *Inflammation* 35, no. 6 (2012): 1860–66.

Nishida, S., S. Kikuichi, S. Yoshioka, et al. "Induction of apoptosis in HL-60 cells treated with medicinal herbs." *American Journal of Chinese Medicine* 31, no. 4 (2003): 551–62.

Nishioka, K., T. Hidaka, S. Nakamura, et al. "Pycnogenol, French maritime bark extract, augments endothelium-dependent vasodilation in humans." *Hypertension Research* 30, no. 9 (2007): 775–80.

Nunomura, S., S. Kitanaka, and C. Ra. "3-O-(2,3-dimethylbutanoyl)-13-O-decanoylingenol from Euphorbia kansui suppresses IgE-mediated mast cell activation." *Biological & Pharmaceutical Bulletin* 29, no. 2 (2006): 286–90.

Orea-Tejeda, A., J. J. Orozco-Gutierrez, L. Castillo-Martinez, et al. "The effect of L-arginine and citrulline on endothelial function in patients in heart failure with preserved ejection fraction." *Cardiology Journal* 17, no. 5 (2010): 464–70.

Otsuki, N., N. H. Dang, E. Kumagai, et al. "Aqueous extract of Carica papaya leaves exhibits anti-tumor activity and immunomodulatory effects." *Journal of Ethnopharmacology* 127, no. 3 (2010): 760–67.

Palmer, R. M., D. S. Ashton, and S. Moncada. "Vascular endothelial cells synthesize nitric oxide from L-arginine." *Nature* 333, no. 6174 (1988): 664–66.

Pan, Z., W. Zhao, X. Zhang, et al. "Scutellarin alleviates interstitial fibrosis and cardiac dysfunction of infarct rats by inhibiting TGFbeta1 expression and activation of p38-MAPK and ERK1/2." *British Journal of Pharmacology* 162, no. 3 (2011): 688–700.

Pandey, A., S. Bani, P. Sangwan, et al. "Selective Th1 upregulation by ethyl acetate fraction of Labisia pumila." *Journal of Ethnopharmacology* 132, no. 1 (2010): 309–15.

Park, B. K., M. Y. Heo, H. Park, et al. "Inhibition of TPA-induced cyclooxygenase-2 expression and skin inflammation in mice by wogonin, a plant flavone from Scutellaria radix." *European Journal of Pharmacology* 425, no. 2 (2001): 153–57.

Park, C., D. O. Moon, C. H. Rhu, et al. "Beta-sitosterol induces anti-proliferation and apoptosis in human leukemic U937 cells through activation of caspase-3 and induction of Bax/Bcl-2 ratio." *Biological & Pharmaceutical Bulletin* 30, no. 7 (2007): 1317–23.

Park, E. J., J. N. Chung, S. H. Kim, et al. "Schisandrin B suppresses TGFbeta1 signaling by inhibiting Smad2/3 and MAPK pathways." *Biochemical Pharmacology* 83, no. 3 (2012): 378–84.

Park, E. Y., K. W. Lee, H. W. Lee, et al. "The ethanol extract from Artemisia princeps Pampanini induces p53-mediated G1 phase arrest in A172 human neuroblastoma cells." *Journal of Medicinal Food* 11, no. 2 (2008): 237–45.

Park, Y. H., I. H. Son, B. Kim, et al. "Poria cocos water extract (PCW) protects PC12 neuronal cells from beta-amyloid-induced cell death through antioxidant and antiapoptotic functions." *Die Pharmazie* 64, no. 11 (2009): 760–64.

Peng, L., N. Khan, F. Afaq, et al. "In vitro and in vivo effects of water extract of white cocoa tea (Camellia ptilophylla) against human prostate cancer." *Pharmaceutical Research* 27, no. 6 (2010): 1128–37.

Pokrovskii, M. V., T. G. Pokrovskaia, V. V. Gureev, et al. "[Correction of endothelial dysfunction by L-arginine under experimental pre-eclampsia conditions]." *Eksperimental'naia i Klinicheskaia Farmakologiia* 75, no. 2 (2012): 14–16.

Prajapati, M. S., J. B. Patel, K. Modi, et al. "Leucas aspera: A review." *Pharmacognosy Review* 4, no. 7 (2010): 85–87.

Prati, C., A. Berthelot, B. Kantelip, et al. "Treatment with the arginase inhibitor Nw-hydroxy-nor-L-arginine restores endothelial function in rat adjuvant-induced arthritis." *Arthritis Research and Therapy* 14, no. 3 (2012): R130.

Prommaban, A., K. Kodchakorn, P. Kongtawelert, et al. "Houttuynia cordata Thunb fraction induces human leukemic Molt-4 cell apoptosis through the endoplasmic reticulum stress pathway." *Asian Pacific Journal of Cancer Prevention* 13, no. 5 (2012): 1977–81.

Qu, Z. H., Z. C. Yang, L. Chen, et al. "Inhibition airway remodeling and transforming growth factor-beta1/Smad signaling pathway by astragalus extract in asthmatic mice." *International Journal of Molecular Medicine* 29, no. 4 (2012): 564–68.

Quan, H., and Li, H. "[Effects of rad ix astragali on hemopoiesis in irradiated m ice]." *China Journal of Chinese Materia Medica* 1994-12. http://en.cnki.com.cn/Article_en/CJFDTotal-ZGZY412.017.htm. [Note: You'll have to replicate the odd spacing in this article's title in order to find it with an online search.]

Rajan, A., and U. Bagai. "Antimalarial potential of China 30 and Chelidonium 30 in combination therapy against lethal rodent malaria parasite: Plasmodium berghei." *Journal of Complementary and Integrative Medicine* 10 (2013).

Rajasekaran, D., E. A. Palombo, T. Chia Yeo, et al. "Identification of traditional medicinal plant extracts with novel anti-influenza activity." *PLoS ONE* 8, no. 11 (2013): e79293.

Ren, C. A., F. L. Zhang, X. L. Zhao, et al. "[Role of glycycrrhizin on bone marrow hematopoiesis in immune induced aplastic anemia mice]." *Journal of Shandong University (Health Sciences)* 2006-01. http://en.cnki.com.cn/Article_en/CJFDTOTAL-SDYB200601002.htm.

Rios, J. L. "Chemical constituents and pharmacological properties of Poria cocos." *Planta Medica* 77, no. 7 (2011): 681–91.

Rosenblatt-Bin, H., A. Klein, and B. Sredni. "Antibabesial effect of the immunomodulator AS101 in mice: Role of increased production of nitric oxide." *Parasite Immunology* 18, no. 6 (1996): 297–306.

Roudi, H., and F. Ganji. "Effect of Althaea officinalis on cough associated with ACE inhibitors." *Pakistan Journal of Nutrition* 6, no. 3 (2007): 256–58.

Sachdeva, H., R. Sehgal, and S. Kaur. "Studies on the protective and immunomodulatory efficacy of Withania somnifera along with cisplatin against experimental visceral leishmaniasis." *Parasitology Research* 112, no. 6 (2013): 2269–80.

Saklani, S., A. P. Mishra, B. Sati, et al. "Pharmacognostic, phytochemical and antimicrobial screening of Aphanamixis polystachya, an endangered medicinal tree." *International Journal of Pharmacy and Pharmaceutical Sciences* 4, no. 3 (2012): 235–40.

Salama, A. A., M. Aboulaila, A. A. Moussa, et al. "Evaluation of in vitro and in vivo inhibitory effects of fusidic acid on Babesia and Theileria parasites." *Veterinary Parasitology* 191, nos. 1–2 (2013): 1–10.

Salama, A. A., M. Aboulaila, M. A. Terkawi, et al. "Inhibitory effect of allicin on the growth of Babesia and Theileria equi parasites." *Parasitology Research* 113, no. 1 (2014): 275–83.

Salvatore, P., A. Casamassimi, L. Sommese, et al. "Detrimental effects of Bartonella henselae are counteracted by L-arginine and nitric oxide in human endothelial progenitor cells." *Proceedings of the National Academy of Sciences of the United States of America* 105, no. 27 (2008): 9427–32.

Setchell, K. D., M. S. Faughnan, T. Avades, et al. "Comparing the pharmacokinetics of daidzein and genistein with the use of 13C-labeled tracers in premenopausal women." *American Journal of Clinical Nutrition* 77, no. 2 (2003): 411–19.

Shao, P., L. H. Zhao, Zhi-Chen, et al. "Regulation on maturation and function of dendritic cells by Astragalus mongholicus polysaccharides." *International Immunopharmacology* 6, no. 7 (2006): 1161–66.

Sher, H., and M. N. Alyemeni. "Ethnobotanical and pharmaceutical evaluation of Capparis spinosa L, validity of local folk and Unani system of medicine." *Journal of Medicinal Plants Research* 4, no. 17 (2010): 1751–56.

Sheu, M. J., G. J. Huang, C. H. Wu, et al. "Ethanol extract of Dunaliella salina induces cell cycle arrest and apoptosis in A549 human non-small cell lung cancer cells." *In Vivo* 22, no. 3 (2008): 369–78.

Shi, Q. Z., L. W. Wang, W. Zhang, et al. "Betaine inhibits toll-like receptor 4 expression in rats with ethanol-induced liver injury." *World Journal of Gastroenterology* 16, no. 7 (2010): 897–903.

Siedle, B., A. Hrenn, and I. Merfort. "Natural compounds as inhibitors of human neutrophil elastase." *Planta Medica* 73, no. 5 (2007): 401–20.

Singh, S. M., N. Singh, and P. Shrivastava. "Effect of alcoholic extract of Ayurvedic herb Tinospora cordifolia on the proliferation and myeloid differentiation of bone marrow precursor cells in a tumor-bearing host." *Fitoterapia* 77, no. 1 (2006): 1–11.

Singh, S. S., S. C. Pandey, S. Srivastava, et al. "Chemistry and medicinal properties of Tinospora cordifolia (Guduchi)." *Indian Journal of Pharmacology* 35 (2003): 83–91.

Song, D., Z. He, C. Wang, et al. "Regulation of the exopolysaccharide from an anamorph of Cordyceps sinesis on dendritic cell sarcoma (DCS) cell line." *European Journal of Nutrition* 52, no. 2 (2013): 687–94.

Song, J. Y., S. K. Han, K. G. Bae, et al. "Radioprotective effects of ginsan, an immunomodulator." *Radiation Research* 159, no. 6 (2003): 768–74.

Song, J. M., J. C. Xin, and Y. Zhu. "[Effect of Cordyceps cicadae on blood sugar of mice and its hematopoietic function]." *Chinese Archives of Traditional Chinese Medicine* 2007-06. http://en.cnki.com.cn/Article_en/CJFDTOTAL-ZYHS200706021.htm.

Spelman, K., J. J. Burns, D. Nichols, et al. "Modulation of cytokine expression by traditional medicines: A review of herbal immunomodulators." *Alternative Medicine Review* 11, no. 2 (2006): 128–50.

Staniforth, V., L. T. Chiu, and N. S. Yang. "Caffeic acid suppresses UVB radiation-induced expression of interleukin-10 and activation of mitogen-activated protein kinases in mouse." *Carcinogenesis* 27, no. 9 (2006): 1803–11.

Subeki, H. Matsuura, K. Takahasi, et al. "Antibabesial activity of protoberberine alkaloids and 20-hydroxyecdysone from Arcangelisia flava against Babesia gibsoni in culture." *Journal of Veterinary Medical Science* 67, no. 2 (2005): 223–27.

Subeki, H. Matsuura, K. Takahasi, et al. "Anti-babesial and anti-plasmodial compounds from Phyllanthus niruri." *Journal of Natural Products* 68, no. 4 (2005): 537–39.

Subeki, H. Matsuura, K. Takahasi, et al. "Screening of Indonesian medicinal plant extracts for antibabesial activity and isolation of new quassinoids from Brucea javanica." *Journal of Natural Products* 70, no. 10 (2007): 1654–57.

Subeki, H. Matsuura, M. Yamasaki, et al. "Effects of central Kalimantan plant extracts on intraerythrocytic Babesia gibsoni in culture." *Journal of Veterinary Medical Science* 66, no. 7 (2004): 871–74.

Subeki, S. Nomura, H. Matsuura, et al. "Anti-babesial activity of some central Kalimantan plant extracts and active oligostilbenoids from Shorea balangeran." *Planta Medica* 71, no. 5 (2005): 420–23.

Takei, M., M. Kobayashi, D. N. Herndon, et al. "Glycyrrhizin inhibits the manifestations of anti-inflammatory responses that appear in association with systemic inflammatory response syndrome (SIRS)-like reactions." *Cytokine* 35, nos. 5–6 (2006): 295–301.

Tang, B., H. Qiao, F. Meng, et al. "Glycyrrhizin attenuates endotoxin-induced acute liver injury after partial hepatectomy in rats." *Brazilian Journal of Medical and Biological Research* 40, no. 12 (2007): 1637–46.

Tang, Y. J., J. S. Yang, C. F. Lin, et al. "Houttuynia cordata Thunb extract induces apoptosis through mitochondrial-dependent pathway in HT-29 human colon adenocarcinoma cells." *Oncology Reports* 22 (2009): 1051–56.

Tayarani-Najaran, Z., S. H. Mousavi, N. Vahdati-Mashhadian, et al. "Scutellaria litwinowii induces apoptosis through both extrinsic and intrinsic apoptotic pathways in human promyelocytic leukemia cells." *Nutrition and Cancer* 64, no. 1 (2012): 80–88.

Tonnetti, L., A. M. Thorp, H. L. Reddy, et al. "Riboflavin and ultraviolet light reduce the infectivity of Babesia microti in whole blood." *Transfusion* 53, no. 4 (2013): 860–67.

Torres Acosta, J. A., L. C. Fowke, and H. Wang. "Analyses of phylogeny, evolution, conserved sequences and genome-wide expression of the ICK/KRP family of plant CDK inhibitors." *Annals of Botany* 107, no. 7 (2011): 1141–57.

Tseng, J., and J. G. Chang. "Suppression of tumor necrosis factor-alpha, interleukin-1 beta, interleukin-6 and granulocyte-monocyte colony stimulating factor secretion from human monocytes by an extract of Poria cocos." *Zhonghua Min Guo Wei Sheng Wu Ji Mian Yi Xue Za Zhi* [Chinese Journal of Microbiology and Immunology], 25, no. 1 (1992): 1–11.

Tyagi, A., C. Agarwal, G. Harrison, et al. "Silibinin causes cell cycle arrest and apoptosis in human bladder transitional cell carcinoma cells by regulating CDKI-CDK-cyclin cascade, and caspase 3 and PARP cleavages." *Carcinogenesis* 25, no. 9 (2004): 1711–20.

Ullmann, U., J. Metzner, T. Frank, et al. "Safety, tolerability, and pharmacokinetics of single ascending doses of synthetic genistein (Bonistein) in healthy volunteers." *Advances in Therapy* 22, no. 1 (2005): 65–78.

Vogl, S., P. Picker, J. Mihaly-Bison, et al. "Ethnopharmacological in vitro studies on Austria's folk medicine—an unexplored lore in vitro anti-inflammatory activities of 71 Austrian traditional herbal drugs." *Journal of Ethnopharmacology* 149, no. 3 (2013): 750–71.

Wang, H. F., X. C. Lin, X. J. Li, et al. "[Protective effect of polysaccharides of Tricholoma matsutake on hematopoietic function of X-rays irradiated mice]." *Journal of Jilin University (Medicine Edition)* 2008-05. http://en.cnki.com.cn/Article_en/CJFDTOTAL-BQEB200805009.htm.

Wang, I. K., S. Y. Lin-Shiau, and J. K. Lin. "Induction of apoptosis by apigenin and related flavonoids through cytochrome c release and activation of caspase-9 and caspase-3 in leukaemia HL-60 cells." *European Journal of Cancer* 35, no. 10 (1999): 1517–25.

Wang, J. H., M. K. Choi, J. W. Shin, et al. "Antifibrotic effects of Artemisia capillaris and Artemisia iwayomogi in a carbon tetrachloride-induced chronic hepatic fibrosis animal model." *Journal of Ethnopharmacology* 140, no. 1 (2012): 179–85.

Wang, L., and C. L. Weller. "Recent advances in extraction of nutraceutical from plants." *Trends in Food Science & Technology* 17 (2006): 300–312.

Wang, L., F. Zhao, and K. Liu. "[Induction of apoptosis of the human leukemia cells by arctigenin and its mechanism of action]." *Yao Xue Xue Bao* 43, no. 5 (2008): 542–47.

Wang, Y., and B. Zhu. "[The effect of angelica polysaccharide on proliferation and differentiation of hematopoietic progenitor cell]." *Zhonghua Yi Xue Za Zhi* 76, no. 5 (1996): 363–66.

Wang, Y. P., and B. D. Zhu. "[Effect of angelica polysaccharide on granulopoiesis and monocytopoiesis in mice]." *Journal of Experimental Hematology* 1993-01. http://en.cnki.com.cn/Article_en/CJFDTOTAL-XYSY199301018.htm.

Wang, Y P., and B. D. Zhu. "[Effect of angelica pelysaccharide on megakaryocytopoiesis and platelet production]." *Pharmacology and Clinics of Chinese Materia Medica* 1992-04. http://en.cnki.com.cn/Article_en/CJFDTOTAL-ZYYL199204004.htm

Weinl, C., S. Marquardt, S. J. Kuijt, et al. "Novel functions of plant cyclin-dependent kinase inhibitors, ICK1/KRP1, can act non-cell-autonomously and inhibit entry into mitosis." *Plant Cell* 17, no. 6 (2005): 1704–22.

Woosung, Shin, J. Yoon, G. T. Oh, et al. "Korean red ginseng inhibits arginase and contributes to endothelium-dependent vasorelaxation through endothelial nitric oxide synthase coupling." *Journal of Ginseng Research* 37, no. 1 (2013): 64–73.

Wu, H., et al. "[The effect of mobilization of ginseng polysaccharide on murine hematopoietic stem/progenitor cell]." *Journal of Chongqing Medical University* 2007-06. http://en.cnki.com.cn/Article_en/CJFDTotal-ZQYK200706006.htm.

Wu, H., R. Jiang, M. Zheng, et al. "[Experimental study on effect of ginseng polysaccharide and angelica polysaccharide in inducing hematopoietic growth factors in human endothelial cells]." *Chinese Journal of Integrated Traditional and Western Medicine* 2002-09. http://en.cnki.com.cn/Article_en/CJFDTOTAL-ZZXJ200209020.htm.

Wu, L. W., Y. M. Chiang, H. C. Chuang, et al. "A novel polyacetylene significantly inhibits angiogenesis and promotes apoptosis in human endothelial cells through activation of the CDK inhibitors and caspase-7." *Planta Medica* 73, no. 7 (2007): 655–61.

Xenos, E. S., S. L. Stevens, M. B. Freeman, et al. "Nitric oxide mediates the effect of fluvastatin on intercellular adhesion molecule-1 and platelet endothelial cell adhesion molecule-1 expression on human endothelial cells." *Annals of Vascular Surgery* 19, no. 3 (2005): 386–92.

Xiangjin, G., X. Jin, M. Banyou, et al. "Effect of glycyrrhizin on traumatic brain injury in rats and its mechanism." *Chinese Journal of Traumatology* 17, no. 1 (2014): 1–7.

Xiao, A. Q., and B. Q. Dong. "[The observation of Astragalus membranaceus injection in leucopenia patients induced by ticlopidine]." *Journal of Taishan Medical College* 2007-09. http://en.cnki.com.cn.Article_en/ CJFDTOTAL-TSYX200709011.htm.

Xing, X., S. Ping, Y. Cuie, et al. "[Effect of astragalus polysaccharide on supporting hematopoiesis in long term bone marrow culture]." *Chinese Journal of Information on TCM* 2003-04. http://en.cnki.com.cn/Article_en/ CJFDTOTAL-XXYY200304012.htm.

Xingyu, L., L. Dandan, W. Liqing, et al. "[Effect of Agaricus blazei polysaccharide on hematopoietic stem cell and progenitor cells]." *Chinese Journal of Clinical Pharmacy* 2004-04. http://en.cnki.com.cn/Article_en/ CJFDTOTAL-LCZZ200404005.htm.

Xuan, L., G. Tao, L. Chunli, et al. "[Effect of total saponins of Panax ginseng on irradiation-induced bone marrow hematopoietic cell injury and senescence]." *Journal of Third Military Medical University* 2012-22. http:// en.cnki.com.cn/Article_en/CJFDTOTAL-DSDX201222014.htm.

Yamada, K., Subeki, K. Nabeta, et al. "Isolation of antibabesial compounds from Brucea javanica, Curcuma zanthorrhiza, and Excoecaria cochinchinensis." *Bioscience, Biotechnology and Biochemistry* 73, no. 3 (2009): 776–80.

Yan, Z., G. Xuejing, W. Hong, et al. "[Effects of angelica polysaccharides on expression of adhesion molecules and cell cycle in bone marrow mononuclear cells of radiation injured mice]." *Chinese Journal of Histochemistry and Cytochemistry* 2010-06. http://en.cnki.com.cn/Article_en/ CJFDTOTAL-GGZZ201006012.htm.

Yang, H., and H. Wu. "[Effect of APS on recoverable ability from cryopreservation damage of UCB hematopoietic cells]." *Chinese Traditional and Herbal Drugs* 2008-11. http://en.cnki.com.cn/Article_en/CJFDTOTAL-ZCYO200811030.htm.

Yang, M., G. C. Chan, R. Deng, et al. "An herbal decoction of radix astragali and radix angelicae sinesis promotes hematopoiesis and thrombopoiesis." *Journal of Ethnopharmacology* 124, no. 1 (2009): 87–97.

Yang, W., Y. Wang, J. Rong, et al. "[Experimental studies on the hematopoietic growth factor production induced by total saponins of Panax ginseng]." *ACTA Anatomica Sinica* 1997-03. http://en.cnki.com.cn/Article_en/CJFDTOTAL-JPXB703.020.htm.

Yang, X. Y., G. S. Park, M. H. Lee, et al. "Toll-like receptor 4-mediated immunoregulation by the aqueous extract of mori fructus." *Phytotherapy Research* 23, no. 12 (2009): 1713–20.

Yang, Z., K. Kulkarni, W. Zhu, et al. "Bioavailability and pharmacokinetics of genistein: Mechanistic studies on its ADME." *Anticancer Agents in Medicinal Chemistry* 12, no. 10 (2012): 1264–80.

Yanxia, C., Z. Wu, X. Liu, et al. "Preparation, safety, pharmacokinetics, and pharmacodynamics of liposomes containing Brucea javanica oil." *AAPS PharmSciTech* 11, no. 2 (2010): 878–84.

Ying, Z., Z. Qixin, and L. Shu. "[The effects of Bletilla striata polysaccharide on proliferation of hematopoietic cells]." *Pharmacology and Clinics of Chinese Materia Medica* 2009-04. http://en.cnki.com.cn/Article_en/CJFDTOTAL-ZYYL200904013.htm.

Yong, W., Z. Bide, and W. Yaping. "[Effect of total saponins of Panax ginseng (TSPG) on the production of hematopoietic growth factors]." *Immunological Journal* 1996-01. http://en.cnki.com.cn/Article_en/CJFDTOTAL-MYXZ601.005.htm.

Yong, W., W. Shali, W. Yaping, et al. "[Effect of total saponins of Panax ginseng on the bioactivity and mRNA expression of hematopoietic growth factors]." *ACTA Anatomica Sinica* 1999-04. http://en.cnki.com.cn/Article_en/CJFDTOTAL-JPXB199904023.htm.

Yong, W., W. Yaping, and Z. Bide. "[Effect of total saponins of Panax ginseng on proliferation of hematopoietic cells in mice]." *Chinese Journal of Anatomy* 1995-02. http://en.cnki.com.cn/Article_en/CJFDTOTAL-JPXZ199502019.htm.

Yu, S. J., and J. Tseng. "Fu-ling, a Chinese herbal drug, modulates cytokine secretion by human peripheral blood monocytes." *International Journal of Immunopharmacology* 18, no. 1 (1996): 37–44.

Yu, X. F., J. Deng, D. L. Yang, et al. "Total ginsenosides suppress the neointimal hyperplasia of rat carotid artery induced by balloon injury." *Vascular Pharmacology* 54, nos. 1–2 (2011): 52–57.

Yunhe, F., L. Bo, F. Xiaosheng, et al. "The effect of magnolol on the toll-like receptor 4/nuclear factor kB signalling pathway in lipopolysaccharide-induced acute lung injury in mice." *European Journal of Pharamacology* 689, nos. 1–3 (2012): 255–61.

Zavoi, S., F. Fetea, F. Ranga, et al. "Comparative fingerprint and extraction yield of medicinal herb phenolics with hepatoprotective potential, as determined by UV-Vis and FT-MIR spectroscopy." *Notulae Botanicae Horti Agrobotanici Cluj-Napoca* 39, no. 2 (2011): 82–89.

Zeng, J., Y. Duo, J. Guo, et al. "Paeoniflorin of Paeonia lactiflora prevents renal interstitial fibrosis induced by unilateral ureteral obstruction in mice." *Phytomedicine* 20, nos. 8–9 (2013): 753–9.

Zhang, D., G. H. Xu, G. X. Jiang, et al. "[Effects of soup with angelica, astragalus and pig's trotters on hematopoietic function of myelosuppressed model rats]." *Nursing Journal of Chinese People's Liberation Army* 2012–11. http://en.cnki.com.cn/Article_en/CJFDTOTAL-JFHL201211005.htm.

Zhang, J., W. Dou, E. Zhang, et al. "Paeoniflorin abrogates DSS-induced colitis via a TLR4-dependent pathway." *American Journal of Physiology. Gastrointestinal and Liver Physiology* 306, no. 1 (2014): G27–36.

Zhang, S., J. Deng, Y. Gao, et al. "Ginsenoside Rb1 inhibits the carotid neointimal hyperplasia induced by balloon injury in rats via suppressing the phenotype modulation of vascular smooth muscle cells." *European Journal of Pharmocology* 685, nos. 1–3 (2012): 126–32.

Zhang, S., L. Qiu, and M. Y. Li. "[Effects of radix astragali on expression of transforming growth factor beta 1 and Smad 3 signal pathway in hypertrophic scar of rabbit.]" *Zhonghua Shao Shang Za Zhi* [Chinese Journal of Burns] 26, no. 5 (2010): 366–70.

Zhang, Y., et al. "[Compared study of hematopoietic recovery of angelica polysaccharides dosaged pre-irradiation and post-irradiation on radiation injured mice]." http://en.cnki.com.cn/Article_en/CJFDTOTAL -ZQYK201007005.htm.

Zhang, Y. W., D. Xie, B. Xia, et al. "Suppression of transforming growth factor-beta1 gene expression by danggui buxue tang, a traditional Chinese herbal preparation, in retarding the progress of renal damage in streptozotocin-induced diabetic rats." *Hormone and Metabolic Research* 38, no. 2 (2006): 82–88.

Zhao, L., J. Y. Lee, and D. H. Hwang. "Inhibition of pattern recognition receptor-mediated inflammation by bioactive phytochemicals." *Nutrition Reviews* 69, no. 6 (2011): 310–20.

Zhao, L., V. D. La, and D. Grenier. "Antibacterial, antiadherence, antiprotease, and anti-inflammatory activities of various tea extracts: Potential benefits for periodontal diseases." *Journal of Medicinal Food* 16, no. 5 (2013): 428–36.

Zhao, M. R., and J. Zhou. "[Effect of astragalus polysaccharide on suppression of bone marrow after chemotherapy in patients with malignant tumor]." *Tianjin Journal of Traditional Chinese Medicine* 2007-02. http://en.cnki .com.cn/Article_en/CJFDTOTAL-TJZY200702012.htm.

Zheng, M., and Y. P. Wang. "[Study on biological mechanism of angelica polysaccharide regulation on human early multipotential progenitor cell]." *Chinese Journal of Anatomy* 2002-02. http://en.cnki.com.cn/ Article_en/CJFDTOTAL-JPXZ200202001.htm.

Zhong, L., C. M. Li, X. J. Hao, et al. "Induction of leukemia cell apoptosis by cheliensisin A involves down-regulation of Bcl-2 expression." *Acta Pharmacologica Sinica* 26, no. 5 (2005): 623–28.

Zhou, W. B., and Z. L Xu. "[Protective effect of Angelica sinenisis injection on bone marrow histology and ultrastructure damnified by cyclophosphamide.]" *Journal of Xianning College (Medical Sciences)* 2007-01. http://en.cnki.com.cn/Article_en/CJFDTOTAL-XNYB200701005 .htm.

Zhou, Y., F. Wang, L. Hao, et al. "Effects of magnoline on P-selectin's expression in diabetic rats and its reno-protection." *Kidney and Blood Pressure Research* 37, nos. 2–3 (2013): 211–20.

Zhu, B. D., Y. LV, and X. M. Feng. "[The effect of total saponin of Panax ginseng and panaxquinquefoliuml saponin on hematopoiesis in anemic mice]." *Journal of Chengdu University of Traditional Chinese Medicine* 2005-02. http://en.cnki.com.cn/Article_en/CJFDTOTAL-CDZY200502012.htm.

Zhu, T., S. H. Kim, and C. Y. Chen. "A medicinal mushroom: Phellinus linteus." *Current Medicinal Chemistry* 15, no. 13 (2008): 1330–35.

Zhu, X., Y. Pan, L. Zheng, et al. "Polysaccharides from the Chinese medicinal herb Achyranthes bidentata enhance anti-malarial immunity during Plasmodium yoelii 17XL infection in mice." *Malaria Journal* 11 (2012): 49.

Zhu, X. L., and B. D. Zhu. "Mechanisms by which Astragalus membranaceus injection regulates hematopoiesis in myelosuppressed mice." *Phytotherapy Research* 21, no. 7 (2007): 663–67.

Zuo, C., X. S. Xie, H. Y. Qiu, et al. "Astragalus mongholicus ameliorates renal fibrosis by modulating HGF and TGF-beta in rats with unilateral ureteral obstruction." *Journal of Zhejiang University Science B* 10, no. 5 (2009): 380–90.

Septic Shock

Alleva, L. M., H. Yang, K. J. Tracey, et al. "High mobility group box 1 (HMGB1) protein: Possible amplification signal in the pathogenesis of falciparum malaria." *Transactions of the Royal Society of Tropical Medicine and Hygeine* 99, no. 3 (2005): 171–74.

Andersson, U., H. Erlandsson-Harris, H. Yang, et al. "HMGB1 as a DNA-binding cytokine." *Journal of Leukocyte Biology* 72, no. 6 (2002): 1084–91.

Andersson, U., and K. J. Tracey. "HMGB1 as a mediator of necrosis-induced inflammation and a therapeutic target in arthritis." *Rheumatic Disease Clinics of North America* 30, no. 3 (2004): 627–37.

Angeletti, D., M. S. Kiwuwa, J. Byarugaba, et al. "Elevated levels of high-mobility group box-1 (HMGB1) in patients with severe or uncomplicated Plasmodium falciparum malaria." *American Journal of Tropical Medicine and Hygiene* 88, no. 4 (2013): 733–35.

Bae, J. S. "Role of high-mobility group box 1 in inflammatory disease: Focus on sepsis." *Archives of Pharmacal Research* 35, no. 9 (2012): 1511–23.

Balosso, S., J. Liu, M. E. Bianchi, et al. "Disulfide-containing high mobility group box-1 promotes N-methyl-d-aspartate receptor function and excitotoxicity by activating toll-like receptor 4-dependent signaling in hippocampal neurons." *Antioxidants & Redox Signaling.* Published electronically ahead of print January 3, 2014.

Behrendt, J. H., A. Ruiz, H. Zahner, et al. "Neutrophil extracellular trap formation as innate immune reactions against the apicomplexan parasite Eimeria bovis." *Veterinary Immunology and Immunopathology* 133, no. 1 (2010): 1–8.

Camicia, G., and G. de Larrañaga. "[Neutrophil extracellular traps: A 2-faced host defense mechanism]." *Medicina Clínica* 140, no. 2 (2013): 70–75.

Chen, X. L., L. Sun, F. Guo, et al. "High-mobility group box-1 induces pro-inflammatory cytokines production of Kupffer cells through TLRs-dependent signaling pathway after burn injury." *PLoS ONE* 7, no. 11 (2012): e50668.

Chen, X. L., X. D. Zhang, Y. Y. Li, et al. "Involvement of HMGB1 mediated signalling pathway in diabetic retinopathy: Evidence from type 2 diabetic rats and ARPE-19 cells under diabetic condition." *British Journal of Opthamology* 97, no. 12 (2013): 1593–603.

Chen, Y., W. Sun, R. Gao, et al. "The role of high mobility group box chromosomal protein 1 in rheumatoid arthritis." *Rheumatology* (Oxford) 52, no. 10 (2013): 1739–47.

Dacey, M. J., H. Martinez, T. Raimondo, et al. "Septic shock due to babesiosis." *Clinical Infectious Diseases* 33, no. 5 (2001): e37–38.

Deng, Y., Z. Yang, Y. Gao, et al. "Toll-like receptor 4 mediates acute lung injury by high mobility group box-1." *PLoS ONE* 8, no. 5 (2013): e64375.

Denk, S., M. Perl, and M. Huber-Lang. "Damage- and pathogen-associated molecular patterns and alarmins: Keys to sepsis?" *European Surgical Research* 48, no. 4 (2012): 171–79.

Ding, H. S., J. Yang, F. L. Gong, et al. "High mobility group [corrected] box 1 mediates neutrophil recruitment in myocardial ischemia-reperfusion injury through toll like receptor 4-related pathway." *Gene* 509, no. 1 (2012): 149–53.

Ding, H. S., J. Yang, P. Cheng, et al. "The HMGB1-TLR4 axis contributes to myocardial ischemia/reperfusion injury via regulation of cardiomyocyte apoptosis." *Gene* 527, no. 1 (2013): 389–93.

Fu, J., H. Cao, N. Wang, et al. "An anti-sepsis monomer, 2',5,6',7-

tetrahydroxyflavanonol (THF), identified from Scutellaria baicalensis Georgi neutralizes lipopolysaccharide in vitro and in vivo." *International Immunopharmacology* 8, no. 12 (2008): 1652–57.

Gao, X. H., X. X. Xu, R. Pan, et al. "Qi-shao-shuang-gan, a combination of Astragalus membranaceus saponins with Paeonia lactiflora glycosides, ameliorates polymicrobial sepsis induced by cecal ligation and puncture in mice." *Inflammation* 34, no. 1 (2011): 10–21.

Gao, X. H., X. X. Xu, R. Pan, et al. "Saponin fraction from Astragalus membranaceus roots protects mice against polymicrobial sepsis induced by cecal ligation and puncture by inhibiting inflammation and upregulating protein C pathway." *Journal of Natural Medicines* 63, no. 4 (2009): 421–29.

Garcia-Arnandis, I., M. I. Guillén, F. Gomar, et al. "High mobility group box 1 potentiates the pro-inflammatory effects of interleukin-1beta in osteoarthritic synoviocytes." *Arthritis Research and Therapy* 12, no. 4 (2010): R165.

Gardiner, E. E., and R. K. Andrews. "Neutrophil extracellular traps (NETs) and infection-related vascular dysfunction." *Blood Reviews* 26, no. 6 (2012): 255–59.

Girard, J. P. "A direct inhibitor of HMGB1 cytokine." *Chemistry and Biology* 14, no. 4 (2007): 345–47.

Griffin, K. L., B. M. Fischer, A. B. Kummarapurugu, et al. "2-O,3-O-desulfated heparin inhibits neutrophil elastase-induced HMGB-1 secretion and airway inflammation." *American Journal of Respiratory Cell and Molecular Biology* 50, no. 4 (2014): 684–89.

GuoQian, C., W. GuoRong, Z. Qi, et al. "Effect of berberine on extracellular release of HMGB1." *China Journal of Traditional Chinese Medicine and Pharmacy* 24, no. 11 (2009): 1530–32.

Hayakawa, K., K. Irie, K. Sano, et al. "Therapeutic time window of cannabidiol treatment on delayed ischemic damage via high-mobility group box1-inhibiting mechanism." *Biological and Pharmaceutical Bulletin* 32, no. 9 (2009): 1538–44.

He, Z. W., Y. H. Qin, Z. W. Wang, et al. "HMGB1 acts in synergy with lipopolysaccharide in activating rheumatoid synovial fibroblasts via p38 MAPK and NF-κB signaling pathways." *Mediators of Inflammation*, 2013: 596716.

Higgins, S. J., K. Xing, H. Kim, et al. "Systemic release of high mobility group box 1 (HMGB1) protein is associated with severe and fatal Plasmodium falciparum malaria." *Malaria Journal* 12 (2013): 105.

Jun, M. S., H. S. Kim, Y. M. Kim, et al. "Ethanol extract of Prunella vulgaris var. lilacina inhibits HMGB1 release by induction of heme oxygenase-1 in LPS-activated RAW 264.7 cells and CLP-induced septic mice." *Phytotherapy Research* 26, no. 4 (2012): 605–12.

Kalechman, Y., U. Gafter, R. Gal, et al. "Anti-IL-10 therapeutic strategy using the immunomodulator AS101 in protecting mice from sepsis-induced death: Dependence on timing of immunomodulating intervention." *Journal of Immunology* 169, no. 1 (2002): 384–92.

Kamo, N., B. Ke, A. A. Ghaffari, et al. "ASC/caspase-1/IL-1beta signaling triggers inflammatory responses by promoting HMGB1 induction in liver ischemia/reperfusion injury." *Hepatology* 58, no. 1 (2013): 351–62.

Karlsson, S., V. Pettilä, J. Tenhunen, et al. "HMGB1 as a predictor of organ dysfunction and outcome in patients with severe sepsis." *Intensive Care Medicine* 34, no. 6 (2008): 1046–53.

Kawahara, K., T. Hashiguchi, K. Masuda, et al. "Mechanism of HMGB1 release inhibition from RAW264.7 cells by oleanolic acid in Prunus mume Sieb. et Zucc." *International Journal of Molecular Medicine* 23, no. 5 (2009): 615–20.

Kirchner, T., E. Hermann, S. Möller, et al. "Flavonoids and 5-aminosalicylic acid inhibit the formation of neutrophil extracellular traps." *Mediators of Inflammation*, 2013: 710239.

Kohka Takahashi, H., H. Sadamori, K. Liu, et al. "Role of cell-cell interactions in high mobility group box 1 cytokine activity in human peripheral blood mononuclear cells and mouse splenocytes." *European Journal of Pharmacology* 701, nos. 1–3 (2013): 194–202.

Kumar, K., A. Singal, M. M. Rizvi, et al. "High mobility group box (HMGB) proteins of Plasmodium falciparum: DNA binding proteins with pro-inflammatory activity." *Parasitology International* 57, no. 2 (2008): 150–57.

Laird, M. D., J. S. Shields, S. Sukumari-Ramesh, et al. "High mobility group box protein-1 promotes cerebral edema after traumatic brain injury via activation of toll-like receptor 4." *Glia* 62, no. 1 (2014): 26–38.

Lee, W., T. H. Kim, S. K. Ku, et al. "Barrier protective effects of withaferin A in HMGB1-induced inflammatory responses in both cellular and animal models." *Toxicology and Applied Pharmacology* 262, no. 1 (2012): 91–98.

Lee, W., S. K. Ku, J. W. Bae, and J. S. Bae. "Inhibitory effects of lycopene on HMGB1-mediated pro-inflammatory responses in both cellular and animal models." *Food and Chemical Toxicology* 50, no. 6 (2012): 1826–33.

Lee, W., S. K. Ku, T. H. Kim et al. "Embodin-6-O-beta-glucoside inhibits HMGB1-induced inflammatory responses in vitro and in vivo." *Food and Chemical Toxicology* 52 (2013): 97–104.

Li, B., R. Zhang, J. Li, et al. "Antimalarial artesunate protects sepsis model mice against heat-killed Escherichia coli challenge by decreasing TLR4, TLR9 mRNA expressions and transcription factor NF-kappa B activation." *International Immunopharmacology* 8, no. 3 (2008): 379–89.

Li, G., X. Liang, and M. T. Lotze. "HMGB1: The central cytokine for all lymphoid cells." *Frontiers in Immunology* 4 (2013): 68.

Li, J., F. P. Wang, W. M. She, et al. "Enhanced high-mobility group box 1 (HMGB1) modulates regulatory T cells (Treg)/T helper 17 (Th17) balance via toll-like receptor (TLR)-4-interleukin (IL)-6 pathway in patients with chronic hepatitis B." *Journal of Viral Hepatitis* 21, no. 2 (2014): 129–40.

Li, W., M. Ashok, J. Li, et al. "A major ingredient of green tea rescues mice from lethal sepsis partly by inhibiting HMGB1." *PLoS ONE* 2, no. 11 (2007): e1153.

Li, X., L. K. Wang, L. W. Wang, et al. "Blockade of high-mobility group box-1 ameliorates acute on chronic liver failure in rats." *Inflammation Research* 62, no. 7 (2013): 703–9.

Marik, P. E., and J. Lipman. "The definition of septic shock: Implications for treatment." *Critical Care and Resuscitation* 9, no. 1 (2007): 101–3.

Maroso, M., S. Balosso, T. Ravizza, et al. "Interleukin-1 type 1 receptor/toll-like receptor signalling in epilepsy: The importance of IL-1beta and high-mobility group box 1." *Journal of Internal Medicine* 270, no. 4 (2011): 319–26.

Maroso, M., S. Balosso, T. Ravizza, et al. "Toll-like receptor 4 and high-mobility group box-1 are involved in ictogenesis and can be targeted to reduce seizures." *Nature Medicine* 16, no. 4 (2010): 413–19.

Mersmann, J., F. Iskandar, K. Latsch, et al. "Attenuation of myocardial injury by HMGB1 blockade during ischemia/reperfusion is toll-like receptor 2-dependent." *Mediators of Inflammation*, 2013: 174168.

Muñoz Caro, T., C. Hermosilla, L. M. Silva, et al. "Neutrophil extracellular traps as innate immune reaction against the emerging apicomplexan parasite Besnoitia besnoiti." *PLoS ONE* 9, no. 3 (2014): e91415.

Nadatani, Y., T. Watanabe, T. Tanigawa, et al. "High-mobility group box 1 inhibits gastric ulcer healing through toll-like receptor 4 and receptor for advanced glycation end products." *PLoS ONE* 8, no. 11 (2013): e80130.

Nawa, Y., K. Kawahara, S. Tancharoen, et al. "Nucleophosmin may act as an alarmin: Implications for severe sepsis." *Journal of Leukocyte Biology* 86, no. 3 (2009): 645–53.

Saukkonen, K., P. Lakkisto, V. Pettilä, et al. "Cell-free plasma DNA as a predictor of outcome in severe sepsis and septic shock." *Clinical Chemistry* 54, no. 6 (2008): 1000–1007.

Shu, Q., X. Fang, Q. Chen, et al. "IL-10 polymorphism is associated with increased incidence of severe sepsis." *Chinese Medical Journal* 116, no. 11 (2003): 1756–59.

Sun, Q., F. Wang, W. Li, et al. "Glycyrrhizic acid confers neuroprotection after subarachnoid hemorrhage via inhibition of high mobility group box-1 protein: A hypothesis for novel therapy of subarachnoid hemorrhage." *Medical Hypotheses* 81, no. 4 (2013): 681–85.

Tadie, J. M., H. B. Bae, S. Jiang, et al. "HMGB1 promotes neutrophil extracellular trap formation through interactions with toll-like receptor 4." *American Journal of Physiology. Lung Cellular and Molecular Physiology* 304, no. 5 (2013): L342–49.

Tang, D., R. Kang, W. Xiao, et al. "Quercetin prevents LPS-induced high-mobility group box 1 release and proinflammatory function." *American Journal of Respiratory Cell and Molecular Biology* 41, no. 6 (2009): 651–60.

Tsoyi, K., H. J. Jang, Y. S. Lee, et al. "(+)-Nootkatone and (+)-valencene from rhizomes of Cyperus rotundus increase survival rates in septic mice due to heme oxygenase-1 induction." *Journal of Ethnopharmacology* 137, no. 3 (2011): 1311–17.

Valdés-Ferrer, S. I., M. Rosas-Ballina, P. S. Olofsson, et al. "High-mobility group box 1 mediates persistent splenocyte priming in sepsis survivors: Evidence from a murine model." *Shock* 40, no. 6 (2013): 492–95.

Valdés-Ferrer, S. I., M. Rosas-Ballina, P. S. Olofsson, et al. "HMGB1 mediates splenomegaly and expansion of splenic CD11b+ Ly-6C (high) inflammatory monocytes in murine sepsis survivors." *Journal of Internal Medicine* 274, no. 4 (2013): 381–90.

Velegraki, M., E. Papakonstanti, I. Mavroudi, et al. "Impaired clearance of apoptotic cells leads to HMGB1 release in the bone marrow of patients with myelodysplastic syndromes and induces TLR4-mediated cytokine production." *Haematologica* 98, no. 8 (2013): 1206–15.

Venereau, E., M. Schiraldi, M. Uguccioni, et al. "HMGB1 and leukocyte migration during trauma and sterile inflammation." *Molecular Immunology* 55, no. 1 (2013): 76–82.

Vitali, R., F. Palone, S. Cucchiara, et al. "Dipotassium glycyrrhizate inhibits HMGB1-dependent inflammation and ameliorates colitis in mice." *PLoS ONE* 8, no. 6 (2013): e66527.

Wang, C., H. Nie, K. Lie, et al. "Curcumin inhibits HMGB1 releasing and attenuates concanavalin A-induced hepatitis in mice." *European Journal of Pharmacology* 697, nos. 1–3 (2012): 152–57.

Wang, F. P., L. Li, and J. Li. "High mobility group box-1 promotes the proliferation and migration of hepatic stellate cells via TLR4-dependent signal pathways of PI3K/Akt and JNK." *PLoS ONE* 8, no. 5 (2013): e64373.

Wang, H., M. F. Ward, and A. E. Sama. "Novel HMGB1-inhibiting therapeutic agents for experimental sepsis." *Shock* 32, no. 4 (2009): 348–57.

Wang, L., X. Zhang, L. Liu, et al. "Tanshinone IIA down-regulates HMGB1, RAGE, TLR4, NF-kappaB expression, ameliorates BBB permeability and endothelial cell function, and protects rat brains against focal ischemia." *Brain Research* 1321 (2010): 143–51.

Wang, Y., J. Shan, W. Yang, et al. "High mobility group box 1 (HMGB1) mediates high-glucose-induced calcification in vascular smooth muscle cells of saphenous veins." *Inflammation* 36, no. 6 (2013): 1592–604.

Wiersinga, W. J., S. J. Leopold, D. R. Cranendonk, et al. "Host innate immune responses to sepsis." *Virulence* 5, no. 1 (2014): 36–44.

Williams, M. A., S. A. White, J. J. Miller, et al. "Granulocyte-macrophage colony stimulating factor induces activation and restores respiratory burst activity in monocytes from septic patients." *Journal of Infectious Diseases* 177, no. 1 (1998): 107–15.

Yamaguchi, H., Y. Kidachi, K. Kamiie, et al. "Structural insight into the ligand-receptor interaction between glycyrrhetinic acid (GA) and the high-mobility group protein B1 (HMGB1)-DNA complex." *Bioinformation* 8, no. 23 (2012): 1147–53.

Yang, E. J., S. K. Ku, W. Lee, et al. "Barrier protective effects of rosmarinic acid on HMGB1-induced inflammatory responses in vitro and in vivo." *Journal of Cellular Physiology* 228, no. 5 (2013): 975–82.

Yang, E. J., W. Lee, S. K. Ku, et al. "Anti-inflammatory activities of oleanolic acid on HMGB1 activated HUVECs." *Food and Chemical Toxicology* 50, no. 5 (2012): 1288–94.

Yang, H., D. J. Antoine, U. Andersson, et al. "The many faces of HMGB1: Molecular structure-functional activity in inflammation, apoptosis, and chemotaxis." *Journal of Leukocyte Biology* 93, no. 6 (2013): 865–73.

Yang, J., L. Chen, J. Yang, et al. "High mobility group box-1 induces migration of vascular smooth muscle cells via TLR4-dependent PI3K/Akt pathway activation." *Molecular Biology Reports* 39, no. 3 (2012): 3361–67.

Yang, Q. W., J. Xiang, Y. Zhou, et al. "Targeting HMGB1/TLR4 signaling as a novel approach to treatment of cerebral ischemia." *Frontiers in Bioscience (Scholar Edition)* 2 (2010): 1081–91.

Zawrotniak, M., and M. Rapala-Kozik. "Neutrophil extracellular traps (NETs)—formation and implications." *Acta Biochimica Polonica* 60, no. 3 (2013): 277–84.

Zhang, S., X. Shu, X. Tian, et al. "Enhanced formation and impaired degradation of neutrophil extracellular traps in dermatomyositis and polymyositis: A potential contributor to interstitial lung disease complications." *Clinical and Experimental Immunology* 177, no. 1 (2014): 134–41.

Zhang, W., L. W. Wang, L. K. Wang, et al. "Betaine protects against high-fat-diet-induced liver injury by inhibition of high-mobility group box 1 and toll-like receptor 4 expression in rats." *Digestive Diseases and Sciences* 58, no. 11 (2013): 3198–206.

Zhang, Y., W. Li, S. Zhu, et al. "Tanshinone IIA sodium sulfonate facilitates endocytic HMGB1 uptake." *Biochemical Pharmacology* 84, no. 11 (2012): 1492–500.

Zheng, Y. J., B. Zhou, Z. F. Song, et al. "Study of Astragalus mongholicus polysaccharides on endothelial cells permeability induced by HMGB1." *Carbohydrate Polymers* 92, no. 1 (2013): 934–41.

Zhu, S., W. Li, M. F. Ward, et al. "High mobility group box 1 protein as a potential drug target for infection- and injury-elicited inflammation." *Inflammation and Allergy Drug Targets* 9, no. 1 (2010): 60–72.

Index